THE SECOND LIFE

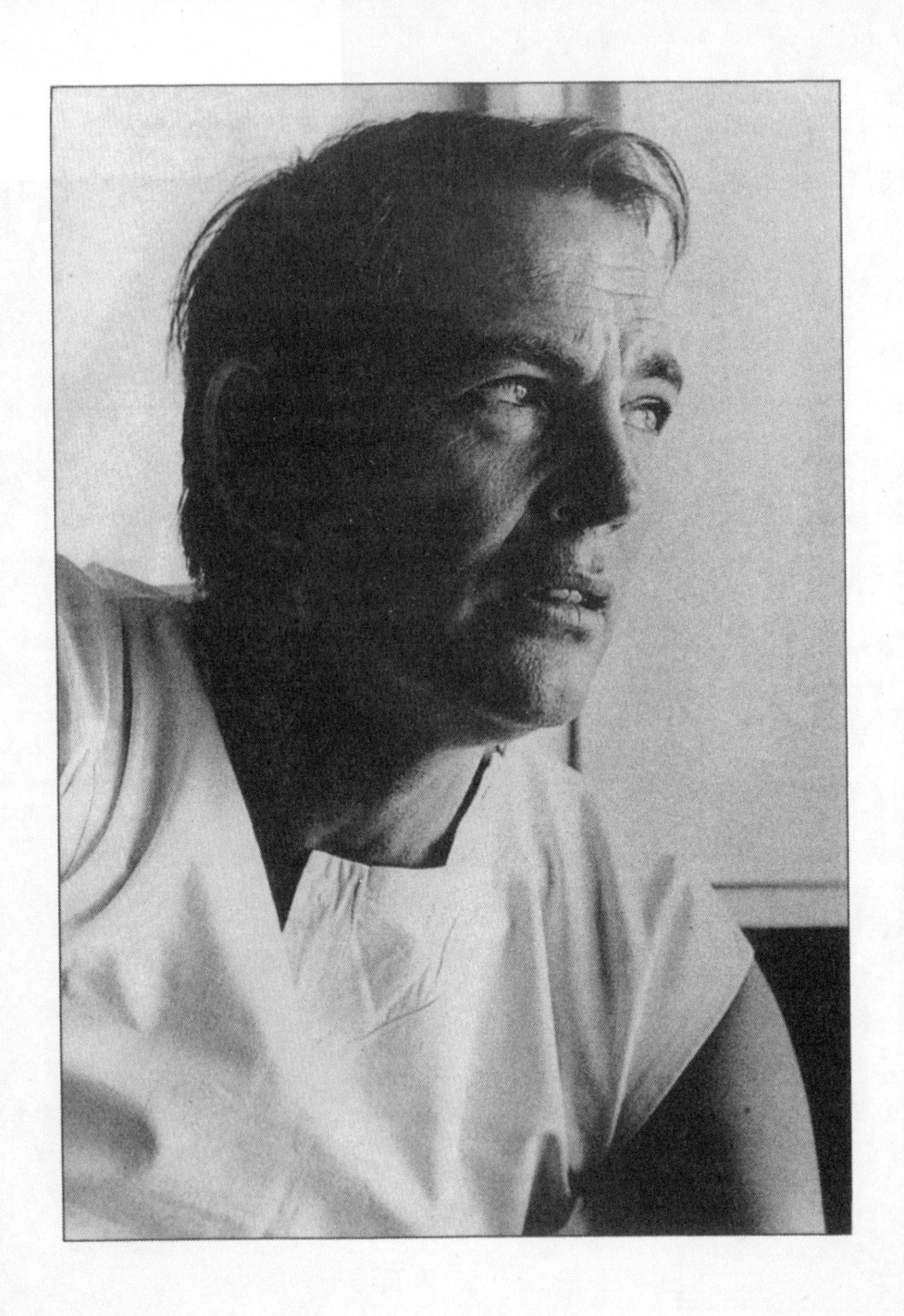

CHRIS BARNARD
THE
SECOND LIFE

MEMOIRS
EDITED BY CHRIS BREWER

Hodder & Stoughton
SYDNEY AUCKLAND

Copyright © Vlaeberg Publishers, 1993

First published in 1993
by Vlaeberg Publishers
P.O.Box 15034
Vlaeberg 8018
South Africa

First published in Australia in 1993
by Hodder & Stoughton (Australia) Pty Limited
10-16 South Street
Rydalmere NSW 2116

This book is copyright. Apart from any fair dealing for the purposes of private study, research, criticism or review as permitted under the Copyright Act, no part may be reproduced by any process without written permission. Enquiries should be addressed to the publisher.

Barnard, Christiaan, 1922-
   Chris Barnard: the second life.

ISBN 0 340 60529 4.

1. Barnard, Christiaan, 1922-   . 2. Heart-
Transplantation. I. Brewer, Chris, 1947-   . II. Title.

617.092

Cover design by Abdul Amien
Typography and production by Wim Reinders & Associates, Cape Town
Typeset by 4-Ways DTP Services, Cape Town
Printed and bound in Australia for Hodder & Stoughton (Australia) by Griffin Paperbacks, Netley, South Australia

ACKOWLEDGEMENTS

I wish to convey my sincere thanks and appreciation to The Argus reference library, The Beaufort West Museum, Philip Blaiberg (*Looking at my heart*), Dr David Cooper, Frikkie Erasmus, Groote Schuur Hospital, David Harrison, David Jones, Bob Molloy (*The Chris Barnard Column*), Alan Palmer, Prof. Jannie de Villiers and everyone who helped in assembling all the reference material.

I also wish to express my gratitude to Chris Brewer. Without his encouragement and help this book would never have been completed.

THE AUTHOR

1

The naked body of Louis Washkansky was lying on the white marble slab. The last beat of his heart in the early hours of the morning had transformed him from a deeply loved, meticulously cared-for patient, to a pathological specimen. The first human ever to receive a transplanted heart from a human cadaver was dead.

The only interest left was what could be learned from his death. Where had I made a mistake? How could I improve the operation next time?

I stood there in deep sorrow. A great sadness overwhelmed me and it was impossible to speak to my colleagues in the morgue – for fear that I would start crying. I have always been easily moved emotionally and I laugh or cry quite spontaneously.

The events of the past 18 days had sapped my strength completely. There were no reserves left and I struggled to get a grip on how I felt. Success had been denied us all. Failure had always been an enemy – an enemy I had conquered many times. But now Louis Washkansky was dead.

What happens through death to change the relationship between Doctor and Patient, Father and Son, Wife and Husband? I had refused to see my father, and later my mother, after they died. I wanted to remember them as they were in life. I knew that the presence of death would change my image of them – might even dull some of my love for them.

The only interest in my patient now was what the pathologist would expose inside the dead body. So why all the sadness and sorrow?

Fear of failure – or what people would say about my failings – has never really bothered me. The only important issue was to be sure that what I'd done was right.

I knew that I'd exhausted every available means to prepare

myself adequately for the first transplant – and this had meant months and years of trials in the laboratory. But sooner or later one had to have the courage to move from the laboratory to the hospital.

I had made such a move when I inserted the first low-profile artificial heart valve in the treatment of patients with severe valvular disease. I'd introduced a new surgical approach for the complete correction of Transposition of the Great Vessels and Ebstein's Abnormality – which were, until then, severely debilitating and terminal conditions. With the same motive I took out the diseased heart of Louis Washkansky and replaced it with the healthy heart of Denise Darvall. I felt I was adequately prepared and I honestly believed it was going to work. I was deeply saddened because Louis had died – he was a brave, very likeable man with whom I lived and suffered and laughed for 18 days and nights. This misery was made worse because I had failed in the end and the belief in myself had been seriously undermined.

'Can we start?' It was Professor James G. Thomson, head of pathology. He hadn't been enthusiastic about the possibility of a heart transplant and was never really committed to the programme – in fact when I discussed it with him he often cut me short and showed no encouragement whatsoever. But now he'd decided to do the post-mortem himself. I nodded my head.

Professor Thomson wasn't alone. I had been amused, the night after the operation – when a foreign television crew came in to Groote Schuur Hospital to interview the transplant team – to see how the interest in this event had increased among the medical staff. When the 'team' later posed for a picture there was hardly any space for me and I had to squeeze in at the back of the room.

He made a long incision down the middle of Washkansky's body. Although we knew that he had died from respiratory failure due to extensive infection of both lungs, there were still several unanswered questions. In the laboratory we had transplanted many hearts over the past three years, but always in normal recipients. Now, in the hospital, it would be different because our recipient would be a patient whose body had been subjected to an increase in venous pressure and poor arterial circulation for months, or even years. The question was, would the functional and pathological changes that had resulted be reversible in future transplants?

We had already found some of the answers in the short 18 days that Louis Washkansky had lived. From the moment the heart of Denise Darvall started to take over his circulation his kidneys had secreted litres and litres of urine – without the use of diuretics. His waterlogged lungs had dried and, where we previously had to resort to the extreme measure of putting small stainless steel tubes in the subcutaneous tissue of his legs to drain off the retained fluid, the swelling in his legs had lessened visibly every day until they were normal. The functions of the kidney and liver had also returned to normal. The operation itself had definitely worked.

The clinical observations convinced me that this operation would be very successful one day because it would result in a tremendous improvement in the quality of life of terminally ill heart patients. They would no longer be invalids but able to live virtually normal lives.

Professor Thomson was ready to give us the pathological answers. He had exposed both the thoracic and abdominal organs and was dictating a commentary as he worked.

'Kidneys appear normal,' I heard him say.

How can they be normal? They're dead. They're unable to purify the blood any more, unable to secrete urine and remove the oedema.

I remember the histology practical classes in my second year as a young medical student – looking through the microscope at slides of kidney, liver, heart muscle, brain and other organs and tissues – all labelled *'normal'*. Even at that early stage of my medical career I was puzzled by the fact that under the high magnification of a microscope there was no distinction between live and dead cells. Yes, it was easy to distinguish between diseased and normal cells, but the mystery of death was invisible.

By now Professor Thomson had removed all the organs. My patient had been reduced to an empty shell of bone, muscle and skin.

'There's no evidence of rejection that I can see. The problem is definitely the lungs. The appearance is typical of a *Pseudomonas pneumoniae.*' We knew that already. The question Professor Thomson couldn't answer is why we had not been able to control this infection.

Professor Forder had reported four days previously that there was a heavy growth of *Pseudomonas* and *Klebsiella* in the cultures from the sputum. He said that these organisms were sensitive to drugs such as carbenicillin, gentamicin and cephaloridine. We used all three and monitored their blood levels to be sure that we reached a concentration that Professor Forder's tests showed would kill these bacteria. Yet, they had not only survived but flourished and killed my patient.

The tests done were applicable to bacteria growing on culture plates but of no value in patients whose natural defence against infection was severely jeopardized by the drugs that were used to prevent rejection.

The goal would be to administer the immunosuppressive drugs, which were available then, in doses that would prevent rejection but would not suppress the immune system to the extent that the body would be defenceless against all the deadly bacteria, viruses and fungi around. Would that ever be possible?

We were encouraged by the success of kidney transplantation, but the heart was altogether different. It was not possible to use living family members as donors, as we did in the case of kidneys – obviously because there is only one heart. Related donors significantly reduce the dangers of rejection because of the genetic compatibility between members of a family. Heart transplantation was further complicated in that we had no artificial heart to fall back on if the transplant failed. In kidney transplantation the surgeon could keep immunosuppressive drugs at a relatively low level and accept the risk of rejection because he had an artificial kidney he could revert to. This approach would give him enough time either to reverse the rejection or to remove the rejected kidney and wait for another donor.

Then the awful reality hit me. I had overlooked two very important factors.

Professor Forder had reported, before the operation, that he had isolated *Pseudomonas aeruginosa* from the swabs taken of the puncture wounds where the metal tubes had been inserted in the patient's leg to drain the oedema. It was now obvious to me that I should not have operated until this infection had cleared. The treatment to prevent rejection had lowered his resistance to such an extent that these deadly organisms had simply invaded the body at will. Of further importance was the finding that Louis suffered from diabetes, a condition which also reduces the body's ability to deal with infection.

We had been wrong in assuming that there were no contra-indications for selection of patients. Maybe some patients are just too ill to benefit from the improvement in circulation provided by the transplanted heart? Maybe the critics were right. Maybe we did not know enough. Maybe I should stop?

Suddenly the room was oppressive and claustrophobic. The realisation of what we'd done was just too much to bear. I turned my back on the dead body and quickly left the room.

Outside the building the dawn was beginning to floodlight Cape Town with the start of another hot summer's day. I took several deep gulps of fresh morning air, steadied myself as best I could and made my way up the slope from the laboratory to the hospital.

The tall man walked slowly through the parking-lot, shoulders stooped and head down, as he made his way towards the main building. Eileen Blaiberg watched him through a window as she stood next to her husband's bed.

'Why are you so early today – aren't you working?' Philip Blaiberg asked.

'No,' she smiled thinly. 'I just felt I wanted to see you.'

'The nurses say that Professor Barnard is also coming to see me this morning.'

She continued watching the professor make his way towards them. He'd stopped and was gazing at the building. She knew that Washkansky was dead. So did the nurse who busied herself in the room, but neither looked at the patient.

Philip Blaiberg lay back in his bed at Groote Schuur Hospital waiting. Waiting for the miracle of heart transplantation to save his life as it had done with Louis Washkansky, unaware of the morning's tragedy.

I climbed the steps to the third floor and Ward D1 deep in thought, mumbling to myself. There was no need to stop on the second floor to look in on wards C2 and C3 because I knew Louis' bed would be empty and freshly made-up with clean white linen, ready for the next patient.

Why do I get so upset when a patient dies or develops complications? Why do I raise hell with the nurses and doctors for not doing enough? Was I pushing myself – and everybody around me – to the limit for the patient's sake or for my own ego?

Let me be honest. I've always been a bad loser – I've always wanted to be the best. At medical meetings I was proud to report my results that were as good as, or even better than those of other surgeons. That was the real driving force.

And after all, was that so bad? If I *was* the best it meant I'd be giving my patient the best too.

Many in the medical profession will disagree and say their first concern is for the patient. A noble sentiment perhaps – but nonsense. A doctor, like anyone else – from the playing field to the pulpit – wants above all, to satisfy his own ambition and ego. It's perfectly human and doctors are, after all, only human.

Eileen Blaiberg rose to excuse herself when the dishevelled surgeon walked into the room.

'No, don't go,' Professor Barnard said to her. 'I want to speak to you together.'

Philip Blaiberg looked more closely at his doctor. He was haggard and drawn, as though he hadn't slept all night. He felt a twinge of pity for the man when he saw the pain in his face and his eyes.

'So, when do I get the same chance as Washkansky?' He looked up at him very slowly. Philip Blaiberg knew something was seriously wrong.

'But don't you know that Louis Washkansky is dead?' he asked. 'He died this morning, of pneumonia.'

It dawned on him why his wife and Professor Barnard had made this unexpected visit. Now he knew the reason for the distress.

Chris Barnard felt his patient's pulse and said that he'd just been to see the post-mortem. 'The heart was strong until the end – but the body couldn't cope with the pneumonia,' he said gently.

Afraid that future transplants might be stopped after the failure on Washkansky, Philip Blaiberg insisted, 'Professor Barnard, I don't want to live the way I am now. The quality of my life is worthless. I can't breathe. I'm sitting up day and night gasping desperately for air and I'm suffering so much that death would be better than this sort of life.

'So if there's any hope that, through this operation, my life can be improved then I'm prepared to take the chance.'

In case there was any misunderstanding he added, 'I want to go through with it more than ever now. I know that you're upset because Louis Washkansky died and you're probably unsure of yourself as well, but Professor, you gave him hope and, from what I've heard, he had a few wonderful days after the operation when he was relieved of the misery of total heart failure. I want that hope too. I also want those few days.'

Both men smiled. 'I will operate on you,' said Professor Barnard. 'I will give you a new heart, and this time it's going to be successful.'

'Professor Barnard, there's a call for you.' It was my secretary, Ann

Levett. I walked into the corridor where a nurse handed me the black phone. 'Yes?' My voice sounded hollow and far-away. 'Prof, the people from CBS are here. You and your wife will be leaving for the United States later this afternoon.'

Two weeks previously I had been invited by Gordon Manning of CBS, to appear on America's most popular programme, *'Face the Nation'*. Five minutes before I couldn't face anybody, but my conversation with Philip Blaiberg had helped me substantially to regain my confidence. I knew we were on the right road and had to continue. I knew that, one day, heart transplantation would become a very successful and routine procedure.

Meanwhile many questions were being asked and had to be answered.

Why was the first transplant done in South Africa of all places? Dr Gould, who interviewed me from London soon after the operation, suggested that I did the first transplant in South Africa to 'improve the bad image of my country overseas' – which had been the first suggestion that politics were involved.

There were a lot of uncertainties about the ethical, moral and legal issues – as if they were different from kidney transplantation. The newspapers made the most of the suggestion by somebody that I should be tried for murder by the World Court as I had removed a *live* heart from a human being.

I was in the middle of cross-fire from critics and accusers alike because the concept of brain death was not generally accepted and not clearly understood. There were those whose opinion was that we'd jumped the gun – that heart transplantation was still an experimental procedure and should only be done in the laboratories.

Everybody felt qualified to address these questions – especially theologians, lawyers and, of course, politicians. It was a sure way to get one's name and photograph in the newspapers.

I discussed the CBS invitation with Professor Louw, head of the department of surgery and with Dr Burger, the medical superintendent of Groote Schuur Hospital. They said I should go.

If Washkansky was still alive I would never have considered leaving the country, but Louis was dead. Now there was Blaiberg – waiting. What would happen if I was in America and his condition suddenly deteriorated? Professor Velva Schrire, who was head of the cardiac clinic, assured me that he would look after him until I returned. Vel also said that I owed it to the people of the

United States. After all, I had used a grant from the American National Institute of Health to pay for the first heart-lung machine which I used to start open heart surgery in Cape Town in 1958. In fact I used the same heart-lung machine in the first transplant operation.

It was also in Minneapolis, at the University of Minnesota, that Doctors Lillehei and Varco taught me open-heart surgery. He said it would be correct and polite to show my gratitude by reporting back to the people of the United States and to show them that their money had been well spent. I went back to Dr Blaiberg. He was desperately short of breath and the nurse was holding the oxygen mask over his face. 'What's happening?' I asked in alarm.

Mrs Blaiberg turned to me, 'Philip has just had one of his coughing spells. He's always very short of breath afterwards but he'll soon be better.'

'I just wanted to tell you that I'm going to be out of the country for a few days but when I come back we'll do your operation.'

Dr Blaiberg lifted the mask off his face. 'I'll still be here and waiting,' he said with a smile.

I went back to the morgue but by that time everybody had left except for Professor Thomson who was cutting up various tissues and organs for histology. We briefly discussed his findings and he was quite sure that the main problem was the extensive pneumonia that had caused the death of Washkansky.

On my way out I met an old friend of mine, Jacques Roux. We had been together at medical school and had remained very good friends – he'd just come down to say how sorry he was to hear that Louis Washkansky had died and he said something that I've always remembered, 'Chris, your life is going to change drastically and you'll never look back again.' I didn't quite know what he meant at that stage but I was soon to find out. My life certainly would change – but I would still, often, look back.

I went to my office and there were three men from CBS there including Frank Manitzas – who was determined to keep me away from the other media and take me as his 'prisoner' to the US. We made arrangements that a car would come to Zeekoevlei and collect us that afternoon. ('Zeekoevlei' is a lake-side suburb of Cape Town about 30 minutes from Groote Schuur and means 'sea cow lake' – hippopotamus lake.)

But there was still one more press conference. We all gathered in a noisy room, around a table covered with bunches of microphones taped together, and squinted under the television lights. I hoped I'd be able to keep my emotions in check.

I read a prepared statement confirming that Louis Washkansky had died from respiratory failure due to pneumonia and that there was no morphological evidence to suggest that rejection had caused death.

'Does this mean the end of the heart transplant experiment?' someone asked.

'It wasn't an experiment,' I snapped, 'it was the correct treatment for a sick man – and there's no evidence that will convince me to discontinue such treatment for patients with these terminal heart diseases. When the next occasion arises we will definitely transplant again.' How different now from the morning when I left the hospital after the first operation. Then there was not a single reporter, photographer or television camera waiting for me in the parking-lot. We hadn't even taken a single photograph then. It wasn't important.

The radio news on December 4th had simply said 'a team of doctors did the first human heart transplant in Groote Schuur Hospital today.'

Within hours there had been phone calls from Australia, Sweden, Britain, America, Europe and even Russia. Within the next few days there was a mass migration from all over the world of reporters, photographers and television teams. The hospital, medical school and my home were overrun by them.

We had been totally unprepared for dealing with the situation. There were days when I spent more time giving interviews and posing for photographs than caring for my patients.

If one of the journalists wanted an exclusive interview or a special picture and I couldn't accommodate them they were upset – and wrote bitter stories which inevitably made headlines. So when I didn't have a few minutes for a reporter from Istanbul the headlines read: *'Barnard not Turkish Delight any more!'*

Then, when I went out of my way to tell them about our work and posed for pictures, I was accused of being a publicity-seeker – an accusation which was especially prevalent among my colleagues, unfortunately.

Whatever I did seemed to be wrong and it would take me many years of embarrassment and heartache to learn how to cope with the press.

After reading the statement and answering some questions I

introduced Professor Thomson who described the post-mortem findings while I excused myself.

I went home and Louwtjie, my wife, was busy packing and getting things ready. She was very excited about the trip. I was extremely tired and decided to lie down for a while before we left. ('Louwtjie' is an Afrikaans nick-name, taken from her maiden name – Louw – pronounced 'low-key'.)

It has always been a great relief to me that I can rest and sleep virtually anywhere. Perhaps it's a result of the years spent studying and the 24-hour-a-day internship – or from being on call and delivering babies at all hours of the day and night.

At about 3 pm, I took a shower and got dressed. I had never been particularly fussy about clothes. They just didn't interest me at all. After our divorce Louwtjie even said, truthfully, that she insisted I wear underpants! So, dressed in my least-frayed shirt and a blue suit I'd bought 15 years before when my daughter, Deirdre, was baptized, I joined my wife in the lounge and waited for the car.

Louwtjie looked beautiful in a navy-blue and white dress which she had made herself. She was a wonderful woman. She made all her own and Deirdre's clothes – in a tiny room up in the attic of our house that you could only reach with a ladder.

We'd had some difficult times in the past – either living-in at the hospital or moving from one rented house to another. Money was also tight and, on my salary in those days, every penny had to be accounted for. She'd lived through all the hardships of being married to a medical student, had worked as a nursing sister herself and had even found time to bear us two children – Deirdre and André. Our marriage had been rocky at the best of times, especially recently; maybe things would be better now?

Eventually our transport arrived and, to my surprise, the biggest black limousine I'd ever seen stopped outside our little house in Zeekoevlei, so off we went to the airport – and America.

At DF Malan airport in Cape Town I wanted to take my suitcases and book them in but no; nothing like that would be allowed. The senior South African Airways officials made sure there were people to help us carry our suitcases and coats. We were shown into the VIP lounge where they fussed around us and kept the reporters away.

I thought about what Jacques Roux had said and realised that life certainly *was* changing.

We left for Johannesburg where we changed planes for London and, for the first time in our lives, we were flying first class – sitting in row 1 – seats A and B – on a new Boeing 707. As soon as the seat-belt lights went off drinks were served. I asked for a glass of French champagne for myself and a tomato juice for Louwtjie. It was the first time that I had tasted French champagne and I found it very enjoyable!

The stewardess then brought the dinner menu. It was a whole page, listing items I'd never heard of, like canapés and *foie gras* – which I didn't order because I wasn't sure what they were. We could choose from a variety of South African red and white wines, but I stayed with the French champagne. Throughout the meal Louwtjie watched me enjoying myself with little expression on her face. She wouldn't answer me when I asked what she was thinking about. I reclined the back of my seat, took off my shoes, tie and jacket and closed my eyes. I had come a long way from the days of my childhood at Beaufort West – a small town 573 kilometres from Cape Town in the semi-desert area of South Africa called the Karoo. In those days my evening meal consisted of a few slices of home-made brown bread on which I spread dripping-fat, sprinkled with salt and pepper. On special occasions we had golden syrup which we mixed with the lard before spreading it on the bread.

I had a choice of drinks then too – either black coffee with sugar or black coffee without sugar and it was the best coffee I've ever tasted – made by my mother from coffee beans that she roasted in an iron pot on the Dover stove. Roasted beans were ground by one of the children with a coffee mill turned by hand. The coffee was percolated by placing the coffee grounds in a sock made by my mother (from the same material that she used to make our pyjamas) which was suspended on the neck of the black kettle with a wire ring.

Reliving the carefree days of my youth I fell asleep. It must have been a deep sleep because I was woken by the voice of the captain announcing that we were approaching Heathrow Airport.

We were to catch a TWA flight from London to Washington but we didn't have to go through the airport as they took us by car from the South African Airways flight to the TWA plane.

I only then learned that because the SAA flight was late, the TWA flight had been delayed by several hours so that I could make it. Just for Me! I suddenly felt very important.

When we boarded the TWA plane I laughed when the pretty stewardess asked me to autograph that week's edition of *Time* magazine – there was a picture of me on the cover. Three short weeks previously I couldn't even afford to *buy* a copy, I reflected wryly.

Instant fame is an intoxicating experience.

The flight from Johannesburg to London had been overnight but now, to Washington, it was daylight. I felt refreshed and ready to enjoy every minute. Louwtjie was reading a monthly publication, *Path of Truth*, to which she subscribed, so I made my way to the galley and chatted with the two stewardesses.

I had always enjoyed the company of American girls. They usually oozed self-confidence and took great pride in their appearance and were almost always friendly and vivacious. It may sound strange but I also liked the fact that they always smelled clean – and shaved their legs. Nothing is a bigger turn-off to a man than hair on a woman's body where it shouldn't be.

These two stewardesses were typically American – Julie was a blonde from Florida and Anne a brunette from Washington. They kept telling me how much they admired my work and what a wonderful man I must be, which was very flattering and, better still, they made it clear that they were willing to take care of *any* of my needs. I'd heard about this kind of service but never thought it really existed.

The call-bell rang and it was the captain inviting me to the flight deck. Anne showed me the way and I followed her undulating bottom down the aisle to the front of the plane. We passed Louwtjie, who looked up from her *Path of Truth* without any expression.

Captain John Cunningham must have been about my own age. I was expecting him to explain flight procedures and show me some of the instrumentation – but what he really wanted was some free medical advice. He had been flying for 20 years and like some other pilots I've met he was worried about the yearly check-up they were subjected to. What could he do to prevent heart problems? He knew his blood pressure, his blood cholesterol, triglycerides and even the ratio between low density and high density lipoproteins! I told him I was a surgeon and was only called in once the patient had developed serious heart problems. The physician was more involved in advising people about the prevention of heart disease.

It was time for lunch so I was saved from further queries about his health and went back to my seat. I left him feeling his own pulse.

During lunch Louwtjie asked, 'How long do you think this charade will last?' There was a bitter edge to her clipped voice and she made no attempt to hide the fact that this was not the world for her.

'I don't know,' I answered carefully – I had no intention of being drawn into an argument and, after a sip of Mouton Rothschild 1959 (which I knew from my limited knowledge of wines was hailed as the 'vintage of the century'), I added, 'I thought the transplant would make the headlines once or twice and then be over.'

Perhaps it would be over very soon – but, in the meantime, I thought, kicking off my shoes and lounging back in the first class seat, 'If this is what they call life-in-the-fast-lane then I want to enjoy every last second of it.' Maybe when we reached the United States the dazzle would already have begun to fade?

But our arrival in America proved the opposite – there were even more cameras and journalists – but the Americans are very well organised at that sort of thing and, within moments, we were whisked away from the airport. Soon we were unpacking in our suite at the Washington Hilton.

Even Louwtjie was enjoying herself – suddenly transported from our humble house at Zeekoevlei to the presidential suite at the Hilton. We stood at the window and looked at the monuments we'd visited 11 years ago with our children, Deirdre and André. That had been on our way to New York when they'd taken a boat back to Cape Town and I returned alone to Minneapolis to continue my studies.

There was a bottle of champagne 'with compliments from the management and staff' waiting for us on ice and I couldn't help but smile – my month's salary back in South Africa would hardly cover the cost of the wine, let alone the room.

And so we discovered America again – but how very different it was now!

Any thoughts of relaxing in our new-found luxury were quickly dismissed by the CBS aides suddenly invading our rooms and outlining my immediate itinerary.

They talked about my appearance on *Face the Nation* and other commitments – as well as our visit to Lyndon B. Johnson's ranch.

It's hard for me to recapture now, what I felt then. I must have had experiences like that a thousand times since, but I was new to publicity of any kind and all the fussing and attention seemed too good to be true.

I acknowledged all their instructions with, what I thought at the time, a fair imitation of a seasoned professional.

Professional? We didn't even *have* TV in South Africa then – I had hardly seen 'live' interviews let alone been the central figure in one. I recognized the first feelings of panic when someone on the CBS staff reminded me that the programme was America's biggest by far – and that millions of people would be closely watching me.

After a while they left us alone. We explored what was to be our home for the next three days. The suite was much bigger than our entire house in Cape Town – with two large bedrooms, two bathrooms, two toilets and a huge lounge.

'What's this, Louwtjie?' I asked, turning the tap. The water squirted straight up into my face.

'I've seen pictures of them in magazines,' she said, doubling up with laughter. 'I think it's called a bidet, but don't ask me what it's used for,' she added, leaving me to dry my face and the front of my shirt.

We wandered through the lounge. It was at least thirty paces long with large windows overlooking Washington. Everywhere there were fresh flowers arranged in expensive-looking vases.

Louwtjie fixed us some biscuits and cheese and we sat down at the bar counter. We were alone at last.

She looked at me with her big brown eyes and said, 'Let's make love Chris. It's been such a long time.'

I woke up completely disorientated about time and place. Where was I? What was I supposed to do? It dawned on me that today was the day I 'faced the nation'.

Louwtjie was still fast asleep and I covered her with a blanket and walked to the window. I gazed out over Washington, the capital of the United States with its monuments, the White House and Arlington Cemetery. I wondered whether they had already buried my patient – whom I'd come here to talk about now.

I tried to imagine the concept of millions of people all over the country getting ready to watch me being interviewed. This doctor from Africa who'd taken out the heart of a young girl and put it into the chest of a man.

What were they expecting? Some kind of Frankenstein creator? A mad scientist? I'd seen some of the American reactions in print already. I remember the *Daily News* headline: *'It's going to work! Dying African gets girl's heart and lives!'* and the *Washington Evening Star*: *'South Africa scores a first; grocer lives with transplant heart'*. These were fairly typical of the reactions – except for one paragraph which was a bad omen for things to come, 'There are some signs of professional heartache in the comments of top American heart specialists who had hoped for a "first" themselves in the heart transplant field.' Professional jealousy wasn't something I had anticipated.

Although this was just media hype I couldn't help but wonder how they thought of the people involved – what did they think of Denise Darvall? Would anyone remember her? The pretty girl whose brain had been smashed in a road accident – and her father, who gave permission for me to remove her heart? And what about Louis Washkansky? They knew him only as a 'grocer from Cape Town' – I knew him differently.

Absent-mindedly I opened the bottle of champagne as I gazed out at the frozen landscape – so very different from where I'd been only 24 hours ago.

Most of the critics had been right. Dr William Mustard had been out by only a few weeks when he said 'This heart transplant will last two or three months' and he was 100% correct when he said that 'anyone can transplant a heart'. The difference was that nobody else had – and I couldn't help smiling when I remembered my history teacher telling us about Columbus – which seemed relevant as I was now standing fairly close to where he had landed – when his discovery of America was dismissed by courtiers with 'but anyone could have done it'. His reply was to ask them all, sitting round a long table, to take an egg and make it stand on its end. One by one they tried and failed. When the egg was finally passed back to him he simply cracked the base so that the shell broke enough to allow him to make it stand on its end. 'Oh, we could have done that!' they cried. 'Yes,' he said, 'anyone *can* do it but I *did* it.'

Yet still the American press statements bothered me. The president of the American Heart Association, Dr Irvine Page, had said, 'You simply can't go round taking people's hearts out,' and another prominent doctor in Washington had said, 'I have a horrible vision of ghouls hovering over an accident victim with long knives unsheathed, waiting to take out his organs as soon as he is pronounced dead.'

Was that what the American public were expecting – a ghoul? The fact that I was from South Africa probably wouldn't help matters either.

I poured two glasses of champagne and Louwtjie joined me at the window. We toasted each other and, as if reading my thoughts, she showed me newspaper quotes of Dr Michael de Bakey – who would be on *Face the Nation* with me and who was the doyen of heart surgeons – 'The only question remains our ability to prevent rejection,' he'd said and, responding to a question about my own hospital in Cape Town, 'They have a very fine group of people there. I have a very warm feeling for them. They are doing wonderful work and it really is a very great achievement.'

Those were kind and reassuring words from a man I really admired. Doctors who worked with him always told me what a real bastard he could be. There were stories that he used to make his assistants stand in a corner of the operating room when they didn't assist him properly. I'd also been on the receiving end of his anger once.

When I was in training in Minneapolis Professor Wangensteen, the head of the department of surgery, thought it would be a good idea to send me to Houston to observe the work of Doctors De Bakey and Cooley.

I had been watching him resecting an abdominal aneurysm – leaning over to get a proper view into the abdominal cavity. Dr De Bakey was struggling to control bleeding from the inferior vena cava. He suddenly looked up at me.

'Get out!' he bellowed 'You're contaminating my operating area!'

Maybe I was leaning over too much and getting in the way, but I was young and eager to learn.

I would have felt more at ease if Dr Denton Cooley was to be on the programme instead. He had always been very kind to me. I remembered the cable that he sent on the Monday morning after the Washkansky operation, 'Congratulations on your first transplant, Chris. I will be reporting on my first hundred soon.'

'Adrian Kantrowitz is the other surgeon who will be with you on *Face the Nation*', Louwtjie reminded me.

I didn't know Dr Kantrowitz very well. He worked at the

Maimonides Hospital in New York. I'd read some of his work on assisted circulation with mechanical devices and also on his work where he used puppies as donors to study the growth of the heart after transplantation. He was a good choice, as he was the first to do a heart transplant in the United States – three days after I did mine.

At that time I felt that his choice of a recipient was a bad one. It was a small baby with a very complex congenital heart abnormality. The selection of an anencephalic baby as the donor was also a controversial one. Although these unfortunate children are born without the higher senses of the brain – specifically the cortex and medulla – the brain stem is still present and therefore they can breathe spontaneously.

Before Denise Darvall was declared brain-dead by the neurosurgeons they insisted that there should be no brain activity detected by all the tests available at normal temperature, and that there should be *no spontaneous respiration* for three minutes before she was disconnected from the respirator.

I wondered at what stage Dr Kantrowitz felt legally and ethically prepared to take out the heart of this donor? I thought that if I had an opportunity I would ask him this question on the programme.

It seemed like no time at all before there was a call from the concierge to tell me the studio car had arrived. Louwtjie had decided not to come along and was going to watch the programme on one of the three television sets in the suite.

When I arrived at the studio I was immediately taken to a room full of mirrors, brushes, combs, pots of cream, powders and puffs. A young man (or was he a girl?) asked me to sit in a chair. The process of make-up started. First he put on base with a wet sponge, then powder with a puff. He combed my hair and even my eyebrows!

When this embarrassing experience was over I was taken back into the studio where Doctors De Bakey and Kantrowitz were sitting. They both stood up and greeted me most enthusiastically.

The three of us first had to pose around a plastic model of the heart and great vessels for pictures as no photographs were allowed during the programme.

The floor was a sea of cables, there were television screens everywhere and the whole place was, generally, in a state of total chaos – except for one small corner, where we would be sitting.

Before the red light came on and we were live on the air I gazed in total bewilderment at the scenes behind the camera – I'd always thought the operating theatre to be a tense place – but this was frenetic! I wondered how many of the people working here would end up with a heart attack themselves.

I tried to wriggle myself into a more comfortable position on the chair – succeeding only in disconnecting one of the microphone wires. A girl shrieked in horror and skidded across the floor to make a connection as a man counted 'ten, nine, eight ...' in front of the cameras as Martin Agronsky checked his fly zipper once more.

Suddenly the room went quiet and a voice boomed out *Face the nation* presents a special one hour interview with the South African ...'

I tried to peer beyond the cameras and the lights but all I could see was a bank of newspaper reporters behind the cameras – it did remind me, in a strange way, of an operating theatre – all the urgency, the tension, the underlying dynamism of the occasion.

I was jolted back to reality by the announcer, 'Here is CBS news correspondent, Martin Agronsky!' Suddenly, rather like a marionette jerked to life by its strings, Agronsky turned to one of the cameras and started talking about transplants and Louis Washkansky and me.

Me! My mouth went dry and I felt a small bead of perspiration trickle down the contour of my spine. My hands were clammy. What on *earth* was I going to say? Surely there should have been a rehearsal?

Martin Agronsky was looking at me and smiled. He had obviously finished a long introduction and I could only remember one word, 'Welcome'.

So I smiled. He smiled back and I said, 'Thank you.'

I heard him introduce Earl Ubell, the science editor of WCBS-TV News in New York, Dr Michael de Bakey and Dr Adrian Kantrowitz and I was aware that he was chatting to them but I was still trying to adjust my eyes to the glare of the lights.

I think that one of the most valuable 'talents' I have is the ability to focus my mind very sharply on any given problem and, after clarifying what must be done, I find it easy to channel my thoughts in that direction and am very seldom distracted. This myopic ability has been a great asset to me – from writing exams to standing at the operating theatre for several hours on end. So I turned to my hosts and concentrated on what it was they wanted to hear. I now felt very comfortable and not in the least nervous.

Dr Kantrowitz also welcomed me to the programme and asked me at what stage I had thought the transplant was going to work.

'Well, I think we knew all along it was going to work,' I said. 'We've had nine years of experience with open-heart surgery, having performed well over a thousand open-heart operations. My team, therefore, has a great deal of experience preparing very ill heart patients for major surgery. We also know how to monitor and care for the patient during open-heart procedures using the heart-lung machine. And, more important, how to care for them in the post-operative period. So it wasn't as if we were operating on the heart for the first time. We perfected the surgical technique by doing transplants in dogs in the laboratory. I feel these two aspects ensured that the operation would be a success. But, to answer your question, I only thought it would work when, finally, I had stopped the circulatory support of the heart-lung machine and the transplanted heart maintained a good circulation according to the readings of the blood pressure, the venous pressure and urinary output.'

Michael de Bakey was introduced, and he asked, 'We would all be very interested to know what the factors were that contributed to your decision to perform the procedure on Mr Washkansky. Were there some factors, in terms of medical knowledge, that were available then that were not available, say, a year ago when, from a technical stand-point, you were certainly able to perform the operation. Why did you decide at this time to do it?' I agreed that, from a technical point of view, we could have done the operation well over a year previously and that in my mind there was never a race to be the first. We had prepared ourselves by first doing a kidney transplant. This gave us the opportunity to get experience in human donation of a vital organ, under South African law, and also on the use of the immunosuppressive drugs.

They looked amazed when I told them that I could have done the transplant several weeks earlier when I was presented with a very suitable black donor. We turned down this opportunity because Dr Schrire and I decided that we would not use a black recipient or a black donor for the first transplant in case we, as South Africans, were accused of 'experimenting' on black people.

I asked them to show a slide I'd brought of Washkansky's heart and showed them where the main pumping chamber had been destroyed.

Dr Kantrowitz added, 'Looking at that slide it's obvious that it's enormously enlarged – it looks like it could weigh 600 or 700 grams whereas a normal heart should weigh 300 grams.'

'Yes, that's true,' I replied, 'The heart had become enlarged because of its injuries and couldn't stand up to the normal pressure inside the chamber. The only other option was to remove the diseased part of the heart which, in Louis Washkansky's case, would have been impossible because about 90% would have had to have been cut away.'

To stop the debate becoming highly technical Martin Agronsky asked a question I'd faced before, 'Did you, Dr Barnard, tell Mr Washkansky the chances he had in such an operation and, when you discussed it with him, what did he say?'

I replied, 'In any treatment one has to be totally honest with the patient. We told Mr Washkansky that we thought the only way to help him was to do a transplant – which had never been done on a human before – and he said, "You don't have to tell me anything further, go ahead and transplant the heart."'

And so the interview continued, discussing the ability of the transplanted heart, which was without a nerve supply, to respond to varying demands of the body. A mechanical device which Dr De Bakey and Dr Kantrowitz appeared to favour would not be able to do this. We all agreed, at this stage, that there was no mechanical device available that could be totally implanted to take over the full function of the circulation.

I briefly dealt with the legal and moral aspects.

In South Africa the neurosurgeons and coroner stipulated that three criteria should be fulfilled to declare the patient brain-dead. First there must be no brain activity on clinical examination at normal temperatures. Secondly, there must be no spontaneous breathing when the respirator is disconnected for 3 minutes and thirdly, there must be no electrical activity in the brain as monitored by the electroencephalogram.

I also stressed that in the case of Denise Darvall I had discontinued the respirator and that we had not opened her chest until her heart had gone into ventricular fibrillation.

'As far as the moral side is concerned, to me this is very straightforward. My duty as a doctor is to treat the patient. Now, as far as the donor is concerned, I could treat her no more. She was beyond the realms of medical knowledge for treatment – so there my duty had ended. She was dead.

'As far as the recipient is concerned, I had one way of treating him, and that was to transplant a heart, which is what we did. I have no moral dilemma over this.'

Suddenly it was over and although the programme seemed to last only a few moments it was, in fact, an hour long.

As the lights were being turned off and microphones removed I carefully stepped over the spaghetti of wires and thought that this television business was not so bad after all. I thought it had gone quite smoothly in fact.

It was fleeting comfort – I was to face very many aggressive interviewers in the years to come – and I wouldn't always come off so well.

Louwtjie Barnard was one of the millions watching the programme and later, said, 'With confidence, knowledge, wit and charm, he captured the hearts of millions and once more the world cheered and congratulated him. He accepted it with dignity and a smile. I thanked God for the privilege of being married to this brilliant man. Watching him on Face the Nation *I admired and loved him silently. But little did I know that my husband would change beyond recognition in the next few years. Had I not witnessed it from start to finish, I wouldn't have believed it possible.'*

She strolled around their suite in the luxurious Hilton Hotel in Washington idly thinking how much she was enjoying the celebrity treatment but when she opened the closet door she smiled thinly and thought to herself, 'We don't really belong here.' The three suits belonging to her husband and her own four dresses looked out of place, lost.

It was bitterly cold outside. She realized she was homesick.

Monday was Christmas. Louis and I often discussed how he was going to celebrate the first Christmas with his new heart but he hadn't made it. He was lying in his coffin in the cemetery and I was now in the Plaza Hotel overlooking New York's Central Park.

After the interview in Washington, Louwtjie and I had flown in the CBS private jet to New York where we spent Christmas Day at the home of the network's boss, Gordon Manning.

I had a full schedule the next day: first an interview with Walter Kronkite who was, at that stage, the most popular newscaster in America – a very highly respected man. We became good friends and met again often in the years to come.

There was also an important interview with a reporter from the *New York Times*. CBS had had their scoop and were now willing to allow the other media to talk to me.

27

The science writer from this influential newspaper sat down in the lounge of my suite and opened his notebook. 'It was on the wire this morning that Dr Blaiberg has had a very severe setback and that he is dying,' he said without showing any emotion. I sat bolt upright and was obviously startled. Looking at me carefully, he continued, 'Yes, the bulletin from the hospital said that your patient has suffered a pulmonary embolus and gone into severe right heart failure while you are here.'

That was exactly what I was afraid of. But why hadn't Vel Schrire phoned me? How did the media get the news before me?

I was to learn in the years to come that reporters often knew more about my patients than I did. They had an uncanny way of getting news about patients and especially donors before the information reached me. I often wondered how much it cost them.

I had to know what was happening back in Ward D1 before continuing this interview, so I excused myself and used the phone in the bedroom. I hoped I'd find Vel. It must be about 5 pm in South Africa. He was probably studying electrocardiograms in the cardiac clinic.

I dialled 027 for South Africa, 21 for Cape Town and, finally, 55-1111 for Groote Schuur Hospital. Almost instantly I could hear the phone ringing at the other end but why was there no damned reply? It just kept on ringing and ringing. After about two minutes the exchange operator answered, 'Groote Schuur Hospital.' His voice sounded so clear that he could have been speaking from next door.

'This is Dr Barnard – I'm calling from New York – please put me through to the cardiac clinic – quickly.'

'Hi Doc, are you having a good time in the States?' The operator obviously wanted to have a little chat before he put me through.

I was very short with him. 'Listen to me, I've already waited two bloody minutes for you to answer! I desperately need to speak to Professor Schrire – now!'

'Okay, hang on.' He was obviously disappointed. I didn't care but silently prayed, please God, let Vel be in the clinic.

'Schrire speaking,' it was the voice of the man whom I idolised so much.

'Vel, this is Chris. How's Dr Blaiberg? What's wrong? They tell me he's dying, must I come back immediately?' The words gushed out in a torrent of anxiety.

'Absolute nonsense, he's had a minor setback – a small pulmonary embolus – but he's in no immediate danger. He'll hold until you get back.' That was Vel, always cool and so sure of himself. I still think he was the best clinical cardiologist in the world – ever.

'Are you sure, Vel?'

'Of course I'm sure. By the way I heard you did very well on *Face the Nation*.'

'Thanks – it wasn't nearly as bad as I expected. What can I bring you from America?' I was so grateful and relieved I would have taken him the Statue of Liberty if I could.

'Just bring yourself back; we still have a lot to do.'

I virtually ran back to the reporter. 'You are badly informed, I have just spoken to the cardiologist who is looking after Dr Blaiberg. He said things are well under control.'

It was soon clear that the so-called science writer from the *New York Times* was not interested in the medical aspects of our work – I suspect he was keener to get something sensational or controversial.

'Dr Dwight E. Harken from Boston claims you stole the technique from Dr Shumway?' he said with a sardonic smile. It was a statement rather than a question.

'I know Dr Harken. I have great respect for his work and he's entitled to his own opinion.' I was definitely not in the mood for an argument – I felt so relieved and happy that Blaiberg was okay.

The reporter wouldn't give up. 'Dr Shumway said in an interview, and I quote: "The surgical technique Barnard used was based on the work done by Doctors Lower and Hurley at Stanford."'

I summoned all the composure I could and, refusing to lose my temper, I explained, 'Let's get this clear once and for all. The surgical technique of orthotopic heart transplantation became a very simple procedure when it was suggested that portions of the right and left atria into which the veins drain should be left in the recipient. The systemic and pulmonary venous systems of the patient could now be connected to the donor heart by simply joining these atrial cuffs to the back wall of the corresponding atria of the donor heart.

'This technique was discussed by Cass and Brock in the Guy's Hospital Report in 1959. In 1960, in *Surgical Forum*, Lower and Shumway reported their results in canine transplantation using the same technique. I'll leave it to you to decide whose technique I used.'

'Dr Barnard, are you implying that Dr Shumway made no contributions in this field?'

Now I was really beginning to lose my temper.

'No, I'm not saying that at all,' I sighed. 'Dr Shumway and his colleagues did excellent research in this field and I have never hesitated to give them full credit.

'What I don't understand is why some American doctors feel that I stole his ideas and that *he* should have done the first heart transplant. I'm the first to admit that I made use of a lot of his findings. Surely he published them in medical journals so that other doctors could learn from his experience? That's what I did because, as you should know, doctors share information – which, incidentally, is also why I'm in America right now.'

The reporter finally gave up. He switched off his tape recorder and, with a half-hearted good-bye, he left. It was obvious that he had not got what he came for – which was unimportant because he'd write what he wanted to anyway. But the criticism was, by far, outweighed by the support I received in America so the bad press and sensational reporting didn't really upset me very much at all.

I was far more concerned about my marriage which, while I had hoped the excitement of travel might bond it together, was actually breaking apart.

Louwtjie always said that I was a 'difficult' man to live with – and I agree with her. As a matter of fact, all three of my wives are of the same opinion. I am a moody, selfish, irritable perfectionist. I am never wrong and modesty isn't my strong point. But apart from that I'm really quite a nice guy.

In fact a BBC reporter once asked me, 'Why are you so popular?' and I replied, 'Because I'm a nice guy.'

I'm not sure he understood what I meant because he said, 'Can we have a serious answer?'

So I said, 'That was a serious answer.'

I think now, looking back, that Louwtjie's biggest problem was that she married a medical *student* – and never adjusted to my becoming a doctor. I don't think we'd have lasted even if I'd stayed a GP in Ceres – a small town two hours away from Cape Town. She blamed the fame but I think there were far more complicated reasons.

She was a wonderful mother and a good wife – in the true Afrikaner tradition. She liked to sew and cook and keep house. She never wanted to be anything more than a 'boere meisie' (farm girl) and, being married to someone like me who wanted much, much more from life, the marriage never really stood much of a chance. Of course when the world opened its doors to me, with all the fanfare and bright lights, it was probably her worst nightmare.

Unfortunately Louwtjie never had much of a sense of humour. She was a happy person generally, with a quick smile – but serious. And such a severe outlook on life can become excruciatingly dull. After years of study and hard work I needed some *fun*.

My life was missing that *spark*, that extra *something* that makes living a joy. That's the reason I started looking at other girls – a long time before the transplant. It's the old story of doctors and nurses – and true in my case. I have regrets but I make no excuses.

Louwtjie wasn't to blame but nor was I when I think about it. We just sort of drifted. I'd grown with my career and she was still married to the medical student. The first few sips of success were so sweet and I wanted to enjoy every last drop – but that very success and publicity we were now enjoying in America had every prospect of bringing our marriage to a very painful end. She knew it and I knew it.

We left New York and arrived at San Antonio airport late the same afternoon – on our way to meet the most powerful man in the whole world, the President of the United States. The reporters wanted to know what the president and I were going to discuss; was I going to examine him? At that stage I wasn't even aware of the fact that President Johnson had a heart problem.

Dr Reid, a senior general surgeon who at the age of 70 was still in the operating theatre every day, was going to look after us during our stay in San Antonio. I could see he was highly respected in this town because he cut the interview short without a murmur from the members of the media. He obviously had a lot of clout.

On the way to our hotel he told us they had heard about my love for Dixieland music and had arranged dinner for us that night at the Riverside Club where an excellent Dixieland band was playing.

Louwtjie said she was tired and would rather stay and have something to eat in our hotel room so I went on my own with our hosts.

I had a wonderful evening and even agreed to sing with the

band – a ballad called 'Release me', the words of which, I thought at the time, were a portent for my marriage. The audience seemed to like it although one guy suggested I shouldn't think seriously about giving up my daytime job.

When I returned to the hotel it was past midnight. There was a message that Dr Reid's daughter would fetch us just after breakfast to visit a few of the historical sites of San Antonio and, at about 10 o'clock, a car would take us from the hotel to the LBJ ranch.

The lights in our room were still on but Louwtjie was already asleep. She looked so vulnerable and lost in the king-size bed as she lay curled up with her face turned to the dark side of the room.

How sad, I thought, recalling the fun and laughter I'd had that evening at the club.

The next morning was bright and crisp as we set out with Dr Reid's daughter to the Alamo that had been built as a Catholic mission station. She became quite emotional when she told us how 150 Texans, under Lieutenant Colonel William Barret Travis, withstood the attack of 5 000 Mexican soldiers under General Antonio Lopez de Santa Anna from the 23 February to 5 March 1836. Eventually these brave men had exhausted their ammunition and the Mexicans scaled the walls. The Texans, she told us with real tears in her eyes, fought on using their rifles as clubs until the last man was killed. Among those who died were the border heroes, James Bowie and Davy Crockett.

We then left the Alamo for the president's ranch. I was surprised that there were no photographers or reporters following us. The driver of the limousine assured me that I would still see them before the day was over. 'There ain't no place to hide from them,' he added with a chuckle.

After the assassination of President Kennedy I thought the farm would be bristling with armed guards and that both Louwtjie and I would be thoroughly searched, but we weren't even stopped and drove straight through the gates up to the front of a quite ordinary farmhouse. Two men came out and led us in to a modestly furnished room.

President Johnson was sitting on one of those chairs with a lever at the side which, when you pushed it forward, the back of the seat reclined and a foot rest came out at the front. He was dressed in an open-neck shirt and a lumber jacket. I, on the other hand, was toffed up in a blue suit and tie while Louwtjie was in one of her prettiest self-made dresses. The president had his grandson on his lap.

This man, who could upset the world's stock exchanges within a few hours and who had the lives of half a million young Americans in Vietnam in his hands, at that very moment could easily pass for a sheep farmer back in the Karoo – a desert area in the northern Cape of South Africa.

After the introductions were completed Mrs Johnson asked Louwtjie to join her and the president and I were left alone. I was ready for a barrage of questions on heart transplantation but no. In fact President Johnson wasn't interested in my work at all and couldn't stop telling me about all his achievements since he'd become president.

'I'm a Texan,' he drawled, 'and since Jack's death we've done a lot of good things here. I brought in the civil rights bill – something your government could take some lessons from – as well as introduced Medicare so our old folk have full access to medical treatment.

'A lot of people say I'm not a popular guy – but did you know that, in the 1964 election I got 61% of the popular vote? That's a bigger majority than any president ever got.' And he leaned back with a smile.

After listening to this for about 15 minutes I tried to steer the conversation on to the Vietnam War. After all, he was commander in chief of the American armed forces, but that was one of his activities he obviously had no intention of discussing.

I wonder now, if he knew then, that the Vietnam War would make him one of the most *un*popular presidents ever?

After a lunch of wild turkey President Johnson invited us for a chopper-ride over the ranch. This was the first time that Louwtjie and I had ever flown in a helicopter and we were thrilled that this should be with the President of the United States and his wife. We couldn't wait to get home and tell our friends.

Back at the ranch, before we left, President Johnson took me aside and reminded me not to forget to tell the press about all his achievements – it still didn't dawn on me that our meeting would be such a closely watched event and such a big media opportunity for him to regain some of his popularity: I didn't help him much however.

So he told me again how much money he'd spent on social welfare, hospitals and health programmes. I was tempted to ask him how much money he had spent on killing people, but thought better of it.

So that was the President of the United States. What a disappointment!

Perhaps it's unfair to judge a man after such a short time, but I have to say he was far from being the formidable leader I expected. His size and height were impressive – his intellect wasn't.

At the press conference the first question they asked me was 'How did you find the president?' I said that when we first met he looked rather tired but, after we started talking, he brightened up and was full of life.

The next day the newspaper front pages were headlined, 'Heart specialist, Dr Barnard, says President looks tired'. I hadn't realized my casual remarks would have been taken so seriously or given such prominence. I was still getting used to the fact that *everything* I said was recorded and reported.

A few weeks later I had a letter from Lyndon Johnson with clippings from the newspapers telling me how much my press statements had harmed his image. Politicians, the world over, are obsessed with their media image. I'd naively thought he was genuinely interested in my work – but his main concern seemed to be to use my current celebrity status for his own political ends.

Blaiberg was waiting back in Cape Town so we left for South Africa the following morning.

The task ahead was crystal clear to me. Although the American people and medical profession, on the whole, were enthusiastic and fascinated by the operation on Louis Washkansky they were not as confident as I was about future transplants.

Our first operation showed only that a heart transplanted in a patient with severe heart failure could be technically successful but, and this is what we would have to prove in the case of Dr Blaiberg, could such a patient live more than 18 days? Could he eventually be discharged from hospital? And, at home, would he be an invalid in a wheel chair taking a handful of pills every day or could he play ball with his kids, visit friends and enjoy a normal life?

Blaiberg would have to provide the answers to these questions. The world was waiting. I planned and re-planned the Blaiberg operation in my mind many, many times on our return flight home.

We stepped off the plane at Cape Town's DF Malan airport on New Year's day and went home. Two hours later my registrar, Dr 'Bossie' Bosman phoned, 'Prof, we've found a donor for Blaiberg.'

Eileen Blaiberg knew that Dr Barnard was due back in Cape Town any day now and gently squeezed her husband's hand in encouragement.

'Do you remember,' he asked, 'when we first heard I was going to get the transplant?'

'Yes, very well.'

'There we were – the two of us, married for over thirty years and with a grown-up daughter, laughing and crying like children!'

She handed him a glass of water as he started coughing again.

Looking out of the hospital window at the mob of newsmen gathered outside she marvelled at how they'd tracked Phil down as the next transplant patient. Word had somehow leaked out that an operation was imminent and someone had mentioned that a 'retired dentist' was being considered. With that information it didn't take local reporters long to discover Blaiberg's name – simply a process of elimination – paging through the telephone directory and making a few calls.

It was the last thing Groote Schuur Hospital had wanted – after the chaos following the Washkansky operation. Eileen wondered how she was going to avoid them when she left – she'd run out of answers.

Her husband had just fallen asleep when Dr Bosman asked her into the waiting room.

'Great news!' he said. 'It looks like we'll be doing the transplant tonight – probably within the next few hours.' The tears coursed down her pale cheeks. She felt near to collapse and held onto Bossie Bosman for support.

Meanwhile, in another part of the hospital, the Haupt family were grieving the loss of Clive – a man who, only a few hours before, had been playing on the beach when a massive brain haemorrhage ended his life.

Now his heart would give new life to Philip Blaiberg.

In those evil days, when the apartheid laws were ravaging South African society, Clive Haupt was treated in a different part of the hospital.

Philip was 'white' and Clive 'non-white' but now that didn't matter and the two men lay in adjacent rooms of a theatre for a very special performance.

The two principal actors were already on stage. One was dead and one was dying.

In the drama to unfold in the Charles Saint operating suite on this, the 2nd of January 1968, the whole world would be the audience and would witness the dead give life to the dying.

The various members of the supporting cast were also arriving and taking their places. One of them was me – waiting impatiently and nervously before the lights went on – especially as there had been only one previous performance. I hoped I'd remember my lines.

I took a slow, deep breath to steady my nerves and tried to dismiss the arthritic ache in my hands. I strode into the room and, with a grim smile, nodded briefly to my colleagues.

'Lights on!'

I blinked as the operating lights were turned on to spotlight the small area of Blaiberg's chest.

He had already been anaesthetized and lay prone on the table – his body violated by a host of tubes and pipes.

A tube which passed through his mouth into the main windpipe, or trachea, was connected to a mechanical ventilator.

From his left nostril the nasogastric tube was connected to a machine for slight suction to prevent overdistension of the stomach during surgery.

From his right nostril there was an electric thermometer the sensor of which was positioned in his oesophagus, behind the heart, allowing an accurate monitoring of the heart temperature.

From his anus, a second electric thermometer, had been positioned in the rectum to give us an idea of his body temperature.

From his penis, a catheter passed into the bladder and was connected by a tube to a bottle standing under the operating table. The rate of urine flow is a good indication of the blood flow to the kidneys and thus of the circulation in general.

There was an intravenous line into each forearm through which fluids, drugs and blood would be given during the operation as well as in the post-operative period.

There was also a metal cuff around his left leg from which an electric wire ran to the diathermic machine.

My patient's arms were secured at his side with a bandage and he was strapped down with a leather belt so that the operating table could be tilted.

All this apparatus was necessary because we were about to deny the body its ability to control many of its natural functions.

The healthy, warm-blooded animal has the amazing ability to

keep the internal environment or *milieu interieur* (defined about a century before by Claude Bernard) within the limits of a normal lower and normal upper range. It does this through its own sensors that regulate the function of organs such as the kidneys, lungs, the cardiovascular system and sweat glands.

In normal circumstances the human body adjusts itself naturally. If, for example, there is a rise in body temperature it will result in an increase in the metabolic flame and, therefore, in metabolic demand. The heart and respiration rate will immediately increase to take care of the increased demand for oxygen and fuel demanded by the various organs and tissues of the body. At the same time perspiration will increase, which will result in an increase of water evaporation from the surface of the body, thus cooling it down. If this continues for any length of time, resulting in dehydration, the kidneys will retain water and secrete a smaller, but more concentrated, volume of urine, reducing fluid loss but still expelling the waste products.

During the transplant operation, however, there would be at least two hours during which the lungs would not be working. The heart would either not beat or not be present in the chest at all.

The functions of these two vital organs would be taken over by the heart-lung machine, which would not obey commands of body sensors.

During the operation, 'Ozzie' Ozinsky, the anaesthetist, would be the guardian of the constancy of the body's internal environment.

Frequent blood samples taken from the body would be rushed to the biochemical laboratory to be analysed for salt content, acidity and oxygen levels. These results indicated how the internal environment was changing and any corrections necessary could be made by Ozzie. Thus, if the acidity increased, sodium bicarbonate would be given intravenously – if the potassium dropped then potassium chloride would be administered.

The surgeon relies completely on the anaesthetist and heart-lung technicians to see to these extremely important matters.

While Johan van Heerden and Dene Friedmann, both excellent technicians, did final checks on the heart-lung machine Dr Hitchcock and Sister Peggy Jordaan prepared the operating field by painting the body with an iodine solution and then covering it with a sterile, transparent, plastic sheet through which an incision would be made.

Finally the entire body was draped with sterile green towelling so that only the right groin and the front of the chest and upper abdomen were exposed. As he would be immunosuppressed from then on, extreme precautions had to be taken to avoid the introduction of bacteria or viruses during the operation.

I left Blaiberg in A-Theatre and walked through the connecting room to B-Theatre to see what was happening to Clive Haupt – the donor.

Dr Cecil Moss, an anaesthetist, and one of my registrars, was checking some lab results which had just been received.

Although Clive was dead he had to be checked and monitored with the same meticulous care as Philip. This was even more difficult than in a living patient as two of the main sensors, the brain, and the pituitary – that peanut-sized gland at the base of the brain and conductor of the orchestra of endocrine glands – were dead.

Serious changes in the internal environment can lead to extensive damage to the donor's heart. As there was no artificial device to fall back on, as in the case of the kidneys, once the heart-lung machine had been stopped after the transplant, success would be dependent entirely on the adequate function of Clive's heart.

'How are things going?' I asked.

'I think this is a very strong heart,' Marius, my brother, answered. He and Dr Terry O'Donovan, as with the first transplant, were the surgical team looking after the donor.

Cecil Moss, the anaesthetist, gave me details of the vital signs. 'The mean arterial pressure is 95, pulse 86 and venous pressure 2 and he's putting out buckets of urine – and that's without any cardiac stimulants. I've already stopped the isoprenaline – about twenty minutes ago.'

'Potassium?'

'It was 3 but I've given another 2 grams.'

'I think we should raise the venous pressure a bit despite the good circulation,' I said – because the patient, due to pituitary death, couldn't regulate his blood volume. 'Terry, you and Marius take the heart out.' At the first transplant I had done that myself.

During Washkansky's operation I had disconnected the respirator on Denise Darvall and waited until her heart had gone into ventricular fibrillation before allowing her chest to be opened. Although this increased the risk of damage to the donor heart – and therefore to the success of the operation itself – we had decided on this approach as we had anticipated criticism for removing a heart which was still beating. This time I thought the precaution was unnecessary.

I could hear the sound of the saw in A-Theatre as it sliced through the breastbone so I went into the scrub-room to prepare myself for surgery.

I'm not a superstitious person but I do believe in following routines which 'work' and have brought me 'luck' in the past – so I'm more a creature of habit than anything else.

Since we started using the heart-lung machine in 1958 I had always used the bubble oxygenator which gave us very good results – while many surgeons were experimenting with disc oxygenators, screen oxygenators and membrane oxygenators.

This habit extended to using the same heart valves, stitching material and post-operative monitoring. I even used the same sink in the scrub-room every time and often wore the same jacket to the hospital when I was going to do a major operation.

I took a piece of soap and a brush and started scrubbing – as I had done a thousand times before – and I went over again, in my mind, the changes in technique I had been planning.

In the first transplant, the donor heart was removed in the way that many surgeons agreed was best – by cutting through the left and right atrial bodies and the wall that divided these two chambers.

We had noticed, however, as others had, that using this method of excision meant there was a risk of damaging the intrinsic nerve supply of the heart, resulting in a type of heart block.

Shumway and his colleagues had even suggested that a mechanical pacemaker should be inserted, as a matter of routine, so that the heart could be paced if necessary in the post-operative period.

But pacing has disadvantages in itself so we devised a technique of our own which would ensure that the nerves could never be damaged during excision. Instead of cutting through the upper chambers and septum, we would remove these two chambers as a whole by cutting the six veins that connected them to the body. Then, small openings would be made later in the back wall of the chambers to connect them to the cuffs of atria left in the patient.

I was certain that this variation in technique would significantly improve results. With arms covered in soap I went to the door of A-Theatre and called out, 'Rodney, is everything okay?'

Dr Rodney Hewitson had a good pair of hands and for years had been my first assistant. Having him there was reassuring.

'I think the arterial blood is a bit dark, but Ozzie says he's satisfied that the patient is well ventilated.'

'Ozzie?' I asked, 'how can he be well oxygenated when arterial blood is dark? I don't understand!'

'I think it must be the poor circulation – he's on 80% oxygen and I've double-checked the intra-tracheal tube – it's in position okay but he's not passing much urine. The venous pressure is 20 but the mean arterial pressure only 50.'

I didn't want to hear that – it meant that he could die before we even had a chance to *begin* the transplant.

I leaned my head back and closed my eyes. Please God help us. Don't let him fibrillate before we connect him to the heart-lung machine! My patient had been waiting so long for a donor – it would be tragic if his life ended moments before we could perform the operation he had been praying for.

'Check the Astrip and increase isoprenaline, Ozzie. Rodney, give the heparin and start cannulating the femoral artery, I'll be with you in a minute.' My voice was strained.

Rodney Hewitson called back, 'Chris, I think we should put the arterial cannula in the aorta.'

He was right and it reminded me that, during the Washkansky operation, we had run into great problems due to cannulating the arteriosclerotic femoral artery. As soon as we went on by-pass Johan, the heart-lung technician, reported an abnormally high line pressure.

This almost certainly meant an obstruction in the femoral or external iliac artery due to the same arteriosclerotic disease that had closed off the coronary arteries.

In the middle of the operation we had had to change to aortic cannulation and, in the ensuing panic, the arterial line had blown off from its connection to the heat exchanger.

It's difficult to change horses midstream and I nearly lost Washkansky even before I had time to give him the new heart I'd promised him. But we were lucky. This time I might not have the same luck and, to make matters even more tense, hordes of reporters were camping outside the hospital waiting for news.

To them, I imagined, it didn't matter very much whether the outcome of the operation was good or bad. They just wanted their headlines to be as sensational as possible and I think a lot of them might even have preferred 'Blaiberg dies on the operating table'.

'You're right Rodney, let's do that,' I said and walked across to B-Theatre.

'Terry, you and Marius can start now and don't forget to give the heparin,' I reminded them.

I turned to the heart-lung technicians in Marius and Terry's team. 'Alastair, as soon as you and Nick are on by-pass, start cooling.' I decided, as with the first operation, to protect the donor heart from anoxic damage by cooling it down with oxygenated blood. This precaution would also protect the kidneys which were going to be transplanted into two other patients dying from incurable kidney disease at another hospital.

I hurried back and finished scrubbing, the nurse poured spirits over my hands and arms and, with forceps, passed me a sterile towel to dry them. I put on my gown and gloves and walked into A-Theatre.

Blaiberg's chest was wide open through a median sternotomy. The heart that had kept him alive for 58 years was still obediently struggling to respond to the demands of the body even after large portions of the main pumping chamber had been destroyed by the extensive disease of the coronary arteries.

The heart – what an amazing pump! No wonder, that over the centuries it has had such a prominent place in religion, poetry and prose. You love with your heart – not with your kidney or liver – two very essential and much more complex organs. You also hate with your heart and, as many believe, it is the very seat of the soul.

It was not so long ago that surgeons believed that if you touched the heart, life would immediately end – oh, how wrong they were!

In the 12 years that I've operated on it I've never ceased to be amazed by the heart's ability to respond immediately to the call of the body for blood – even after being assaulted by disease and by the surgeon's knife. It doesn't give up easily.

I took up my position on the right side of the table and asked Rodney to move to the left side – next to the second assistant, Dr Hitchcock.

'How does it look?' I asked, looking at Blaiberg's heart myself for the first time. The heart that was *still* keeping him alive – the heart that I was about to remove and destroy permanently.

Nobody answered. The air was heavy with tension and anxiety.

Rodney already had the arterial catheter in place high up on the ascending aorta. I needed at least four inches of aorta in order to cross-clamp it below the insertion of the catheter and to anastomose the donor's aorta after the recipient's heart had been excised.

'Let's have the line, Dene,' I asked the second heart-lung technician, the pretty daughter of Captain Friedmann, an old friend of mine.

A length of sterile three-quarter plastic tubing full of red blood was passed from the heart-lung machine to me. I took it around my body and handed the open end back to Dene to be connected to the venous well. The tube would be divided and the portion on my left connected to the arterial catheter and the portion on my right to the two venous catheters I was about to insert. That would complete the extra-corporeal circuit.

As soon as by-pass was started, Blaiberg's venous blood would be prevented from entering the heart and lungs by the two venous catheters. They would divert, or direct, the blood to the venous well. From there the venous pump would force it up the mixing chamber where oxygen from a cylinder would be bubbled into it.

These bubbles function as the alveoli – little air sacs of the lungs. Oxygen then diffuses out of the bubbles into the blood – turning it red – and carbon dioxide diffuses out of the blood into the bubbles.

The circuit then leads to the debubbling chamber where the bubbles burst and liberate the carbon dioxide which would otherwise blow off.

The oxygenated blood is pushed by a second pump via the arterial line back to the circulation of the patient. The body can then be cooled and supplied with oxygenated blood, without the use of its own heart and lungs.

This technique, discovered by researchers such as Gibbon and De Waal in the mid-1950s, has made successful open-heart surgery possible. We all owe great credit to these pioneers.

'Let's put in the venous catheters.' I extended my right hand and Sister Jordaan gave me a needle holder into which was clipped a curved needle with a three-o silk thread.

She had been assisting me for many years and could anticipate every move – even before it was requested. That was why I preferred to work with the same team every time.

It was also the reason that I refused requests to operate in unfamiliar circumstances in other countries – except once in Delhi – and after that, never again.

Rodney took a wet swab, placed it on the right atrium and

gently pulled it towards himself so that I could position the purse-string suture, through which the venous catheters would be introduced as low down as possible on the body of the right atrium. As the two catheters had to remain in place after the heart was excised, their position far back would leave enough atrial wall in front for the anastomosis of the donor's heart.

'The arterial pressure is right down,' Ozzie warned with little emotion. He was calmly doing his job.

'Well, what are you doing about it?' I snapped. I was certainly far from calm.

'I can't do anything about it while you're pushing on the heart like that.' The tone of his voice didn't change as he studied the dials.

But I had to see what I was doing and the heart was in the way. 'Rodney stop pushing on the atrium.'

There was a minute of silence.

'Blood pressure's coming up, give the heart a bit of a chance to recover, then you can go on,' said Ozzie.

'If we carry on like this we'll be here the whole day,' I said contritely – but I knew he was right, as pressure on the right atrium had interfered with the venous return and immediately dropped the cardiac output. As soon as we relieved the atrial pressure the situation returned to normal.

'How far is Marius?'

It was the floor nurse who replied. 'They've just sent in a message to say that Clive is on by-pass and the cooling has fibrillated his heart. They are ready whenever you want them to take out the heart, Prof.'

'Tell them to hold on for a while, I'll be ready as soon as Ozzie allows me to continue with surgery,' I said tersely.

Ozzie didn't credit the sarcasm with any response – we knew each other so well that remarks like those didn't mean anything.

'Okay, you can carry on now,' Ozzie confirmed as he checked all his readings.

The two purse-string sutures were placed without any further drop in the blood pressure.

I introduced the inferior vena cava catheter first, through a stab wound in the centre of the purse-string made with a stiletto-bladed knife and secured it by tightening the purse-string suture. Then, in a similar way, the superior vena cava catheter.

'Blood pressure down again,' Ozzie warned.

'Okay, let's connect the venous line – Y-piece, Sister.' But Peggy had already anticipated this and had connected the one limb of the Y to the venous line.

My hands were so painful from a flare-up of rheumatoid arthritis after my American trip that I struggled to push the ends of the venous catheters over the other two limbs of the Y.

Oh Lord, please help me through this operation, I prayed silently. It's so human to turn to God only when there's trouble – if all else fails, pray for help.

'Okay. Pump on.'

'We can't, Prof!' was Johan's immediate cry. 'You haven't connected the arterial line yet!'

Dear God, what in heaven's name was I doing! My brain was so tired I couldn't have been thinking straight. I silently cursed myself for going on the American trip before the operation.

'You usually connect the arterial line first,' Rodney quietly reminded me.

'Why didn't you bloody-well say so then! What the hell are you here for?' I shouted – trying to conceal the panic I was feeling.

I grimaced as I took the arterial line with a metal connector firmly in my left hand and the end of the aortic catheter in my right hand. Pain was shooting violently through my fingers.

'Slowly release the arterial clamp.' As the blood welled up, replacing air, I tried to push the end of the catheter over the metal connector but the pain had sapped my strength. I couldn't control the two ends with my shaking hands.

Then the *very* worst thing that could have happened did happen. The metal connector slipped off and, overcompensating, I jerked the arterial catheter out of the aorta. This was a deadly mistake.

Blaiberg's struggling heart, finding an easier passage for its load, pumped the blood in a gushing arc out of the resulting hole left in the aorta. Soon the heart and aorta were obscured by a well of red blood and I was in serious trouble – not to mention Philip Blaiberg.

Fortunately, years of experience with major bleeding since I lost a little girl patient when I was a registrar taught me that you can nearly always control bleeding with finger pressure.

I immediately started searching in the well of blood for the aorta with my right index finger. I found it and applied firm pressure.

'Blood pressure is right down.' Ozzie's alarmed, but calm, voice sounded far away.

'That's good! The lower pressure will slow down the bleeding,' I countered petulantly, realizing immediately that it was a stupid, supercilious remark and I regretted having said it.

'Sucker on, Johan.'

As the patient was heparinized I could suck the blood back to the heart-lung machine.

There was a slurping sound as the pericardial sac emptied.

I could now see the aorta. The finger pressure had stopped the bleeding completely but the aorta was soft. The heart, with such a reduction in blood volume, was not able to generate much pressure.

I *must* calm down. I could *not* afford to make any more mistakes as speed was now critical – to prevent Blaiberg from suffering brain damage.

'The purse-string suture hasn't torn out.' Rodney tried to encourage me with some good news.

'Okay, release the suture slowly so I can slip the catheter back into the aorta.'

Still applying pressure I searched for the hole under my finger with the tip of the catheter.

'Release a bit more – it's still too tight.' I felt nauseous with tension. I *had* to get the damned catheter back in place – quickly – or my patient's brain would die.

I slowly moved the tip of the catheter in small circular movements under my finger – where *was* that bloody hole?

Suddenly, to my great relief, the catheter's tip slipped securely into the aorta.

'Okay, tighten the purse-string suture and give me the arterial line again,' I said, trying to sound as relaxed as possible, and then I thought again for a second. 'No, I think it's better if you do the connection, Rodney, my hands hurt too much.'

Rodney quickly and confidently made the connection.

'Right! Release the clamps and start the pump so Ozzie can stop panicking,' I said lightly, hiding my anxiety with a poor attempt at humour.

'Who's panicking?' retorted Ozzie, but I could hear the relief in his voice.

I looked up at the clock on the wall. It felt as if I had done a day's work already but it was only 30 minutes since Rodney had started cutting. It was 11:53.

'I think the worst is over,' I sighed – little realizing what still lay ahead.

'Start cooling – and tell Marius they can take the heart out.'

There was no further need for Blaiberg's heart. We would soon be at the point of no return – the moment when we would stare into the empty cavity of a man without a heart – but a man who would still be alive.

'Everything running smoothly, Johan?'

'Yes Prof, I'm on full-flow and the line pressure is 120, oesophageal temperature 32 and rectal temperature 36.'

'Ozzie? On your side?'

'No problems, Chris.'

I felt much more relaxed; nothing more can go wrong I assured myself. But, of course, I was always wary of being overconfident.

'Cross-clamp.' Sister Jordaan handed me the arterial clamp which I placed across the aorta just below the arterial catheter and closed it. Now those diseased coronaries could be closed off, there was no further need for them either.

I detached the left ventricle from the aorta by cutting through it just above the aortic valve. The wall was sickened and the lumen dilated by the disease. Stitching was going to difficult, I reminded myself.

The pulmonary artery was detached from the right ventricle in a similar way. This vessel was even more dilated because of the abnormally high pressure it had had to tolerate as a result of the severe failure of its left-side partner.

Although the muscle of the old heart was now deprived of life-giving blood it continued struggling as if it still felt responsible for providing oxygen and nourishment to the body that had shielded and protected it for so long.

A lot of blood was coming back from the lungs but I didn't want to cross-clamp the pulmonary artery as well – in case pressure built up in the lungs and damaged the small capillaries.

'Put the small sucker into the pulmonary artery, Dr Hitchcock. Rodney, you lift up the end of the aorta and pulmonary artery so that I can see the back of the heart. Sister? Scissors please.'

We were ready to cut horizontally through the two top chambers and the wall that divided them.

I began transecting the atria by making an incision into the cavity of the left atrium under the roots of the great vessels and then across the septum and along the outer border of the right atrium close to the groove where it bordered onto the right ventricle. This incision extended down to the diaphragm. In the same way, along the outer border of the left atrium, close to the atrioventricular groove, the incision was extended to meet the right atrial incision. All that remained was to cut down through the septum.

The heart, suddenly severed from its roots, flopped back into the pericardial cavity – its home for so many years – with a final spasm of life. It lay there motionless in the red pool of blood.

I wondered how many times it had contracted and relaxed during its lifetime, and whether it really did respond to every human emotion.

Inserting my hand I removed Blaiberg's heart and placed it in the basin held out by Sister Jordaan.

Had I also removed his soul?

It was four minutes past midday.

Marius was there. 'We left the aortic catheter and vent in place. You can use it for coronary perfusion and suction.'

I looked up from the empty, dark hole as he handed Peggy the round basin in which lay the heart of Clive Haupt – immersed in ice-cold Ringer's lactate solution. The two catheters dangled over the side of the rim.

I removed the heart from the basin and placed it on the fresh green towel Sister Jordaan had opened over Blaiberg's thighs. Before lowering it into its future home I had to create the two holes in the right and left atria approximately the same size of the atrial cuffs left in the patient's chest.

I looked at the heart. It was flabby and sickly pale-blue in colour. There was no evidence detectable by the human eye that it was still alive, but somewhere I knew a spark of life lay dormant which would burst into action as soon as it was woken up by the warm oxygenated blood gushing through the coronary arteries.

These would be the signals to the rest of the heart to come alive and start pumping to save the life of a man Clive Haupt had never known.

Under the master scheme of apartheid the Haupts were classified as 'non-white.' They were not allowed to sit on the park benches labelled 'Whites Only'; nor could they use the buses and trains reserved for whites.

They had been evicted from the houses in which they were born and had lived for generations, because these were in the 'white' area.

Most of the restaurants, hotels and the beaches on the beautiful oceans of South Africa were for whites only.

If Clive Haupt had met the daughter of the man whose life he was about to save, he would not have been allowed to fall in love with her, nor have sex with her, nor marry her.

Yet, when I asked his father to donate his son's heart to Philip Blaiberg he hadn't said, 'My son's heart is for non-whites only.' He agreed without hesitation, without anger and hatred for the whites who had humiliated and degraded and deprived him for so long.

I wondered if this sad blue heart that lay in front of me harboured just that little bit of hate?

Vel Schrire and I had discussed the possible reaction of the Nationalist government if we transplanted a 'black' heart into a 'white' chest. We came to the conclusion that, although some of them might be horrified by the idea, they wouldn't utter a murmur in public as the heart transplant programme was the only positive news coming out of South Africa at that time.

Blaiberg, being Jewish, was no stranger to racism. The Jewish nation had been persecuted for centuries. I was sure that he would have no qualms about having a 'black' heart. As a medical man, he must have noticed a long time ago that, irrespective of skin colour, religious belief or race, once one cuts through the skin all humans are the same.

In fact, I was to tell the press later, 'We have taken the heart from a coloured man, put it in a white Jewish man and we have treated him with a serum made in Germany.'

'Stille's please.'

Sister Jordaan placed the small scissors in my hand.

I carefully cut away the piece of left atrium that remained between the openings where the four pulmonary veins from the lungs had entered – then squinted back into the empty chest to gauge whether the hole created would fit onto the left atrial cuff into which the recipient's four pulmonary veins drained – it had to be judged as accurately as possible without the help of any measurement – a surgeon needs three-dimensional vision.

I peered back into the chest again and trimmed away a little more.

'Do you think it's big enough, Rodney?' I needed some reas-surance.

'Yup, and you can always enlarge it later if you have to.'

Now for the right atrium. This was where our revised technique would make the big difference. A stump of the ligated superior vena cava stuck out from the top of this chamber. It's where the two join that the heart's own 'pacemaker' is located and this area must definitely not be damaged by our incision nor by our stitches later on.

So I opened the atrium with a cut that ran from the inferior vena cava opening towards the base of the right atrial appendage – and steered the incision away from the vital area of the 'pacemaker'.

I found the black stitch that Marius and Terry had left as a marker and lowered the heart into Blaiberg's chest. The time was 12:16.

'Let's start coronary perfusion.' Although the donor heart had been without oxygen for twelve minutes, it had been kept cooled and I doubted whether any damage had occurred.

The catheter left in the aorta was connected to a small separate pump that drew oxygenated blood from the heart-lung machine.

'Okay Johan – coronary perfusion on slowly.'

The stump of the donor's aorta started to fill with blood and once all the air had been expelled I cross-clamped above the catheter.

'Increase flow to about 400 cc a minute.'

Immediately the aortic stump became tense, the heart muscle became firmer and slowly the pale blue colour changed into healthy pink. It looked more beautiful than any sunset I'd ever seen.

'Let's connect the vent.' This would act as a safety valve to prevent overdistension of the main pumping chamber.

Dark blood, almost black, came from the coronary sinus opening. This meant the heart muscle had an oxygen deficit.

'Rodney, with your right hand gently push the ventricle out of my way,' I instructed.

Exposure in surgery is of utmost importance – especially if you have to do anastomosis where any later bleeding would be difficult to reach and could be fatal. The left atrium is one of those areas – as it lies behind the ventricle when the heart is in its proper place.

Once I had located the black marker and judged the middle of the left border of the atrial cuff I joined these two areas with a four-o silk suture that had a needle at either end.

First, using the one needle, I stitched the two atrial halves together towards the head of the patient at a point where the septum divided the right and left chambers. Then, with the second needle, I stitched down again towards the septal area.

'Another stitch please.' This was used to secure the bottom stitch with a knot and a third stitch for the top suture line. Joining the septa was next, with a running suture from the top to the bottom. The right atrial connection was done in a similar way.

The blood returning from the lungs and the body could now enter the pumping chambers of the donor heart.

After I had carefully inspected the suture line and placed a few additional stitches where I felt the gaps were too wide, Rodney lowered the ventricles into the pericardial sac.

It was one hour past midday. The atrial connections had taken me nearly an hour but it didn't matter, as the donor heart was being perfused continuously.

'How are things going at your end, Ozzie?'

'Just fine. Arterial pressure 90, venous pressure zero, oesophageal temperature 22,5 and the rectal 27. He's putting out a large quantity of urine and the Astrip is spot on.'

'Is the brain okay after the period of low pressure?'

'I think so.' Ozzie sounded unsure.

'What do you mean "you *think* so"?' That period of low perfusion was worrying me.

'Well, how can I be sure when he's anaesthetized? I can't ask him.'

'But what about his pupils?'

'They're dilated but it may be the drugs.'

'So we don't know if we're going to end up with a patient with a healthy heart but a damaged brain then, Oz,' I snapped testily.

'You just take care of the healthy heart, Chris, and leave the rest to me.'

'Let's get this finished,' I said to my assistants, irritated by the uncertainty.

The two pulmonary arteries were joined without difficulty, now only the aorta remained, but the catheter used for coronary perfusion made stitching difficult.

'We'd better do this without perfusion.'

Rodney nodded.

'Stop coronary perfusion.' Immediately the aortic stump went soft.

The donor heart was now without blood and speed was essential. I looked at the clock. It was 13:35.

'You can start warming the patient now. Sister, give me the cold saline so we can keep the heart cold.' I was handed a beaker of ice-cold saline which I poured into the pericardial sac, submerging the heart.

'Three-o stitch, please.'

The openings of the two aortas did not match. The patient's aorta was about twice the size of that of the donor. Stitching was difficult and time was passing quickly – very quickly.

Only another centimetre and we'd be done. It was like a long-distance runner rounding the last bend and seeing the finishing line a few steps away. We were home!

Suddenly the operating room lights went out.

'Who switched off the fucking lights? I can't see!' I bellowed.

'Oh my God – we've had a power failure, Prof!' Dene's voice was shaky.

'What about the pumps?' I barked.

'They've also stopped,' Johan told me gravely.

Blaiberg had no heart and the heart-lung machine had stopped – so he was now without circulation – which meant he would die.

'What about the hospital's emergency generator?'

'It hasn't come on yet.'

'Johan, you and Dene hand-crank the pumps!'

'We want to but I can't find the handle of the venous pump!' Johan cried as he scratched furiously through the toolbox.

I had to be calm and think clearly. I closed my eyes briefly and suddenly the dark curtain lifted and I could see perfectly, even in the dim light from the theatre window. I was now in complete control of both myself and the crisis. I knew *exactly* what to do.

I spoke slowly and in measured tones. 'Johan, listen carefully. Take the tubing out of the venous pump so the blood can drain freely by gravity into the venous well and crank the arterial pump. Ozzie, raise the table.'

'Arterial pressure rising – it's back to 90.'

'Let's see whether we can get the heart started. I'll keep this opening in the suture line closed and you release the aortic clamp, Ozzie – keep warming, Johan.'

Rodney slowly released the clamp, allowing air and blood to spill through the opening which was still in the aortic suture line and then I sealed it with my finger.

'Okay, take the clamp off.'

The transplant heart became tense and rapidly turned pink.

'It's fibrillating!' Ozzie observed.

'What's the temperature, Oz?'

'Oesophageal is up to 35,7 but the rectal is still low – 27,1.'

'Keep warming, Johan – and we'd better get a message out to the superintendent that we are having problems – if this is a general power failure the press will be all over him.'

They knew, as we all did, that power supply was vital and my guess was that they would already be speculating about an unfortunate end to the operation.

Then, as if the heart knew that Blaiberg, we, and the rest of the world were depending on it – and without any help – it started to beat spontaneously.

'It's beating!' Several voices rejoiced.

Then the lights came on.

'Start the pumps again – and cancel that message.' I turned around and looked up so that the floor nurse could wipe the sweat from my brow and then, for the first time, I noticed that the observation gallery was filled with onlookers.

I thought, absently, how unusual it was that even Dr Mibashan, head of the department of haematology, was there.

'Start ventilating, Oz.' And, for the first time in two and a half hours, Blaiberg's lung took over its proper function in the exchange of gases.

Using a side clamp, I gently closed the remaining opening in the suture line under my finger and then completed the aortic anastomosis.

'How's the temperature, Oz?'

He's warming nicely, the rectal temperature's up to 31,8.'

'How long has he been without circulation?' Blaiberg had now had two periods of low perfusion – the one when the aortic catheter slipped out and the other when the pump stopped – there was a distinct possibility of serious damage to his brain.

'Just over two minutes, Chris, but at that stage his temperature was 25 degrees and that should have protected the brain.'

'I hope you're right, Oz. Release the venous snares and let's pull the superior vena cava catheter into the atrium and take out the inferior vena cava catheter.'

After this Blaiberg was on partial by-pass. A portion of his circulation was now being carried by the transplanted heart.

The heart showed no evidence of failure. With each beat we could see that the ventricles were emptying the full volume of blood they received from the atria.

'Slow down the pump. Still okay, Oz?'

'Everything looks great, mean arterial pressure 95, venous only 7.'

'Let's give it a chance – say about five minutes – to recover, then we'll turn off the pump.'

I used this period to inspect the suture lines carefully. There was slight oozing but that would stop as soon as we'd neutralized the heparin and the blood could clot again.

'Okay, how does it look? Everything fine?'

Now was the moment of truth – would the new heart take over completely when the pump was stopped?

'Pump off.'

It was 15:25. The operation had taken four hours.

The heart didn't hesitate. It plunged on, strong and sure of itself.

'80...85...90...95. It's holding there – venous only 5 and he's passing lots of urine!' Ozzie confirmed delightedly, his voice filled with emotion for the first time.

We took out the remaining venous catheter and the arterial catheter and closed the hole with the purse-string sutures already in place.

'Ozzie, start the protamine.' This was the drug that would neutralize the heparin.

Outside the hospital, hundreds of media people were waiting for news. There was a strong bond of camaraderie among the reporters and TV cameramen from all around the world who had gathered in the car park. It was like a huge picnic and they lounged on cars and walls or simply sat on the pavement.

'If he fails with this one, people will be calling him a butcher, not a genius,' was one strong opinion.

One reporter laughed as he repeated the current gossip from his newsroom. 'Did you hear that two guys from The Times *were found in the out-patient's department dressed up in women's clothes?*

'I wonder what the hell is happening in there?' said another as he gazed up at the building. 'I've only got an hour before my deadline – if that power failure was all over the hospital then he's up shit creek. Any more of that coffee left?'

I glanced at the electrocardiograph screen. The heart was in perfect sinus rhythm.

'Will you and Hitchcock please close the chest for me, Rodney? I could do with a cup of tea – I suppose we all could.' I handed out

53

the arterial and venous lines and, taking off my gloves, I left Operating Room A.

Clive Haupt had already left Operating Room B, on the way to his lonely grave – without a heart.

Marius and Bossie were already in the tearoom.

'So how did it go?' Marius asked. He knew already, but was looking for some reassurance from me.

'Well, the road was bumpy, but at least we didn't crash.'

'Do you think his brain's okay?'

'We'll just have to wait and see when he wakes up.' As an afterthought I added grimly, '*if* he wakes up that is.' The orderly stuck his head round the door.

'Dr Bosman, phone call for you in the corridor.' Bossie hurried out of the tearoom.

'Chris,' said Marius, 'I've been thinking. This is the best type of donor one can have.'

'What do you mean?' I asked my brother, taking a sip from the steaming cup. Hospital tea is not renowned for its delicate flavour – but this was the most delicious I'd ever tasted.

'I mean a donor who has suffered brain death from a rupture of a berry aneurysm. Unlike accident victims, they don't have extensive injuries with haemorrhage and long periods of low perfusion.'

'I think you're right. This heart took over and maintained a good circulation right from the word go. It got us out of a damned tight corner. You heard what happened?'

'Sure, I was there.' Marius looked at me and I was grateful to see in his eyes the obvious respect he had for me. 'I don't think there are many surgeons who could have got out of that mess. It's true what Ozzie says about you – you *can* think quickly on your feet.'

For brothers, Marius and I got on very well. For several years he had been a GP in Rhodesia – present-day Zimbabwe. When he realized that Ian Smith was going the wrong way he packed up and got an appointment in the department of surgery with Professor Jannie Louw. For one year he did valuable research in my laboratory studying relationships between a low serum potassium and digitalis toxicity in patients undergoing open-heart surgery. I'm quite sure that this work saved many lives.

Then he went to Houston where he trained with Doctors De Bakey and Cooley. After this he came back to Cape Town and joined our transplant team.

'Prof, it's Dr Viviers.' I hadn't noticed Bossie return. 'He says the press are driving him crazy and he's got to send out a report.'

'I swear we work for the press and not the hospital! Tell them the transplant is finished and that Dr Blaiberg is doing very well.'

Both Bossie and Marius looked sharply at me as if to say, Are you *really* sure?

I thought for a moment. 'No, let's rather say, "The transplant is finished, the heart is beating well and maintaining a good circulation".'

Bossie didn't leave – I could see he was embarrassed about something. 'They also want to know how *you* are feeling,' he added cautiously, looking past my shoulder.

That was just too much. 'Tell them I feel I have to go to the toilet. They've kept me so busy the last few days that I haven't had time for a shit!'

'No use getting upset, Chris. You have to learn to live with them.'

Marius was right. 'Okay, tell them I feel very tired – but happy that everything went so smoothly,' I conceded with a sigh.

An exclusive interview with one of the major magazines about the *true* drama of that morning would probably have sold for quite a lot of money then – but possibilities like that never entered my mind. The only thing that was important at that moment was whether my patient's brain had been damaged by my mistakes.

I finished the tea, pulled the mask over my nose and went back to A-Theatre.

Rodney was busy putting wire sutures through the sternum with an awl. These would splint the two halves of the sternum so that there would be no movement with breathing – allowing it to heal.

Two tubes were in place through stab wounds in the abdominal skin. One was positioned behind the heart in the pericardial sac and the other would be just below the sternum once it had been closed.

There's always some oozing after open-heart surgery as some of the elements necessary for blood to clot adequately are destroyed by the foreign surfaces over which the blood flows in the heart-lung machine.

The two suction tubes would be connected to drain this blood out of the pericardial sac and mediasternum in the post-operative period. This would also give us an indication of the quantity of blood lost that would need to be replaced.

'What about the cortisone?' Ozzie was now ventilating by hand to keep the lungs well inflated.

'Let's see,' I said, 'before surgery he received 200 milligrams of Imuran and 100 milligrams of hydrocortisone. You gave him 100 milligrams of hydrocortisone during the operation. So he's had 200 milligrams already. I want him to receive 500 milligrams of hydrocortisone in the first 24 hours. Give him another 100 milligrams right away and then we'll give him another 200 milligrams in the intensive care unit between now and tomorrow morning.'

I was extremely anxious to look under the towel and see whether his pupils reacted to light but I knew Ozzie would get upset – that was his side of the business. So I left again for the tea-room.

Marius was paging through a medical journal as I entered.

'What are you reading?'

'I was just looking at this article in *Circulation* published last year by Lower and his associates on the electrocardiographic changes in dogs which have had heart transplants.'

'Yes, I know the article well – I've studied it several times – but I have a feeling the electrocardiographic changes they describe only show up once rejection is well established. We'll have to find a more sensitive way to diagnose the onset of complications like that.'

I poured myself another cup of tea.

Marius put down the magazine and, with a faint smile, asked, 'Is Norman Shumway really so upset because you pipped him to the post? I've heard he's nearly suicidal.'

'I don't know about that – I didn't see him during my visit to the States – nor did he contact me. All I know is that there's a lot of shit that we "stole" the idea from him.'

'How did that happen? You never worked with him. You only knew what you read in the articles he published!' Marius put his cup down with a loud clatter.

'That's just the point. They've got very strange ideas over there.'

'They want you in A-Theatre, Prof.'

I recognized the floor nurse, even though she still had her mask on. She had a firm, slender body with urgent and inviting young breasts.

Both Marius and I jumped up and hurried back to A-Theatre.

A glance at the monitor showed that the electrocardiogram and heart rate had not changed.

'What's the matter? What's the problem?'

'No problem,' Ozzie replied. I just wanted to know whether you want the patient ventilated afterwards.'

'I'd like to have this tube out of his lungs as soon as possible but maybe we should ventilate him for the first few hours and you can extubate him in the ward.'

The risk of lung complications is always reduced if the patient can breathe – and cough – on his own.

Rodney was putting in the last skin sutures. The wound was then cleaned with an antiseptic solution, covered with sterile gauze strips and closed with an Elastoplast strip.

The green towels were removed and Blaiberg's naked body was covered with a blanket. Johan was stripping the tubes connected to the drains.

'Is there much bleeding, Johan?'

'No Prof, only 25 cc from both drains in the last twenty minutes and there are no clots – probably just a bit of oozing.'

Everything inside the chest appeared to be going well. What about inside the skull?

As if reading my thoughts, Ozzie said 'I'm going to neutralize the scoline and wake him up – is that okay with you?'

Please, dear God, let him wake up, I said in silent prayer as I nodded my head.

Ozzie injected the prostigmine. We waited but Blaiberg didn't move.

I bent over his face, 'Philip, can you hear me?' No response.

I turned to Ozzie, 'What's happening?'

'Give the prostigmine some time, Chris,' he said softly.

But I couldn't wait. My heart was thumping loudly inside my chest. I bent over him again, 'Philip, it's me – Professor Barnard – can you hear me?'

Somewhere deep in the brain something must have registered. My patient opened his eyes. Then he slowly smiled – and winked at me!

On a hot Wednesday afternoon I left Cape Town for Germany. I was glad to get away – I had been feeling like a stallion locked up in a stable and only able to look at the distant green pastures and the fillies over the top of the stable door. I needed to get back out into the new, exciting world I'd found and had arranged to meet some of my colleagues in Rome.

It was already Blaiberg's 10th post-operative day. We had been able to extubate him the day after surgery. In my experience, there's nothing better to prevent post-operative lung complications than to get the patient breathing and coughing on his own as soon as possible.

As a result of the experience we'd had with my first patient, the physiotherapist was working on his lungs twice during the day and once at night. Daily chest X-rays showed that both lungs were clear except for a small shadow at the base of the right lung, which Vel interpreted as the result of the pulmonary embolus he had suffered when I was still in America.

Dr Blaiberg was now out of bed, recovering well and was also enjoying his own celebrity status. There was a post-operative complication, however – but not a medical one.

Without my permission – or that of Philip Blaiberg – Dr Mibashan had quietly been taking pictures during surgery and then he had tried to sell them to the media. I recalled looking up from the operating table and thinking at the time how strange it was for a haematologist to be so interested in the operation.

When the hospital authorities heard about the photographs they immediately accused my friend, Don Mackenzie – a photographer. Threats of legal action eventually sorted the matter out. The pictures, of very poor quality, were confiscated from Dr Mibashan and I've never seen them since – nor have I seen Dr Mibashan. His career at the hospital was brought to an abrupt end – just because of some silly little photographs.

Since we started performing open-heart surgery our policy had been that, as soon as the patient had recovered from surgery, he became the responsibility of the cardiologist. This ensured that a more unbiased assessment of long-term results was published. I always took the results analyzed and reported elsewhere by surgical teams themselves with a pinch of salt – the results and prognoses have so much more credibility when compiled and controlled by a removed third party.

At the invitation of Südwest Rundfunk I made my first European TV appearance in Baden-Baden – and also my first appearance in a film star's bed.

The programme was a question and answer affair and never really got going. With my limited experience, I felt it was an

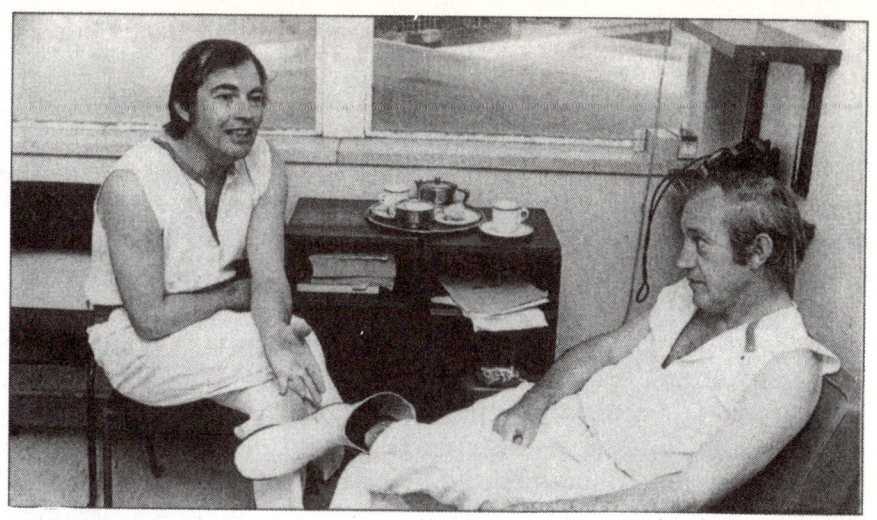

Tea break with brother Marius

extremely unimaginative production – poorly organised and painfully slow. When we left the studio it was already late in the evening and, without an overcoat, I suffered in the German winter. I wondered what the first impression of the German public was of the heart-transplant surgeon from South Africa.

Because it was so late, both the director and producer of the station suggested we should cancel our reservation at the restaurant out of town and rather go to one just across the square.

It's frightening to think how a simple change of plan can often result in a series of unforeseen and drastic consequences.

Crossing the square, I heard some lively music coming from a night club. They asked if I would like to go there and, of course, I didn't see any harm in it – at least it would be warm inside. The problem was that I was not prepared for this new life and I ought to have realized that the *last* place I should be seen in was a night club – especially with photographers skulking around everywhere.

We settled down at a table next to the dance floor. The producer excused himself and, within a few minutes, returned with some female company. One of the girls made my heart lurch. She had a stunning body, brown hair, a Slavic look with high cheek bones and deep brown slanting eyes.

'This is Uta Levka – and this is Professor Barnard.' He made the introductions. I felt gauche in the presence of this beauty and mumbled an awkward greeting. This was a unique and unnerving experience for me – Uta, however, oozed sex, vitality and confidence.

'Would you like to dance?' she purred.

I've never been a good dancer. My mother considered dancing to be form of fornication so, as a child, I was forbidden to go near a dance floor – although I did do so a few times secretly.

While at university I lived with my eldest brother, Johannes, and his wife. He allowed me to take a few dance lessons at an Arthur Murray studio in Cape Town – with a girl at least five years older than I was. I was taught the basic steps of the foxtrot and waltz – and even a few steps of the tango.

Louwtjie just couldn't keep time and, no matter how hard she tried, she always looked uncomfortable on the dance floor. In fact, she didn't even know the difference between a quick-step and a waltz. Dancing, therefore, was not at the top of her list of entertainment so I had had very little opportunity to improve any dancing skills with my wife.

And here, this beautiful girl – probably a model – had asked me to dance! Fortunately the band played a slow number. We walked to the middle of the dance floor and I held out my arms. She glided so naturally in between them and our bodies simply moulded together. Instantly the dance floor was transformed into daylight by the flash bulbs of the photographers – but I was mesmerized by the closeness of her body. We danced for most of the evening – cuddling and laughing as if we were familiar lovers.

Today it's hard to believe my gullibility – it didn't dawn on me that this could mean disaster – after all we were only dancing.

To make matters even worse, when I left, I stupidly signed their visitors' book and wrote: An unforgettable evening in the arms of the most beautiful girl in the world!

I remember lazing in my hotel bed the next morning thinking about how *sexy* the girl had been and what a marvellous evening I'd had – when I saw the newspapers.

A bucket of cold water couldn't have had a more sobering effect.

There were front-page pictures of me dancing and cuddling with this girl – who was, apparently, an actress well known for appearing naked in movies. The story quipped that she usually wore less clothing than any patient on my operating table!

I winced when I saw that they'd printed exactly what I'd written in the visitors' book.

After some strong coffee and a cigarette I began to see the funny side of it and consoled myself with the fact that it was only a local story and I'd probably heard the last of it.

What an idiot! Of course, the story was syndicated and Louwtjie, back in Cape Town, read about it only a few hours after I did – which, naturally, did precious little to strengthen our relationship.

Louwtjie Barnard finished reading the newspaper and threw it on the floor. She ignored the telephone which hadn't stopped ringing all morning – she knew it would be newspapermen. Why, oh why, couldn't Chris just behave normally? Why did he have to be seen in public with a slut?

She lit another cigarette and flounced out of the room into her garden, kicking the newspaper out of the way as she did so.

'Mrs Barnard?' a young man called from the roadside, 'I wonder if I might have a word with you?' He was definitely a reporter.

'No, you may not!' she stormed

'That telephone isn't going to stop ringing until you say something to one of us about today's story,' he said, tilting his head in the direction of the insistent telephone.

He saw her hesitate, 'Come on, I need a break, it'll only take a couple of minutes.'

She flicked the cigarette into a bush and stood quite still, arms crossed and stared down at her feet, her chin tucked into the crook of her arms.

'Please?' the reporter asked again.

She didn't move but raised her eyes slowly to look at him. He seemed like a nice enough young man. She relented. 'Well, only one minute then – but you must promise to tell your friends to keep away from here – and to stop pestering me.'

'Will do,' he smiled, walking briskly across her lawn and joined her on the verandah.

He took a small notebook from his jacket pocket as he sat down, crossed his legs and asked, 'So, what do you think about the stories in today's papers?'

'I'm thoroughly disgusted,' she fumed.

'With your husband?'

'No! With the press! It's utterly despicable for them to insinuate that there is something scandalous about my husband enjoying an innocent evening out.

'As far as I'm concerned the incident was quite innocent. I'm only too happy that my husband enjoyed himself – and I hope they both enjoyed the dance.'

She knew that reporters exaggerated things out of all proportion – just *as she instinctively knew there was more than a grain of truth in the story – but would this reporter believe she was as unconcerned as she pretended to be?*

Chris would be phoning that night or the next. She'd give him an earful when he did!

In fact it *was* an innocent evening and I didn't have anything more to do with her – then – but when your wife sees pictures and stories like these in the newspapers it's difficult to talk your way out of it – and I couldn't blame her for thinking that it was more than just a casual meeting.

Meanwhile, I had the morning free, which was a nuisance as I had time to think about the evening. Why should the newspapers make such a fuss about my dancing with a girl? I'm sure that many of my married colleagues had had the same experience in night clubs without even a hint of scandal.

If it had happened to me two months previously, nobody would have even noticed. Oh well, an opportunity only comes once a lifetime and one must make use of it in the lifetime of that opportunity. I was determined not to let this one pass me by.

After a steaming hot shower I dialled room service and ordered a continental breakfast in preference to English. I've always tried to limit eggs to once or twice a week and, in any case, a heavy breakfast tends to make me feel sluggish all morning.

I had very little on my schedule that day – only a visit to the famous Baden-Baden health spa – and, that evening, a small and private party at the TV director's home.

The following morning Max Schiller, the photographer of *Stern*, would drive me to Munich to be the guest (unnoticed I hoped) at a ball in the Bayerische Hof.

The private party turned out to be a wonderful evening. It was a small affair with senior staff of the station and, of course, Uta.

Of the hundreds of enjoyable evenings I've had since, I remember only a few. This was one of them – perhaps because it was so relaxed and simple. We ate, drank, danced and played house games just like children.

At about 2 o'clock in the morning Uta and I decided to slip out and maybe have a last drink at my hotel.

It had started to snow quite heavily. As I opened the front door there was movement behind some bushes in the garden – so I pushed Uta back into the house.

At least 20 photographers had been waiting all evening in the snow. They looked more like snowmen by this time. Poor bastards – they were only trying to earn a living.

I ended up in bed alone again that night.

At midday, Max called for me at the hotel. It's about a three-hour drive from Baden-Baden to Munich. Uta had promised me she would also be at the ball but the snow was heavy and I started to worry that we wouldn't make it to Munich at all.

Eventually, after slipping and sliding along the autobahn past the magnificent Wagnerian castles built by Ludwig II, I walked into the Bayerische Hof six hours after we left Baden-Baden. I was sure that Uta wouldn't have arrived yet, but enquired of the concierge whether there was a message for me.

'No message, Sir.'

Herr Steinmeyer and Max Schiller, together with what seemed like half the hotel staff, accompanied me to my suite. The manager opened the door with a flourish and showed me around. He was especially proud of the bathroom. It wasn't a bath but more like a small, round, swimming pool with big taps made of solid gold he said – although I thought that was stretching it a bit far.

After fussing around for at least 10 minutes to see that all my needs were taken care of, the management corps left and Max Schiller, Herr Steinmeyer and I had time to discuss the evening.

The problem would be if the press saw me with Uta again, so they suggested that I should go to the ball disguised. That evening, they arrived with a suitcase full of masks.

As I was getting dressed I fooled around, coming out of the bathroom with one mask on after the other – again, not even dreaming that it could later be embarrassing. I thought it was just some harmless fun but, of course, Max Schiller of *Stern* took pictures of me clowning around and, some months later, the magazine published them with a headline, 'The Man Behind The Mask', which succeeded in making me look rather foolish.

Eventually I decided not to wear a mask as Uta probably wouldn't have made it to Munich in all the snow anyway.

The ballroom was very dark – and packed with people. We slipped in and sat down at a reserved table. I tried to spot Uta but, even if she was there, it would have been virtually impossible to find her.

We had arranged that she would meet me on the dance floor –

among the dancers. So, when the music started, I wandered alone onto the floor but couldn't stay there alone for too long, obviously.

After a full minute of anticipating her touch and the smell of her perfume in vain, I went back to my table. I really felt let down. I had been looking forward to the evening so much.

A few glasses of champagne later I felt a little better. To hell with her – I probably wouldn't ever see her again anyway but I thought I'd try once more. So I went out on the dance floor and waited briefly.

I was just about to return to the table, when I heard a voice behind me, 'Here I am darling.' And there she was – looking sexier than a *Playboy* pull-out. We fell into each other's arms and I was delighted to notice she was as excited as I was because her arms were suddenly covered in goose pimples when we embraced.

'What happened to you?' I whispered in her ear.

'I nearly didn't make it but it doesn't matter – we're together now.'

The evening passed far too quickly and the dance floor became less crowded as the people started to leave.

'This will have to be our last dance, Chris,' she said, slipping a piece of paper into my hand.

I said good night to my party and went up to my room to read the note which said: Hope to see you later. There was an address written below the message.

I quickly changed into some casual clothes, went downstairs and, without handing in my room key, walked out into the street and caught a taxi to number 22 Kaiserstrasse.

Uta was dressed in a very flattering and sheer gown which left very little to the imagination. Soft lights and music helped the romantic atmosphere, and there was no doubt in my mind as to why she'd invited me to her apartment.

In the early hours of the morning I went back to my hotel and crept stealthily past the front desk – careful not to wake the doorman.

Gratefully I slid in between the starched sheets and sighed happily. Within seconds I'd drifted off into a dreamless sleep.

I did not see Uta after that until quite recently when I met her with her boyfriend.

2

I had seen some amazing scenes of overeager reporters at South African and American airports but the chaos at Rome airport left me absolutely speechless. Never in my wildest dreams could I have imagined I would be so much in demand. It was impossible to believe that the thousands of people there had come to see me. My first thought was that perhaps the Beatles had been on the same plane.

The crowd was almost uncontrollable and I started to panic slightly as I pushed my way through the mob. An Afrikaans word describes the feeling very well: *benoud* – not exactly claustrophobic but somewhere between stifling and oppressive. It was, I imagine, very much like being packed into a tin of sardines – there was no room to move.

I knew the South African ambassador was there somewhere but I couldn't see him through all the flashing bulbs. There was one photographer who had two Hasselblad cameras on a bar so that he could take 72 pictures without even stopping to change film!

Autograph books and microphones were thrust under my nose and the noise was deafening. One young girl actually opened her blouse to fully expose her left breast and asked me to sign my name over her heart! But, with all the photographers around, I was careful not to make a boob like that.

Finally, with the help of airport security, I was safely ushered into the VIP lounge where an impromptu press conference was set up.

I was so overwhelmed that I can't recall a single question. I just remember meeting the ambassador briefly and then being whisked away to the Hotel Flora on the Via Veneto where I met the rest of my party.

Orilio Cinquegrani, whom we later nicknamed 'pronto-prego', was the head of Alitalia in South Africa and he had organized my visit to Italy as the guest of RAI Television.

There was a large reception committee waiting for me in my suite. My two colleagues, MC and Bossie were there, also the Cape Town photographer, Don Mackenzie, and the owner of the very successful La Perla restaurants in Cape Town, Emiliano Sandri – accompanied by a beautiful South African girl called Cathy Bilton.

Italy was represented by Cinquegrani and three representatives from RAI Television. When I arrived the chianti was already flowing freely. We discussed the activities for the next few days, the most important being a meeting with the Italian president the next morning followed by a private audience with the Pope. In the afternoon there would be a round-table discussion with some of the senior Italian doctors on television.

I've said before that I had no particular interest in fashion but having attended some glittering occasions – with more to follow – I was becoming increasingly embarrassed at my shabby and travel-weary clothes. I had splashed out and bought an off-the-peg suit before leaving Cape Town but it was beginning to sag here and there.

Now I was to meet the Pope and all I had was a suitcase of wrinkled suits. No shops were open on a Sunday – not that I could have afforded Roman fashions anyway. Then, as if in answer to Cinderella's prayer, the telephone rang, and it was my 'fairy-godmother' in the form of a tailor.

The voice, in very broken English, said, 'Professore Barnardi, this is Angelo Litrico and I see pictures of you on the television and, please to forgive me, but the clothes you are having are not good for to meet Il Papa (which is what he called the Pope) and what I am doing is come and measure you and make a fine suit for you which will be suitable for Il Papa. Is okay, Professore?'

It was just incredible! I agreed immediately, of course, and he came to take measurements that afternoon.

He limped into the room majestically – even though he had one artificial leg. He was followed by three assistants.

'I am Litrico,' he said, coming to attention and drawing himself to his full height. 'Angelo Litrico – the tailor of Rome,' he added ceremoniously, as if I should have known perfectly well who he was.

He looked with distaste at the suit I was wearing. He produced a silk handkerchief with a flourish and wiped the sweat from his bald patch. 'What is thees?' he asked, his voice dripping with sarcasm.

'It's a new suit I bought in Cape Town last week.'

He steeled himself to touch the lapels. 'Thees was maybe new, but it is not a zoot, Professore!' He patiently explained, 'A zoot does not look like thees!' And he ceremoniously pocketed his handkerchief again.

Before I had time to figure out just how disparaging the remark was he switched his attention to my tie.

'Thees tie – is also new from South Africa?' he teased.

I had paid a lot of money for the tie and I didn't much care for some stranger criticizing my taste, but before I could reply he flipped open my jacket with his delicate hand to reveal my striped shirt.

He raised his eyebrows, sucked in his breath and pursed his lips. He didn't have to say anything about the shirt.

Before I knew what was happening his assistants, at the flick of his fingers, had removed my jacket – which Angelo took from them, looked at the label, and promptly discarded on the floor.

Magically, he produced a tape measure and, stepping on my rejected jacket, began taking measurements. While he was doing this another of his assistants was asking my opinion about various samples of fabric – not that I believed my opinion mattered very much. All this activity was accompanied by much head-shaking and a torrent of rapid-fire Italian.

'I, Litrico, will not allow your South African tailor to disgrace you like this. You will see!'

And, with that, he was gone.

While 'the tailor of Rome' was making my suit that evening we went to a reception at the home of Signora Capucci – a famous couturier. It was a very glamorous affair in her beautiful home on the Spanish Square. I was introduced to one aristocrat after the other, from politicians to Italian celebrities and movie people.

I really fell in love with Italy on this trip – and it was largely due to their enthusiastic reception and friendliness I think. Italians have such a great *zest* for life! I loved their grand architecture, their wild exuberance and, of course, their food. At around midnight, I collapsed into bed at the hotel.

Litrico was back again just after dawn with a complete wardrobe of specially tailored clothes. He again cast aside my navy-blue suit together with the tie – and *out* went the shoes 'that go clumpa clumpa clumpa when Il Professore walks into a room!'

In their place, was a double-breasted dark blue suit with tie and soft-collared shirt to match. Blue shoes with tapering toes completed the outfit.

The suit fitted as if I had been poured into it. The shirt didn't stick out at the cuffs or ride up out of my trousers and the shoes were so light I had to look down to be sure I was wearing them. With this outfit came the most magnificent velvet-collared overcoat I'd ever seen and enough 'socks Italian' to ensure I would never have to resort to 'socks English' again.

Putting these clothes on was one of the most sensual experiences I'd ever known – and very new to me. I would never have believed clothes could feel so *good* – almost orgasmic. They were absolutely perfect and I preened in front of the mirror.

Such is the excellence of Italian tailors that the suit jacket, no matter which way I turned, always hung exactly right.

I was really beginning to feel, and look, important. I felt as if I *belonged* in them, and it changed my opinion about clothing entirely. I now believe that clothes reflect the man's personality, which doesn't mean they have to be expensive – simply 'right' for the person wearing them.

The best part of all was that he refused to allow me to pay for anything – I guess he thought the publicity was worth it. This was the first time I'd ever received such an expensive gift just for being who I was.

Angelo became a very good friend of mine. He was one of the most generous human beings I've ever known and, until his death, every time I went to Rome he would invite me to his salon and supply me with new suits, shirts, shoes, socks and ties – he made me very aware of how important good clothes are and I was always well dressed while he was alive. I will always remember, with love and respect, my Sicilian tailor.

A car arrived to take me to the Italian president, but leaving the hotel proved to be a great deal more time-consuming than I'd imagined. The press wanted more statements and the hotel lobby was jam-packed with photographers.

Slowly we threaded our way through the foyer answering questions and posing for photographs as we went. Eventually we reached the street. Seldom had the Via Veneto seen such a crowd. Some people just wanted to touch me while others wanted autographs. Girls thrust slips of paper with their telephone numbers into my hand, while older women hugged me and asked me to kiss their babies.

Finally we were in the cars and on our way to President Saragat's official residence. After chatting for about half an hour I asked him whether he had heard the story about the man who wanted a brain transplant. He appeared quite keen to hear about it.

'There was this doctor,' I said, 'who became very famous because he was the only surgeon in the world who could transplant the brain. One day a man consulted him and requested a new brain, but informed the surgeon that he could not pay very much and wanted one of the cheapest ones.'

The president interrupted and wanted to know whether this was a true story or not.

'No, it's only a joke,' I said and continued with the story.

'The doctor took him down to a room where he kept the various brains stored in big glass jars. He offered one to the patient for $1 000. When the patient asked why it was so cheap, the surgeon said that it was taken from a man whose profession was sweeping the streets.

'The patient said that he wanted something a little better so the surgeon pointed to another that cost $10 000 because it came from a mathematician.

'The patient agreed to take that one, but out of interest, asked whether he had anything better. The surgeon pointed to a jar in the corner and said that the brain would cost $100 000.

'"That must come from a very intelligent man!" said the patient. The surgeon replied, "No, it's so expensive because it's never been used – you see it comes from a politician".'

I don't know whether the president couldn't understand my English but he didn't laugh and there's nothing flatter than a flat joke. After a few moments more, we said our good-byes.

We left for the Vatican City, the smallest independent state in the world with a population of 1 000 which has been the residence of the popes since the 14th century. It serves as the spiritual and governmental centre of the Catholic Church.

The Vatican City covers only 44 hectares but it exercises spiritual sway over millions of Catholics all over the world. Its ruler is the Pope who is also the Bishop of Rome.

We turned into an avenue about one and a half kilometres long which leads from the river to the Piazza di San Pietra – a large open space in front of St Peter's basilica, the largest church in the world.

The Piazza, designed by Giovanni Lorenzo Bernini, contains two fountains and two colonnades arranged in semicircles on opposite sides of the Piazza like two outstretched arms of the temple receiving all mankind in one universal embrace.

In the centre stands a red granite obelisk – 26 metres high.

The square is dominated by the dome – conceived by Michelangelo's immortal genius – which rises massively over the glorious tomb of the prince of the apostles, St Peter.

I was still gaping, in a kind of spiritual awe, at the grandeur of St Peter's when our party was met and directed to the Vatican Palace – a group of connecting buildings with well over 11 000 rooms.

The Prima Loggia, the Pope's quarters, was in one part of the palace. We were met by the prefecture of the papal household, who arranges audiences with His Holiness. He informed us that only my interpreter, an Italian doctor, and I could proceed further.

We started mounting the steps of the Scala Regia, designed by Bernini in such a way that the staircase appeared much longer and wider than it really was. We were shown into a waiting room magnificently furnished with priceless paintings on the walls and exquisite rugs on the floor.

After waiting four or five minutes we were led further up the steps to another waiting room. Again we waited five minutes, after which we ascended the steps further and eventually stopped in front of the door of the Scala Regia.

The door opened and in front of the desk stood Pope Paul VI. He was a very frail man of medium height, dressed in white robes and, on his head, wearing a cap that looked like the yarmulke the Jews wear.

My interpreter immediately walked up to the Pope and kissed his ring. I didn't do it because I didn't know if I was supposed to or not. In any case the Pope didn't seem to mind and immediately began asking me for information on the transplant operation – at what stage did we take the heart out of the donor, what was the clinical moment of death, what future did we hope for this kind of operation and so on? He was very interested in even the smallest details of the operation and was very well informed about it too – how very different from the president of the United States.

The audience lasted longer than expected because of his keen interest in medicine – especially the moral and religious aspects of transplantation.

When we were finished his last words to me were, 'Professor Barnard, I am not a medical man and do not have the knowledge to tell you if you're wrong or right – but I do congratulate you on your magnificent achievement. There is one thing I am capable of doing for you, and that I will do; I will pray for you, your patients and continued success in your work.' Then he gave me an inscribed book and a medal, both of which are now in the Beaufort West Museum in South Africa.

I found great comfort and encouragement in his words. I am not a Catholic, I'm a Protestant – my father, being a Calvinist, had been very anti-Catholic – and I'm sure he would have turned in his grave if he had known that I was to become so closely involved with Catholics. In fact he was so against Catholicism that he wrote in his will that his first granddaughter would inherit a certain sum of money on condition that she didn't marry a Catholic or join the Catholic Church.

I have never been definite in my beliefs. There was a time when I thought that medical science could cope with any challenge – given the right knowledge and skill. With experience, I came to see that once medical science has done all it can for a patient, it must stand aside and allow other forces – God – to take over.

With still more experience it became clear that this was the wrong way around. If certain forces, not amenable to ordinary medical intervention, are not *already* working in the doctor's favour, then his skills have little chance of success.

It was with these beliefs that I found such solace in what the Pope had said – confirmation, perhaps, that God was not against heart transplants.

After the visit to the Vatican City I felt so moved that I couldn't face any food served in a restaurant. I still could not believe that Chris Barnard had had a private audience with the Pope, a man who was loved and worshipped by millions of people – even in the furthest corners of the world.

We decided to go to Harry's Bar for a cappuccino and sit outside to watch the activities on the Via Veneto.

Soon the South African contingent found us. This gave me the opportunity to study Cathy Bilton more closely; she was a stunning blonde, tall, with prominent cheekbones, blue eyes and a full mouth. Emiliano Sandri had this reputation of always having beautiful women around him. This girl certainly confirmed that reputation.

Bossie, in the meantime, had phoned Groote Schuur Hospital. He gave me the good news that he had spoken to Vel and that Philip Blaiberg had no temperature, the electrocardiogram voltage, although low, was constant. He was up and about and sent his best wishes.

My day could not have been more perfect and I sent up a silent prayer of gratitude.

Mid-afternoon Bossie, MC and I were taken to the studios of RAI television for the debate. The programme was very much like *Face the Nation* but more crowded and not as well organized.

We were shown into the studio and the floor was a phalanx of people. I recognized two very senior and respected Italian surgeons, Professors Steffanini and Valdoni. I didn't know Steffanini personally but, in 1960, Dr George Sachs, a surgeon in Cape Town, had arranged for me to visit the polyclinico in Rome where Professor Valdoni was head of the surgical unit. As they were also doing open-heart surgery, he invited me to lecture on the surgical correction of the 'blue-baby' abnormality – or 'tetralogy of Fallot'.

This was quite a tricky operation and, in the early days of open-heart surgery, had a high mortality rate. At that stage we had done 35 corrections with 15% mortality. Subsequently I did 100 consecutive cases with only three deaths.

When I'd completed the lecture, Professor Valdoni congratulated me. He said that their results were not nearly as good as ours as they had a 50% mortality.

After the lecture one of his registrars, an American doctor, had driven me back to my hotel. 'You know, Dr Barnard, Professor Valdoni honestly believes that his mortality rate is 50% but I can tell you that, since I've been working for him, I haven't seen *one* case recover. I'm sure the mortality rate is more in the region of 100%.'

'Why doesn't he know that himself?' I'd asked, startled by this revelation.

The American doctor explained, 'You see, Professor Valdoni doesn't really follow the patients post-operatively so, his assistants, to keep in his good books, hide the real results from him.'

Open-heart surgery, with the use of the heart-lung machine, took years to become successful in many European centres, the main reason being that they still adhered to the system of 'Herr Professor' (the big professor – as was the case with Professor Valdoni). He was often an older man and a good general surgeon who ruled his unit like a dictator. When a young doctor returned from several years training at an established heart centre, say in America, he wasn't allowed to perform the surgery himself. The professor, who had probably never seen a beating heart, had to do the operation – assisted by the young doctor. The younger doctor's promotion and future also depended on how well he pleased 'Herr Professor'. This type of formality often had very poor results for obvious reasons.

Thank God for Professor Jannie Louw back in Cape Town who'd handed complete control of heart surgery over to me when I returned from Minneapolis.

After waiting for about half an hour in the television studio – in what could only be described as 'organized disorganization' – we settled down and the discussion started.

This was my first experience with simultaneous translation and I found it very difficult to concentrate when I heard the Italian translation in my ears at the same time as I was talking. I was not quite sure whether the girl who did the translation was saying exactly the same things that I had said.

The questions were virtually the same as had been asked over and over again at previous interviews.

A few doctors tried to score points by severely criticizing our work. This turned out to be a foolish mistake on their part as, in the eyes of the Italian public, I could do no wrong – I wasn't quite sure what I had done to win their favour but it was true that I had a great number of admirers in Italy and enjoyed considerable popularity.

After a brief press interview we were taken back to the hotel to prepare for a small party at the house of Alfredo Beni, the film producer.

That evening, when we arrived at his home, it was anything but a small party. Most of the 'beautiful people', especially in the movie industry, were there.

I remember standing with Franco Zeffirelli and Catherine Spaak and Rosano – Beni's wife – when Alfredo arrived with some drinks and asked me if I would like to be introduced to Gina Lollobrigida.

'Would I like to meet her? Sure!' And I followed him into the next room. She was standing alone and, without much enthusiasm, greeted me with only a ghost of a smile.

Although she was already in her late thirties she looked like a little schoolgirl with dark brown hair covering most of her forehead. Gina used very little make-up because, with her lovely dark eyes, perfectly formed nose, full lips and flawless complexion, it wasn't necessary. I remember that she spoke English very well.

After several requests we posed for some pictures. What could be wrong with that?

The next day, of course, the newspapers reported extensively and sensationally about my 'love affair' with Gina Lollobrigida.

Curiously, although it was wild press speculation, the story was not as wrong as many may have thought at that time – just premature – because as we were talking I realized I was becoming increasingly attracted to her. She really was beautiful. I remembered her in a movie I'd seen called *Trapeze* with Burt Lancaster, and for a boy from the Karoo it was an unbelievable experience to be with such a beautiful actress, discussing the movie she was making at the time in Catania, Sicily, *Buena Sera, Mrs Campbell*.

Even more incredible was being fairly sure that she was just as interested in me as I was in her.

After a while, when the party was in full swing, I said, 'Let's go somewhere for a quiet drink together – there's too much noise here.' But she said she was very sorry as she was with an escort. I said I was sure that an actress with her talents could make the appropriate excuses – but she declined.

It's much the same in the animal kingdom; we were just playing a mating game so I decided to risk a final gambit and said, 'Oh well, what a pity – maybe we'll meet again some time.' With that, I moved off to join another group.

It wasn't long before she was at my side again, squeezing my arm and whispering in my ear, 'Meet me in the car park in about half an hour.' I don't know what she'd told her partner.

So I met her downstairs and, in her chauffeur-driven Rolls-Royce, we went to a night club. I must say she was very discreet. We went to a place where nobody worried us – no photographers or newspapermen.

We had a drink there and when we danced she left no doubt whatsoever about what was on her mind. I was feeling very heady

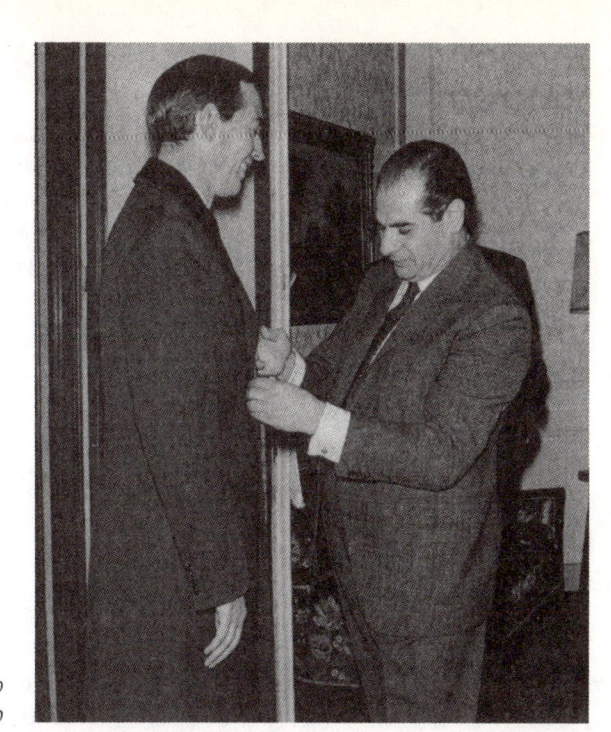

My Italian tailor, Angelo Litrico

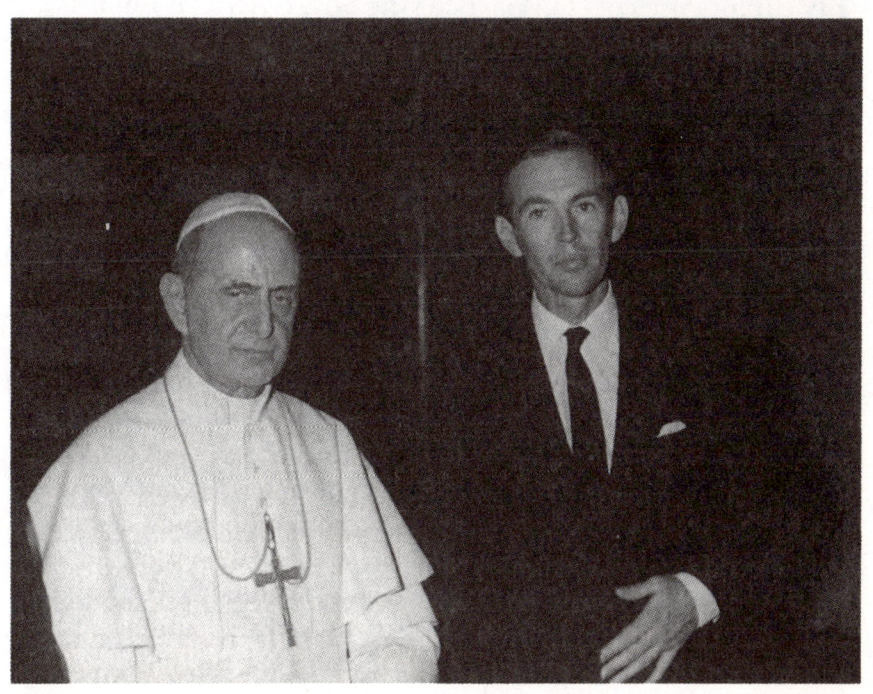

An audience with Pope Paul VI

with excitement when eventually we left and, by mistake I tipped the doorman $100 instead of a $10 bill!

I asked if I could come to her house for a nightcap but she was adamant, 'No, it's impossible, this chauffeur of mine is like my father and I wouldn't like him to see you coming to my house now and probably only leave tomorrow morning.' But she also added with a very naughty grin, 'Tomorrow night he's off duty – why don't you come to my house then?'

The goodnight kiss was just a peck and I agreed to visit her the following evening and went back to my hotel bed alone – feeling very tense, horny and damn sorry about the $100.

I had promised the Pope that I would visit some Catholic hospitals the next day which, after some rescheduling of press interviews, I managed to do.

During the morning I had a message that Sophia Loren wanted to host a lunch for our group the next day.

Time rushed by as we went from one hospital and one press meeting to the next. Early that evening we all trooped off to a typically diplomatic cocktail party at the South African Embassy. I made all the right noises and joined in the general conversation – but my mind wasn't really on it – I was more interested in the unspoken promises of what was to happen later with Gina.

I was very happy when somebody came to take me to her house on the Via Appia – a beautiful property with lights shining in the garden and softer lights glowing inside.

I was wearing one of Litrico's suits and the beautiful coat he had made for me. I waited patiently to be let in.

After a few moments I was ushered into the main living room and my mouth must have gaped – the place was full of people! So much for the romantic and passionate evening I had imagined.

'Gina, I thought you said we would have a quiet evening? I've slept very little and I'm so tired I simply can't have another party. Would you mind if I just rest somewhere? Maybe I can join your party later?' I added lightly, trying to hide my disappointment.

She took me up to her bedroom which was dominated by a huge double bed. I put my Litrico coat on a rack in the entrance to her bedroom and I think it's probably still hanging there because, in my excitement, I left it behind.

I took off my shoes and jacket, loosened my tie and lay down on the bed and fell asleep. Absolutely fast asleep.

I woke up when I heard Gina coming into the room. She was carrying a bottle of champagne and two glasses. Huskily she murmured, 'Now we're going to be alone,' as she sat on the bed next to me and slowly ran her fingers down the side of my cheek. Her long nails traced a faint outline down the front of my shirt and my eyes followed the heaving swell of her breasts as she breathed deeply and leaned across me.

We celebrated with the champagne several times during the night and I left early the next morning. She drove me back to my hotel in her Jaguar – absolutely naked inside a mink coat. I've often wondered what would have happened if we'd had an accident or the car had broken down.

Obviously she was very fond of me – and I found her to be an extremely vibrant and sexually uninhibited woman. Everything had been just *perfect* between us and I was feeling very cock-sure of myself, whistling as I strolled back into the hotel. Had I known the trauma which would follow, I would have kept well clear of the Via Appia that night.

She kept asking me not to go to the lunch party with Sophia Loren because I would embarrass her by being photographed there. In fact she was becoming almost obsessive about it – and the last thing I needed, right then, was a possessive woman.

I couldn't get out of the lunch because I was the guest of honour and, in any event, I didn't want to miss it.

So, after saying *ciao* to Gina I went to my room and shaved, dressed, and left with the rest of our party for Sophia Loren's house – from where we planned to catch a flight to London.

Her home was out in the country – I believe it was once the summer residence of the popes. She and her husband, Carlo Ponti, had a wonderful art collection. There were paintings and sculptures everywhere. They were especially fond of the works of Henry Moore which I personally found rather unattractive – but then, what did I know about art – except for the Bushman paintings in the Karoo?

Sophia was everything I admired in a woman. She was dressed in black with two white flowers above her left breast. Her hair was dark brown, short, and parted in the middle. In her face there was nothing a plastic surgeon could improve upon and, as if that were not enough, there were those big slanting eyes. I could understand

Peter Sellers perfectly for saying, 'Sophia is the most incredible, the most tantalizing, the most beautiful woman I've ever met.' But, then, he was obsessively in love with her.

She spoke perfect English which was made more attractive by her Italian accent. She was highly intelligent with a wonderfully quick and delightful sense of humour.

MC Botha told me, some years later, that when she was showing us around their carefully manicured garden, with sculptures around every corner, he remarked, 'Shouldn't you be walking with Dr Barnard? He's the important man today.'

I was walking further back with Cathy Bilton, Franco Zeffirelli and Valentino.

Smiling, she replied wittily and without taking her eyes off the garden path, 'No, the important man is always the man who walks with me.'

The photographers were falling over each other to take that 'special picture' which would make the headlines and one of them got the shot or, rather, created it. Sophia Loren, Carlo Ponti and I were sitting on a bench and, as she wanted to smoke, I leaned across and lit her cigarette. The camera flashed and the picture was printed – but Carlo Ponti was cut out, leaving only Sophia and me in an 'intimate pose'. No one seeing the photograph could know that we were surrounded by scores of people.

The photographer also managed to take the picture from such an angle that, with her legs crossed, Sophia had exposed some bare thigh above her stockings.

Back in Cape Town the picture also made the front page. All it achieved was to hurt my wife and embarrass my children – but it sold more newspapers, which, it seems, is the main aim of editors, regardless of any personal distress they cause in the process.

Sophia Loren and I became fairly good friends and we met several times afterwards. She's a fantastically beautiful woman – and highly intelligent. I really admire her very much.

She also said something which I've never forgotten. Once, in a hotel room, some thieves broke in and threatened to harm her and her children unless she gave them her jewellery – $200 000's worth. When I said it must have been heartbreaking to lose the jewels she just shrugged and said, 'Never cry over something that can't cry over you.'

We were about to leave for the airport when Angelo Litrico arrived with a trunk full of suits, shirts and matching shoes which

I tried on in Sophia's bedroom. Life was being far too good for me to pay any heed to the warnings of the South African ambassador that I 'was being used'.

I smiled to myself as I took off my trousers – just a few weeks previously I had only ever seen these beautiful Italian film stars in the movies – now I was in and out of their bedrooms as if I'd been doing it all my life.

Emiliano stayed in Rome but Cathy Bilton came with us to London. It so happened that the two of us walked off the plane together. The next day the newspaper fabricated a story that this cute little blonde was my 'secretary' travelling with me – and the insinuations, between the lines, were obvious.

Bossie, MC and I booked in at the Savoy. It became one of my favourite hotels in London and within the walls of several of the bedrooms are some wonderful memories.

I went to bed early that evening as the few days in Rome had been exhausting.

A banging at my door jerked me out of a deep sleep. It was Bossie and MC with the newspapers. They were both upset about the report of me and my 'secretary', Cathy Bilton or, as Bossie called her, Cathy Biltong (a South African stick of dried meat). But, in my eyes, she was anything *but* that!

Bossie thought these reports were not helping us and I agreed to be more careful in future – but a few hours later I put my foot in it again when I was approached by a photographer who begged to be allowed to take some pictures of me with London in the background. All I had to do was walk outside in the street.

My colleagues and I thought this was a good idea – perhaps it would warm the hearts of the British towards me. So I set off immaculately dressed in one of my Litrico suits and a new overcoat.

Slowly we wandered down to Trafalgar Square. This was a typical London scene, the photographer assured me. He gave me a packet of seed to feed the pigeons and soon the birds were sitting and shitting all over my Litrico suit. He had his picture and my image would get the boost we all thought it needed – or so I believed. Wrong again.

A few days later the most ridiculous picture of me and the pigeons made the front page of the *Evening Standard*. I looked like an absolute moron – covered with fluttering birds perched on my head.

When Louwtjie saw the picture she laughed herself silly and said, 'Now at least you look exactly the way you behave – like a clown.'

That evening MC and I were on the BBC programme *Tomorrow's World*, a special edition called 'Barnard faces his critics', the toughest encounter I'd yet had in open public debate.

The programme was chaired by Raymond Baxter and in the audience were over 150 medical men, theologians, lawyers and newspapermen. They all sat in a studio with rows stacked upwards behind each other rather like a university lecture room – it seemed, at the time, more like a public interrogation than a meeting of the minds.

My lasting impression was that they often called each other 'Sir' and spoke such *perfect* (that's 'pah-fekt') English – especially when compared with my South African Karoo accent.

While there were very many distinguished doctors in the audience such as Professor Roy Calne, Professor Arnott, Professor Beaconsfield and Professor Batchelor, it was really a kind of a match between some key players – MC and I on the one side with Malcolm Muggeridge and Dr Donald Gould on the other side.

Raymond Baxter opened the debate by quoting some recent criticism and emphasized that medical opinion in Britain was widely divided. He asked me how I felt about such remarks. My answer was quite simple, 'Everybody's entitled to his own opinion. If people want to criticize our work they are welcome to do so. As long as they have the facts we are willing to answer their criticism.'

From the audience Dr Gould was the first to speak and wanted an explanation of what we meant by the definition of 'success' – waving a copy of the December issue of the *South African Medical Journal*.

Journals like these are produced for the international medical fraternity – and are read carefully all over the world. When a new discovery or surgical technique is done it is usually reported in these publications so that the medical profession can keep abreast of the relevant news.

This issue had been entirely devoted to various aspects of the first operation. He pointed out that, in the leading article, we had said, 'A human cardiac transplant – an interim report of a successful operation, performed at Groote Schuur Hospital in Cape Town.'

With glee he then read the editorial postscript which had been printed with a thick, funereal black border around it, 'We regret to report the death of the patient, Mr Louis Washkansky, on 21 December 1967.'

I pointed out to Dr Gould that we had not said a 'completely successful heart transplant'. This comment brought the house down.

I explained that we thought it 'successful' because we had been able to remove the heart from a desperately ill patient, replace it with a human donor's heart and restart it again, enabling it to recover normally during the post-operative period. So, technically speaking, it had been a success.

Professor Roy Calne attacked us on the way we had handled the publicity – why hadn't we refused to give out the personal details of the donor and so on? 'I feel that if you'd done so you wouldn't be sitting here answering criticism,' he said – which really upset me.

As an experienced transplant surgeon he should have recognized that the publicity had been completely uncontrollable. Although I was upset about his remark I kept calm and replied, 'If that could have been done we would have – but it was just impossible. We tried to stop all publicity from the start. You will remember that the first report contained no names at all. But afterwards it just snowballed.'

MC spoke up in support and said, 'When we chose our second patient the only thing we released was that he was a dentist who could no longer practise and the press identified him by a process of elimination – going through the telephone books. We just can't stop that sort of thing.'

'But if you feel we were out for publicity,' I said, 'then you must credit us with very little knowledge because we made no announcements prior to the operation.'

'In fact, when the first heart transplant was over, we were having a cup of tea and decided to make a call to the medical superintendent and tell him. That's the only call we made,' MC concluded.

Professor Arnott, a highly distinguished man, commented, 'I really must come in on your side, Dr Barnard. I do believe the publicity was utterly beyond your control. You were dealing with a heart, which unlike the kidney, occupies a very ancient place in the arch-psychology of mankind. That is a very important factor in focusing attention in an uncontrolled way that would not be applied to transplantation of the kidney or the bladder or the stomach for example.'

Then Malcolm Muggeridge took up the cudgel, 'Man is made in the image of God. This is the basic Christian notion. And from it, it seems to me, to follow that man's body deserves our deep respect. Now the view of science suggests that, in fact, man's physical necessities must take precedence over all others. And it is in following this notion that I see our society being transformed into a sort of vast broiler house. And it is because I see these heart transfer operations as part of this process that I instinctively find them repugnant. I wonder what the fury of heaven would be at the notion that our bodies are collections of spare parts?'

This was greeted with an outburst of great laughter and cat-calls.

After some further arguing, a woman from Australia who had received a transplanted kidney, spoke up, 'All I can say is that I'm very grateful for my "spare part" because I'm perfectly well again.'

Then a doctor asked, 'Would Mr Muggeridge accept a corneal transplant if he were blind and it were going to restore his sight?'

I thought that might shut him up but he replied, 'I would accept an eye because I'd know that it was removed from a body that was indubitably dead.'

But he knew he was losing favour with the audience when they jeered and heckled him – so he changed tactics and continued: 'Why, Professor Barnard, was this operation first performed in South Africa? Was it because there are more brilliant surgeons? Better equipment? Or was it, as I suspect, that because of the vile doctrine of apartheid in South Africa, life is held cheaper?'

Hearing this ridiculous statement from such a highly respected man infuriated me and my first instinct was to denounce him as a fool – a fool with a weak argument who had to resort to street-fighting tactics in a supposedly 'intelligent' debate. But I thought about it for a moment and didn't fall into the trap. I just told him that we had very good surgeons, excellent equipment and that we set a high value on human life because we'd done the operation to treat a terminally sick man.

Being South African – and one totally opposed to apartheid – I had faced, and would face many times again, attacks like this on my country.

On this occasion, it was a relief when Professor Calne stood up and said, 'May I say, Sir, that I and most of my colleagues disassociate ourselves from the question put to you!' This was met with great cries of 'hear hear!' foot-stamping and loud applause.

And so it went on – ideological philosophizing about definitions of death, the ethics of transplantation, the morals of doctors and so on. What everyone seemed to forget were the patients – that Philip Blaiberg was back in Cape Town *enjoying* his new life. Only the patients, in my opinion, were qualified to respond to these accusations.

The programme could not have ended on a better note, because a surgeon in the audience introduced a patient who had been suffering from a terminal heart condition for eight years and who had had *twenty-five* emergency operations to keep him 'alive' in a wheel chair.

He said, 'I've followed Professor Barnard through the whole business and I've been thrilled because I've been waiting since 1962 to live a life which I hope a new heart is going to give me.'

Raymond Baxter, trying to draw the man on the risks of such an operation, asked, 'Are you entirely happy about taking the major step of accepting this particular surgery?'

'I would take it tomorrow.' And with that simple, concise answer, he effectively denounced all the accusations that we were 'experimenting on unwitting patients'.

The programme ended and we agreed that we'd put up a fairly good show and answered the questions well. It was a pleasant change to read some good reports in the papers the following morning.

A fellow South African, Donald Ross, who had also been a classmate of mine in medical school at the University of Cape Town, did his first heart transplant in England in March that year, at the National Heart Hospital. After the operation the team posed outside the hospital with a big Union Jack. So much for *their* desire to avoid publicity.

Donald continued with the transplant programme but, as they had limited success, the British surgeons placed a moratorium on cardiac transplantation until 1980.

The next day I was invited for lunch at the headquarters of the Royal College of Surgeons. That was the only recognition this prestigious college ever gave me for my achievements. In fact I've received awards and honours from most Western countries – the only exception being Great Britain.

In the late afternoon we left for Paris and, after the usual shambles at the airports, booked in at the Plaza Athenee Hotel.

That evening was set aside for Paris-by-night.

At the famous Lido there was such a crowd that I didn't even get out of the limousine and we decided to try the Crazy Horse instead.

Shows with naked girls have never turned me on. In the first place it's so contrived and artificial and in the second place one is too far removed from the merchandise. But, at the Crazy Horse, they gave me a special treat and invited me backstage to meet some of the girls and, while I didn't think they were particularly attractive, I was intrigued by their total lack of inhibition as they sauntered around with nothing on.

By the time we left the club the press and photographers had caught up with us and there was some aggressive jostling among them – some lost their tempers and it ended up in a free-for-all fight.

The next day several papers said we were to blame and although we strongly denied it I'm sure I saw MC punch a photographer – who probably deserved it anyway.

The next morning we met with Professor Charles du Bost. He was one of the pioneers of vascular surgery and I was pleased to hear that he and his colleagues were preparing to embark on a transplant programme. Professor Du Bost was a highly respected surgeon and would be a powerful ally in our cause.

Claude Terell invited us for lunch at the famous Tour d'Argent restaurant, well-known for its duck. I was served their 113 690th duck – in a black cherry sauce – which didn't impress me very much but the company did, especially the beautiful woman sitting on my right – Mrs Sucarno, the wife of the then deposed Indonesian president.

During my previous visits to Paris, due to tight budgets, I had always had to slum it, but Paris in this style was fantastic and I was very sad to leave.

Next, and the last stop before returning home, was Milan – mainly to meet with the staff of Mondadori Publishing House and discuss the biography they planned on my life. Before even a word was written they'd bought the world rights and so they were keen to get started.

The managing director was Giorgio Mondadori who suggested that I should come to his country home so that we could work quietly without the *paparazzi* bothering us for at least one day.

I flew to the little town in a small private plane and we lost our way. After searching around for about half an hour over the Italian countryside we eventually found the airstrip and, with great relief, finally landed. I was met by Giorgio and his wife, Nara, who took me to their house – which was more like a palace, surrounded by beautiful gardens with cherry trees, immaculate lawns, a tennis court and swimming pool.

Giorgio and I became very close friends – we had some good times together and also some bad times.

I worked deep into the night with his staff on an outline of the book. He was fascinated by stories from my childhood and my struggles as a young doctor, as well as the preparation for the first transplant.

Eventually we came to the topic of my relationship with Gina Lollobrigida. I was quite keen to meet her again and I think there was a possibility that we could have had a future together – but Mondadori would hear nothing of this. He said that the publicity would harm the sale of the book – and also my reputation. I wasn't even allowed to phone her.

The next day we returned to Milan where I had the usual interviews – answering the same predictable questions over and over once more.

Alfredo Beni had heard about the possibility of the book and the press had a field day about the possibility of a movie, but it was only an idea at that stage. They reported that the 'part of Christiaan Barnard' would be played by Gregory Peck, Warren Beatty, Maximillian Schell, Vince Edwards or James Coburn. All this speculation was very amusing – and quite flattering in a way. James Coburn had, apparently, already done a fairly good job of impersonating me in a film that had just been released – *Candy*.

That evening Beni turned up at the party with a gorgeous girl. She was an ex-Miss Italy, in her early twenties. 'What a lucky guy!' I thought although I knew film directors always had beautiful girls with them who were usually aspiring movie stars.

Throughout the entire evening I was pursued insistently by a woman who must have already been through the hands of the plastic surgeon a few times. If anyone ever deserved to be described as mutton dressed as lamb it was she and she was determined to end up in my bed that night.

I was equally determined to avoid such an awful prospect so I slipped away from this clinging ivy and asked Beni if he would mind taking me back to the hotel.

The valet brought his Rolls-Royce to the front of the hotel where he waited with his girlfriend while I hid in the garden to get away from the persistent lady who was now looking everywhere for me. They picked me up and I sighed with relief at having escaped alone.

When we arrived at our hotel – the Cavour – I said good night and got out of the car. I was absolutely amazed when his 'girlfriend' joined me on the pavement. As Jenny couldn't speak English and my Italian wasn't so good in those days, I was having difficulty trying to understand what she was doing or had in mind.

The director laughed loudly from his seat in the Rolls and asked 'Don't you understand? She wants to spend the night with you!'

I really couldn't believe it, so I turned and looked at her. She had dark hair and deep green eyes – absolutely stunning. She smiled broadly with perfectly even and brilliant-white teeth. I raised my eyebrows in an unspoken question which she answered by wrapping her slender arms around my neck and kissing me fully on the mouth. Her teeth gently nibbled my bottom lip while she rhythmically moved her taut body against mine. Not even the cold weather could contain my excitement and she laughed wickedly – throwing her head back while still holding me firmly as she increased the pressure still further against my groin.

'You see!' said my host gleefully as he drove away, 'you are a very popular man in Italy!'

It had been an exhausting trip so far and I wasn't sure I was up to the kind of night I imagined was about to begin. Anyway, I went into the bathroom to clean my teeth – and undressed at the same time. When I came out the room was in darkness, with the only light coming from the moon through the window.

Suddenly she was standing in front of me, her gentle fingers teasing nerve-endings I'd never learned about in medical school as she edged closer still. I reached out and pulled her to me and we kissed long and passionately. She moaned softly as her tongue darted in and out of my mouth. Our bodies were so firmly together it was hard to tell where I left off and she began.

Her breasts were full and firm as they rose and fell impatiently against my chest with each breath. Her perfume mingled with animal lust and she groaned as she nibbled my ears, my neck, my abdomen as she lowered herself to her knees.

It was all over too quickly and we both fell into an exhausted sleep.

I was woken by an appalling noise which came from the corridor.

I quietly opened the door and peeked down the passage. There was one of my colleagues in his pyjamas and a woman in a shirt and jeans – they were both screaming at each other.

What had happened was that someone at the party had organized a girl for him and he didn't know she was a prostitute. In the morning, when she left, she demanded to be paid.

The unfortunate man just couldn't understand because, where we lived prostitution was only active in the docks where ugly, and usually diseased, women plied their trade – he had certainly never been exposed to high class, clean and beautiful call-girls.

After a few words in Italian – one being *stronzo* – which I'm sure even he understood, she flounced down the corridor hurling further abuse over her shoulder as she did so – hardly a romantic ending to a night of passion!

I went back into my room and as Jenny was definitely not in the same business and seemed to have enjoyed herself, we made love again.

Later that day we returned to South Africa.

I was both surprised and delighted to find Louwtjie and Deirdre waiting for me when I arrived at DF Malan airport in Cape Town but before going home I asked them to take me to the hospital where I found Philip Blaiberg in excellent health. My brother, Marius, brought me up-to-date on his condition and the incredible progress our patient had been making.

'The media are no longer interested in you,' Marius told me with a wink. 'They want photographs of Blaiberg.'

'I don't know,' I said. 'Roy Calne criticized us like hell for giving the first patient and donor too much publicity – anyway I'm sick and tired of the press right now.'

'Yes, we've been reading about some of your adventures,' he said with a grin. 'Are they true?'

'Oh, about fifty-fifty' I laughed back. We were brothers and he understood.

'I don't think there'll be a very warm welcome at home,' he added more seriously.

After talking to Philip and Eileen Blaiberg I agreed to one or two photographs being taken and, maybe, some interviews later – provided that strict sterile conditions were maintained – and then I went home to Zeekoevlei with Louwtjie and Deirdre.

Early the next morning Philip Blaiberg greeted his wife and said, 'Do you know, Eileen, I think that man is really fantastic. I mean, he's been phoning the hospital regularly about me while he's been overseas and now, not half an hour after flying all the way from Italy, the very first thing he does is to visit me! I must be quite important!'

'Yes, you're his most famous patient right now so you'd best get ready for the cameraman because they want some official shots of your progress.'

'What, looking like this?'

'No, I think they want to photograph you shaving,' she laughed happily.

'You mean I can shave myself?'

'Yes, you can – you've had it too easy for too long,' joked one of the nurses as she walked into the sterile room. 'And, if you can keep a secret, I think they'll soon be letting you walk about a little more – even out of this room – so you'll soon, at least, be able to look out of the window.'

He roared with delight. 'And then I guess I can get out of here and go home?'

'Don't be so impatient!' the nurse reprimanded him. 'One thing at a time.' He couldn't see her warm smile behind the mask. All his nurses cared very deeply for him and were thrilled with his progress and his new-found joy for life.

And so, forty-three days after his operation Philip Blaiberg, the world's longest-surviving heart transplant patient, faced the cameras for the first time – in his pyjamas and doing what men do, normally, every morning of their lives – standing in front of the mirror, working up a lather with the shaving-brush and using a razor.

Don Mackenzie and his camera had to undergo the entire sterilization process before being allowed close to the glass partition inside the special intensive-care suite to take pictures through an eye-level glass panel into the sterile rooms. The angle was awkward, but he got a famous photograph.

Now the world knew that Philip Blaiberg was alive and well and shaving in Cape Town.

I was expecting Louwtjie to be angry – and couldn't blame her either. She'd been very quiet since she'd collected me at the airport.

When we were alone she confronted me with the newspaper reports. The pornographic actress, Gina Lollobrigida, Sophia Loren, my 'secretary' in London, scuffling with photographers outside nightclubs in Paris and, 'oh yes, the pigeons shitting on your head!'

'I thought you were supposed to be there on medical business – not gadding around from one nightclub and one girl to the next!' she charged.

I didn't want to be totally dishonest so I ignored most of the stories and concentrated on the Sophia Loren headlines and the Crazy Horse incident. I've learned that if you do have to lie then it's best to have some truth in the foundation.

'Lies,' I said. 'You know very well what those guys are like, they'll say *anything* to get a sensational story – I might have been naive but I really couldn't have stopped them saying all that rubbish.'

'It may be all right for you, but I was so humiliated! You spent more time at social engagements than anything else – that's no way for a father and husband to behave!

'The newsmen here nearly drove us insane with their questions and we had to carry on smiling and pretend that we were quite unaffected by those loathsome people!

'And then, at DF Malan airport, Deirdre and I waited patiently and had to be protected by the police.

'We couldn't even leave the car because that mad mob of reporters and photographers made it impossible – and as for that nosey crowd, I just wish they'd mind their own business!'

Anyway, she seemed a bit happier now that she'd let off some steam but I couldn't help myself from thinking how opposite we were. I have to admit I'd found the entire European trip rather exciting.

But, seeing her upset, even though we had been drifting apart for so long, she still made me feel like a real bastard. With great difficulty I shrugged off the guilt – because, what the hell, I was enjoying myself!

It was only a couple of weeks before I was due to give a talk to the American College of Cardiology in San Francisco and Louwtjie would be joining me there so the bad press reports were soon forgotten and we eased back – uncomfortably – into our strained relationship and faltering marriage.

In the meantime, apart from taking care of my patients and catching up on the administration of my department, I had a complete invasion of the international media to contend with.

Television teams flew into Cape Town from the United States and Germany to present me – Philip Blaiberg – to the world 'in person'. Special sterilized lighting apparatus was installed in my rooms. I was to appear, I was told, on TV screens in millions of homes as 'The Man of the Hour' or 'The Man with the New Heart'.

I put on my brightest smile and did my best to answer their questions and, just for fun, I even sang a song or two! My mind still boggles at the thought that I was seen and heard all over the world.

And then, at last, I was allowed out of the sterile room into the other parts of my suite. It sounds insignificant – but it was a major milestone and proof that I was well on the road to full recovery.

Now I could stand opposite the sealed window and gaze on to the street in front of the hospital, wave to passers-by, and pose for photographs. I must have faced a thousand cine cameras and other photographers with telephoto lenses. I used to make the Churchill victory sign for them. World travellers arriving in Cape Town made special excursions to Groote Schuur, on their sight-seeing trips, to wave to me. I was now, it seemed, a tourist attraction as popular as Table Mountain itself.

Then Don Mackenzie, the photographer, had a brilliant idea. One night he persuaded Professor Barnard to cooperate with him by walking into my room, masked and dressed in his usual sterile outfit, carrying a transparent plastic box – inside was my old heart in a preservative solution. Outside, behind the glass panel in the passage, Don Mackenzie was snapping merrily away with his camera.

Professor Barnard and I sat on my bed and examined my heart with cool professional interest. He showed me that more than 90 per cent of the muscle had become functionless scarred tissue. How I had managed to remain alive until the transplant was a miracle in itself.

Professor Barnard looked up from my heart and said, 'Dr Blaiberg, do you realize that you are the first man, in the history of mankind, to be able to sit, as you are now, and look at his own, dead, heart?'

And that photograph appeared all over the world.

Shortly after my return to Cape Town a meeting was called by the chairman of the hospitals board, Mr Lionel Murray, and other officials of both the University of Cape Town Medical School and Groote Schuur Hospital. They were concerned, they said, about the welfare of the Darvall family – whose daughter, Denise, was the donor in the heart transplant for Washkansky and also the only bread-winner in the Darvall family – and so a fund had been set up in case of their need.

Harry Oppenheimer, chairman of De Beers and chancellor of Cape Town University, also had an idea about the Chamber of Mines building a research centre at the medical school – to help continue investigations relating to transplantation and immunology.

The general consensus was that extensive fund-raising be undertaken, primarily by using my name, in order to establish an ongoing cardiac research programme. Would I be prepared to cooperate?

I said I would do whatever I could – but that we should be careful about making my name too 'commercial' as it could have a detrimental effect on the medical institutions in South Africa and the heart transplant programme itself – not to mention my own reputation. I'd been exposed to a great deal of press coverage – some of which was quite good. Those reports which were bad seemed to concentrate on the suggestion that I had an 'obsession with publicity'.

Some donations from private individuals had begun coming in and the Shell Company, together with the Trust Bank, produced one-ounce gold medallions which they sold at a substantial profit.

They pinned most of their hopes for funds on the income of a book to be written on my life. They had already sold the world rights for a substantial amount and were keen to hear of my discussion with the publisher. I told them of my meeting with Mondadori but pointed out that I couldn't possibly write the book on my own because of the demands on my time and so we decided to look for a writer in South Africa to help me.

Everyone was delighted and had, perhaps, far more optimism than I had for the demand such a book might generate. Dr Nico Malan, the administrator of the Cape, was a good friend of mine (then) and he duly issued a press statement: 'The Darvall Memorial Fund has received sufficient funds to meet any foreseeable needs for Mr Darvall and his two sons.

'At the request of the committee I have consented to the establishment of a research fund and that facilities should be made to selected medical practitioners throughout the world for research into heart and organ transplants.

'Mr Darvall has expressed the wish that the fund be associated directly with Professor Barnard and, with his consent, the research fund will be known as "The Chris Barnard Fund." I feel mankind will benefit as a result of what has been and undoubtedly will be achieved in this field of medical science.'

So the hunt for a co-author was on. One writer after another was appointed – and replaced for a variety of reasons.

As I had predicted, there were immediate insinuations about my 'desire for publicity'.

Then there was a series of articles about various ghost writers – a retired news editor, who had made his name by writing about crime in South Africa 'gave up' because I couldn't devote enough time to help him.

Then a professor of physics took over but that didn't work out either because, working on his own, he invented too many details – I remember, for example, that he wrote a great deal about my 'love for trout fishing' – which is actually something I've never done in my whole life. I think he wrote more about his own childhood than mine, in fact.

'When, if ever, will Barnard's book be finished?' the newspapers asked as they reported on how difficult it was to meet me. It was difficult only because I was under a lot of pressure from dozens of other sources. They seemed unable to understand that I was, first and foremost, a *doctor* – not a fund-raiser or writer. My patients were far more important.

Then a 'Mother of 3 reveals herself as Barnard ghost writer' story appeared which was rebutted by another writer and arguments began about who had written what – and when.

Everyone seemed to think I was responsible for these false-starts. Of course, I wasn't – and, in the middle of all this I had operations to perform, conferences to attend, research to monitor – and a department to run.

Finally I went back to the committee (as I guessed I would have to) and told them I would write the book myself and that I would find someone to help me.

Meanwhile, Louwtjie, quite out of character, had agreed to a press interview which appeared in a story with the biggest understatement of the year as the headline, 'Chris is not a saint, says Mrs Barnard.'

Louwtjie Barnard reluctantly opened the door. Why was she doing this? She disliked newspaper reporters intensely. Still, maybe it was better to cooperate rather than rebel. Maybe this reporter would write the truth — without the usual exaggerations or lies?

'What a lovely home,' he said as he entered the small house.

'I'm pleased you like it,' she said, pausing to light a cigarette, 'because that means you approve of my taste. Chris couldn't care less about the place, so he leaves it all to me. I asked him to cut the lawn weeks ago — but, as you know, he has had other things on his mind.

'Still, he says he'll get round to it one of these days. I don't know when'

'So he's kept a very busy man then?' asked the reporter.

'Since the transplant I hardly ever see him. All I can hope for is 10 minutes in the morning when he throws back half a cup of coffee for breakfast, and last thing at night when he's exhausted.

'I tell you — that man is living on his nerves and one day the backwash is going to catch up with him. But, of course, you can't tell him anything. He won't listen. He's so stubborn.

'One thing you ought to know about Chris is what his priorities are. His patients are number one on the list, and his family comes second. Please don't think I'm complaining. With a famous surgeon it can't possibly be any other way.

'But I can be stubborn too,' she said, crushing out the cigarette, 'especially when it comes to this whole business of fame — suddenly the Barnard family is famous — so what? So nothing I say! I refuse to let any of it change a thing around here. I've got a home to run — whether we are famous or not.

'Naturally Chris is very thrilled about what's happened, and he's enjoying all the adulation. But if I allowed myself to be carried away as well we would be in a real mess.

'No, you've got to keep both feet firmly on the ground. When Chris phoned me early in the morning from the hospital after the first transplant to tell me the patient was okay I said "congratulations — that's wonderful" and I went back to sleep.

'Maybe I should show more enthusiasm but we're not a very demonstrative family. The whole world is showering rose petals on Chris. He's getting offered fabulous jobs, and women from all over the world write love letters to him.

'Wherever he goes he is royally treated. Nothing is too much for him. Compliments come pouring in. Suddenly Chris can do no wrong.

'But he can. He is not a saint. And if his own wife were to treat him like one, he would be impossible.

'When Chris enters our front door he walks into reality. And reality is the one element he needs more than anything else in his life now. And I'm the only person who can give him that. If you pat a man on his back too often he eventually loses balance and falls. I'm here to see that that never happens.'

He hesitated momentarily before posing his next question, 'Mrs Barnard, I believe you have a reputation for being a "hard" woman – do you think that's true?'

Pausing only to light another cigarette she quickly replied, 'Not hard. Just honest. I know, for instance, that some people feel that by now I should have visited Mrs Washkansky and Mrs Blaiberg. And I will. But only when I feel the time is right. And I know some unkind things have been said about me because I refuse to cooperate with the press.

'But what it all boils down to is that I don't want to bask in Chris's limelight or draw attention to myself.'

The reporter noticed how hard she was trying to keep the petulance from her voice.

'Good morning Miss Levett, anything interesting in the mail this morning?' Ann Levett had been my secretary for several years. She was not a beauty but was loyal and very efficient. Unfortunately she was having domestic problems and I could see she'd been crying again.

Without looking up from her desk she replied, 'Only the usual – masses of fan mail and invitations.'

I was getting about 200 letters a day from all over the world with all kinds of offers – from women offering me their hearts in marriage to others giving me their hearts as a donor. At that stage I was listed in the *Guinness Book of Records* as the person receiving the most fan mail – whether that was true or not I can't say – but my name was in the book anyway.

I went into my office to prepare for the next overseas trip. This was an important engagement as it would be the first opportunity I would have to report back to my peers – the American College of Cardiology meeting in San Francisco.

At that stage heart transplantation results didn't look encouraging.

Three days after Dr Blaiberg's operation, Norman Shumway had done his first on Mike Kasperak. The post-operative problems they encountered could fill a pathology book and the patient died after fourteen days.

Three days after Shumway, Kantrowitz did his second transplant – this time on a patient 58 years old. The result was not much better than his first attempt, as the patient died eight hours after surgery.

On the 16th of February Dr Sen, of Bombay, operated on a 29 year old patient – who died after three hours.

So when I received the invitation to address the American College of Cardiology in San Francisco, six heart transplants had been done – with my patient, Philip Blaiberg, being the only survivor.

'Where are my slides?' I called to Ann through the open door between her office and mine.

'I haven't mounted them yet, because Don's still got the drawings he had to photograph.'

'Phone him and tell him to bring them back immediately – if necessary I'll have them photographed myself – otherwise I'm going to leave here without any slides at all!'

I walked to the racks holding the lecture slides to see if there were any of the old ones I could use.

As I'd never lectured on clinical transplantation before I needed to prepare some new slides. One of my registrars, Des Fernandez, had made some colour drawings of the surgical technique and, as we had no medical artist, Ann prepared some graphs of the post-operative course of Blaiberg – showing pulse-rate, temperature, respiratory rate, electrocardiogram voltage and immunosuppressive regime.

These graphs didn't look very professional but I was proud of them as it showed a patient alive and doing well 65 days after heart-transplantation.

Eventually Don Mackenzie arrived in his usual disorganized state.

'What the hell happened to you?' I demanded, 'Probably out with a teenage model again I suppose!'

He was a fashion photographer and not a bad guy to know. Since the transplant he had accompanied me a lot. This was mutually beneficial as it paid him better and I had control over all the photographs.

In his staccato speech he began telling me about all the problems he was having with his girlfriends. He talked faster than a racing commentator.

'Never mind *your* problems – have you photographed my stuff?'

I didn't have much time left as Deirdre, my daughter, was leaving for Australia that afternoon and I wanted to see her off at the airport.

'Yes,' he said as he walked across to a viewing box and unrolled a spool of film.

I selected some of the best photographs and asked Ann to mount them. They were certainly not of the same standard my colleagues in the United States used, but were the best I could do. I would also have to write my talk on the plane as I had no time to spare until then, so I placed some notes and a small slide viewer in my briefcase while Don was telling me in lurid detail about his latest conquests.

Ann brought in the slide box and I left the office for a trip that would take me to Portugal, Italy and the United States.

As Deirdre was on her way to a water-skiing championship in Australia and André, my son, was at school in Pretoria, Louwtjie had decided to accompany me – but only on the American leg of the trip. I had arranged to meet up with her at Fiumicino airport in Rome.

The South African Airways Boeing 707 landed early the next morning at Lisbon. This was only going to be a day stop to discuss my visit later to Coimbra University and I had an appointment in Milan that evening to meet the new co-author of my biography.

I was met in the foyer of the hotel by the bitter-sweet refrain of the *fado* singers, all dressed in black cloaks. They had travelled for four hours in the early morning to welcome me. I found their songs beautiful and sad but the gloom was soon dispelled by the enthusiasm of the students who were proud of their traditions at the oldest university in Portugal and discussed, with great excitement, the arrangements for my visit in a few weeks' time.

I had a day room in the hotel so, after the students left, I decided to lie down for a few hours.

Usually I sleep well in a plane but had had severe heartburn the previous night and there were no antacids available – it had been a long and uncomfortable night.

I was taking Indocin for my arthritis then and knew that this could cause stomach ulcers unless I took the capsules after meals – but my life had become so irregular that I often swallowed them in the early hours of the morning on an empty stomach – just so that I could get out of bed early in the morning without the crippling pain.

I had just made myself comfortable in the double bed when the phone rang.

My heart leaped with fear – the call must be from South Africa as I'd left instructions with the hotel exchange not to put any calls through unless they were from Cape Town – I hoped nothing was wrong with my patient.

'Yes?' I asked apprehensively.

'I'm sorry to disturb you but there is a young lady here who says she has an urgent message for you,' the operator apologized.

'Who from?' I demanded irritably.

'She says she cannot tell me – it must be delivered personally – and she won't leave without doing so.'

I thought for a while. The fact that it was a young girl made the interruption tolerable.

'Okay, send her up to my room.'

I usually sleep naked – so I quickly slipped on a track suit and brushed my teeth.

There was a soft, gentle knock at my door a few minutes later.

'Come in – it's open.'

After some hesitation my visitor entered. She was not particularly young – probably in her early thirties – but slender, tall and dressed in slacks with a white blouse and blazer.

She looked uncertain and it was obvious that she wanted to get this visit over with as quickly as possible.

'Hello, what can I do for you?' I smiled as my mood changed and we both sat down.

She replied with an Italian accent, 'Gina sent me here in a private plane to come and fetch you.'

'Fetch *me*?' I nearly fell off my chair.

'Yes, she asked me to give you this letter and wait for you.'

The messenger opened her Gucci handbag and took out a blue envelope.

What a lovely private postal service, I thought! It was a letter from Gina Lollobrigida in which she began by re-living some of the moments of that night spent at her home. She was now in Catania

– shooting *Buona Sera, Mrs Campbell* – but complained that she couldn't concentrate and begged me to join her for a few days.

God, how I would love to accept the invitation! But it was just impossible. There was no way I could rearrange my plans, I explained, but I did the next best thing – I took her friend to bed. 'Well,' I thought, 'It's only polite to tip the postman.'

I did a stupid thing with the letter, however – I put it into my briefcase and forgot about it.

Exhausted, I left that afternoon for Milan.

Giorgio Mondadori met me at the airport with someone who, I assumed, must be my co-author. He had shoulder-length hair, dark-rimmed glasses and was dressed in a white polo-neck jersey, dark trousers and black jacket. Slung over his shoulder was a dictaphone case.

'This is Bill Pepper,' Giorgio introduced him. 'You will be seeing a lot of each other in the next year or so.'

'Hi,' he responded and extended a hand to greet me with a firm grip.

We immediately left for the Principe Di Savoia. My luggage would be taken care of by one of Giorgio's men.

Bill had been with *Time* magazine, but a few years previously he had started to freelance. He was an American but now lived in Rome with his wife, Beverly, who was famous for her enormous steel sculptures.

Mondadori had just published a book called *The Artist and The Pope* written by Bill on the wonderful relationship between the famous Italian sculptor, Giacomo Manzu, and Pope John XXIII.

Giorgio was very impressed by the success of this book. He liked Bill's style and thought he would be just the right one to work with me.

Probably as a result of my ingrained Afrikaner conservatism, he didn't impress me. I was sure he was one of those liberals who wanted to change everything in the world – but didn't know how.

I was wrong. The more we discussed the book the more sure of him I became. He was enthusiastic, sincere and highly intelligent. It was obvious he'd decided to devote all his time and talent to the book.

I went to bed that evening feeling that I had not only met my author but had also made a new friend. As it turned out that impression was correct. We worked many hours together and his wise counselling made me a better man.

His home in Trastevere, Rome, became my home too. I will always cherish the wonderful time I spent with Bill Pepper – working on *One Life* – the title we'd chosen for the biography.

The next morning we left together for Rome. Although it was only a short flight we discussed our programme for the next few months and decided that, as soon as possible, he should come to South Africa and spend a few months with me.

At Rome airport I was told that Louwtjie had arrived earlier that morning and that she was waiting for me in the VIP lounge. When Bill and I entered, she was hidden behind the reporters and photographers. She had probably had a torrid time since she'd put her feet on Italian soil.

I elbowed my way through the mass of people and gave them my usual toothy smile and when I reached my wife her first remark was, 'You smile like a grinning hyena!' It really hurt – but I understood her mood.

At the press conference which followed I answered for both of us and, eventually, with their last few camera flashes, the reporters and photographers were herded out of the room. Louwtjie, Bill and I were left alone – with a few of the airport officials who were waiting to escort us to the plane for San Francisco.

I could see that Louwtjie had immediately summed Bill up as another 'enemy'. The atmosphere was thick and tense and I was relieved when they called us to board the plane.

After a long flight we arrived in San Francisco – the domain of Norman Shumway – he and his team were based in Palo Alto, about 80 kilometres away.

Norman and I were registrars at the same time in Minneapolis. We both studied under Doctors Lillehei and Varco – two of the leading pioneers of open-heart surgery in the late fifties. I was told that Norman would be on the panel after my lecture and I was looking forward to meeting him again.

He had, at that stage, only performed one heart transplant but, unfortunately, had encountered a lot of post-operative problems.

Almost immediately after recovery his patient developed chronic lung problems and, while internal bleeding was stopped with transfusions, liver and kidney complications developed on the second day.

The patient had breathed periodically without an artificial respirator for the next three days but the kidney function had to be handled by dialysis and he lapsed into a semi-coma because of poor liver function. Large blood transfusions were made to remove impurities.

His gall bladder was removed and he was fed through a plastic tube inserted in his oesophagus – but another emergency operation was needed to stop internal bleeding.

He had three major operations in five days and was semi-conscious. His breathing was helped by a respirator while dialysis performed his kidney functions.

And then he died.

Dr Donald Ross, chief surgeon at the National Heart Hospital in London, made the most significant observation when he said, 'It's not surprising that Mike Kasperak has died. I am amazed that they had been able to keep him alive so long.'

Louwtjie and I were escorted through Immigration and Customs and taken, by a member of the college, to the Hilton Hotel where we were staying and where the lecture would take place the following day – in one of the big function rooms on the second floor.

That evening, the College had arranged a function with some movie stars. Louwtjie and I sat with Milton Berle and Jack Lemmon. Their humour certainly helped me forget my problems with Louwtjie – although only temporarily.

The lecture hall was packed to capacity and I was silently amused to see some of the surgeons sitting on the floor in the aisle. I went to the projectionist to put the slides in the carousel myself because it's a harrowing experience to start a lecture when your last slide is projected first – or it's upside down.

Denton Cooley used to play practical jokes and would sometimes slip a slide of a beautiful, scantily dressed girl in among the slides of visiting lecturers.

I once attended a lecture where a surgeon was talking about terminally ill heart patients on whom he was performing valve replacement operations.

'This will give you some idea of how bad these patients are,' he'd said – 'next slide please.'

But, instead of a patient with an oxygen mask sitting upright in bed, gasping for breath – a beautiful blonde in a topless bikini was shown. The lecturer didn't know what to say for a moment – but quickly collected his thoughts and said, 'No, this is the slide of the patient after surgery!'

To my horror, as I was arranging my slides, I noticed that the one of the catheter findings on Blaiberg before surgery and the one after surgery, illustrating the haemo-dynamic correction achieved by the transplant heart, were missing.

I quickly asked for a phone and got through to Louwtjie in our room and asked if she could look for them, 'I'll be up in a moment.'

Louwtjie Barnard relaxed in their suite on the 23rd floor of the San Francisco Hilton Hotel.

The weather was beautifully sunny and her husband had given an extremely well-received press conference and now he was downstairs about to make a speech to his American peers.

She still couldn't admit that she was enthralled with this new lifestyle, 'but it's not bad I suppose,' she murmured to herself.

And, idly thinking about what she would wear to the dinner that evening, her thoughts were interrupted by the telephone.

'Okay,' she answered her husband's question, 'I'll look for them now.'

Sighing she looked in his suitcase but found nothing. Then she saw the briefcase standing next to the bed and, quickly opening it, she began rummaging through its contents.

With a grunt of satisfaction she found, almost immediately, the envelope of slides and notes he was missing and triumphantly retrieved them from the case.

As she closed it she noticed the corner of a pale blue envelope in one of the briefcase compartments. Alarm bells rang loudly. What made it look so out of place was that it looked so feminine – among all the medical and masculine contents.

Slowly, she re-opened the case and stared for a few moments at, what she clearly recognized now, was a letter.

She shouldn't open it. 'Leave it be,' she told herself. 'Don't touch it – pretend it's not there – it's probably nothing anyway.'

'If it's nothing then there's no harm in looking,' she argued with herself as she tentatively gripped the edge of the paper with thumb and forefinger and eased the envelope out.

She sat on the edge of the bed gently tapping the letter against the side of her leg still debating with herself whether or not she should read it. Suddenly she was overwhelmed with a great sadness – and then panic.

Throwing the packet of slides and notes onto the bed she quickly opened the letter and began to read.

Fortunately, the hotel elevators were much more efficient than those at Groote Schuur Hospital – the doors slid open, I touched the button for the 23rd floor and could immediately feel the centrifugal force on my legs as it gathered momentum and hurtled upwards.

I knocked impatiently on the door but there was no reply. Maybe Louwtjie was in the bathroom? I tried the handle and the door opened. I was worried now because Louwtjie was cautious and believed in keeping doors locked at all times. The lounge was also empty.

'Louwtjie!' I called, but there was no reply.

When I walked into the bedroom I saw her immediately and was horrified at the grim tableau which greeted me. She was sitting, dressed in a night-gown, on the ledge of the open window looking out into space – 23 floors below was the street.

'What the *hell* are you doing?' I demanded, inwardly quaking with fear. She turned round to face me and I could see she was crying.

'What's wrong? Couldn't you find my slides?'

She wearily waved the blue envelope at me. 'I can't go on any more, Chris, not with the way you deceive and lie to me. I don't want to live any longer.' There was a total absence of emotion in her voice. Just simple resignation which echoed hollowly against the faint noises from the busy road below.

I stared at the letter as if hypnotized by its damning presence. It was Gina's – the one I'd received in Lisbon telling me about the wonderful few hours we'd spent in her bedroom and how she had wanted me to join her.

Oh, you sentimental bloody *fool*! Why hadn't I destroyed the damned thing? Why, in the name of God, had I kept it in my briefcase? I was never going to reply to it – after all, it meant nothing to me, or did it? Maybe it was some kind of juvenile trophy or talisman – a certificate of competence? A valuable possession?

'Please Louwtjie, don't start now. I have to give a very important lecture.' I decided to be direct, calm and logical, ignoring the suicide threat. I could always change tack if necessary. I'd have gone on my knees if I thought that would have helped.

She looked at me blankly. 'I'm not starting it now, Chris – it started many years ago. I'm going to end it now,' and she looked out of the window. My heart lurched as she edged herself closer to oblivion.

Would she really jump? She was in a strange country, with no friends to turn to – and now she'd found proof of what she'd been suspecting for a long time.

Where did my priorities lie? In this bedroom on the 23rd floor with a wife who had borne me two beautiful children or in the lecture room on the second floor – with strangers who couldn't care less about what happened to me or my family?

This was an emergency – as in the operating room – and it needed an immediate decision, but I'd never encountered this problem before.

I looked at the pathetic figure sitting in the open window and made up my mind. My presence in the room could, I decided, accomplish nothing – she was best left alone and I prayed that she'd either lose her nerve or realize that this wasn't the answer.

'Louwtjie, I'm deeply sorry, please forgive me. I'll explain later.' And, with that, I left the bedroom and my wife and returned to the lecture room without the two slides.

The place was now packed to capacity and the noise subsided as I entered. I carefully made my way to the stage, stepping over the legs of surgeons sitting on the floor.

The president of the American College of Cardiology introduced me, but my thoughts were elsewhere. I was listening for sirens. Will she really do it? Surely, as a good mother, the love for her two children will stop her? Somehow I had to get through this lecture and then back to the room on the 23rd floor.

There was tremendous applause and I realized it was for me. Walking to the podium I was trying to collect my thoughts about how to start the lecture. My head was fuzzy – probably from the adrenalin being pumped into my system as a result of this gathering as well as my wife threatening to commit suicide. I had to clear my mind.

When I give a talk I seldom use prepared notes and prefer speaking off-the-cuff. I knew more or less what I was going to say, but I wasn't clear on how to start.

'Ladies and Gentlemen,' I began, but my throat was so dry that the words didn't come out clearly. I could see some of the doctors looking at each other and grinning. I was aware of their professional jealousy just as I knew there was an element of the circus in the room – like people watching the tight-rope walker and secretly hoping he'll fall off. I'm sure many were hoping I'd freeze during my talk.

Fortunately there was a glass of water on the podium so I took a sip. I closed my eyes and, as if through Louwtjie's eyes, I could see the ground rushing towards me as I plummeted through the air in a deathly spiral, a spinning and twisting body about to be smashed out of recognition on the cars and the tarmac below – the blue envelope still clutched tightly.

I opened my eyes, blinked, and tried starting my speech again.

'It is a great honour to have this opportunity to present our early experiences with clinical heart transplantation to such an illustrious audience and I'd like to thank the American College of Cardiology for inviting me here today.'

It was better, but I was still tense and nervous and the audience could sense it – they were still shuffling, murmuring and coughing.

Then I had an idea – start with something light-hearted – a subject on which I wouldn't have to concentrate, a funny story perhaps?

'A few weeks ago I had a hair-raising experience,' I began.

The audience became much quieter and I was beginning to feel better, the words were flowing more freely and my throat wasn't so dry.

'No, not in the operating room, it was during a lecture in a small village back in South Africa.

'Because of the tremendous demands on my time and requests to lecture every evening in different towns I decided to hire a chauffeur. This luxury would allow me at least to have a rest, or even a snooze, when I was travelling.

'The man I hired as my chauffeur was a typical Afrikaner by the name of Van der Merwe – "Van" for short – and he was very proud of this position. To be appropriately dressed, he bought himself a white coat and white cap.

'Van surprised me because he showed great interest in my work – maybe even more than this audience today', I added for effect and the last of the whispering stopped.

'Every night, when I gave a lecture, he would sit in the back of the hall in his white coat and white cap and listened intently to what I had to say – even though he'd heard it all before.

'While he was driving, he would sometimes ask me questions about my work – how we selected patients for transplantation, when we determined the donor was dead, and he even wanted to know a little bit about the surgical technique – and rejection.'

Now I had their full attention and I was beginning to enjoy myself, which is usually the secret of a good lecture.

'I realized after a few weeks that my chauffeur had learned quite a lot about heart transplantation. One night we were driving to this little town where I was sure they didn't even know what I looked like. I was very tired and wanted to relax.

'I asked him, "Van, do you think you could impersonate me and give the lecture tonight?" Without hesitation he said, "Sure Professor, I've listened to you so many times now – I know your lecture off by heart."

'Okay, that settles it then – we'll stop just outside the town and change clothes. You can put on my Italian suit and I'll put on your white coat and white cap and drive you into town. You can give the lecture and I'll sit at the back of the hall and have a snooze.

'So we did just that – but despite my tiredness I couldn't sleep – I found Van's lecture so interesting that I sat open-mouthed in admiration as I listened to him.

'When he was finished there was tremendous applause and he was asked by the chairman if he would be prepared to answer some questions from the audience – and he immediately agreed.

'He was a little weak on the medical questions but much better on the political questions. Then catastrophe struck.

'A gentleman in the audience stood up. I recognized him even from the back and went cold. It was Michael de Bakey.'

There were peals of laughter from my audience and De Bakey himself was sitting in the front row, also smiling, so I waited a moment before continuing with my story.

'Dr De Bakey must have known there was something on the go and asked Van a very difficult question on the immunological problems.

'Van looked down at his feet and I realized that he didn't know what the hell Dr De Bakey was talking about.

'I was just about to jump up and admit the whole thing to the meeting when Van looked up and smiled. I waited with bated breath to hear what he was going to say.

'He cleared his throat and, pulling himself up to his full height asked, "Excuse me, Sir, but aren't you Dr De Bakey from Houston?" De Bakey acknowledged that he was. "Well Dr De Bakey, I'm surprised that a man with your knowledge and experience could ask such a *stupid* question!"'

The room in the San Francisco Hilton exploded with laughter and I waited until the noise had subsided before finishing my story.

'So Van added, "And to show you just how stupid your question really is, my chauffeur is sitting at the back of the hall and he'll answer it for you."'

It took several minutes for the laughter to die down and I knew then that the rest of the lecture would go well. I just hoped everything was okay upstairs.

I asked for my first slide, the lights were dimmed and the slide listing the three criteria we used to select a patient for cardiac transplantation appeared on the screen. I pointed out that the criteria were:

Extensive, irreversible disease of the heart muscle; the patient must be in total heart failure and must be non-responsive to extensive medical treatment; and the condition must not be amenable to existing surgical procedures.

I also showed how Washkansky and Blaiberg had fulfilled these criteria, by recalling the history of physical findings and special investigations – without the two slides of the haemo-dynamic changes which were still in my bedroom. Briefly, my concentration wavered but I quickly blanked out the thought of what might be waiting for me after the lecture – although I hadn't heard any sirens outside yet.

Next I dealt with the surgical technique and how we had modified it.

My talk passed very rapidly and I didn't want to overstep the time allotted to me – which is another secret of a good lecture; keep it as short as possible.

So I quickly showed the slides which indicated the tests we performed to detect rejection and the slide of the immunosuppressive regime that we had followed.

I ended with a slide of Dr Blaiberg standing next to the washbasin shaving himself and giving the 'V' sign.

'You will all appreciate the significance of this photograph much more than the press have,' I said. 'Before the transplant this man couldn't shave himself because the exertion was just too much and he would quickly run out of breath. So, for my patient – and the cardiac team in Cape Town – this was a major milestone and, in our opinion, proves conclusively that heart transplantation *does* cure because it improves the quality of life of terminally ill patients – which is, I'm sure, the goal of all of us here today. Thank you for your time.' And I sat down.

I walked back to my chair and was thrilled with the standing ovation of about three minutes which followed. It was an extremely high point in my career – the acknowledgement of my peers – it produced a lump in my throat and moist eyes. The lecture had been a greater success than I could ever have wished for. Why couldn't my private life be as successful, I wondered.

The chairman announced that there would be a panel discussion but that, unfortunately, Dr Shumway had sent his apologies and was unable to make it.

I was very disappointed because I was looking forward to seeing Norman. As it turned out we did not speak to each other again until 20 years later at a meeting in Madrid. He didn't even accept my invitation to attend the first ever International Heart Transplant Congress in Cape Town.

He had desperately wanted to be the first to do a transplant and the fact that he wasn't even the first in America was a torment to him, I've since been told.

The situation, based on this professional jealousy, became even more ridiculous when my operating room sister, Miss Rautenbach, visited his unit on a visit to the United States once and his staff didn't want to show her around or extend any of the usual courtesies given to visiting foreign colleagues.

For me, the panel discussion – especially without Dr Shumway – was an anticlimax. One interesting aspect that did, however, emerge was their different approach on the selection of a recipient.

They pointed out that they were afraid of litigation if they selected a patient in total heart failure, took out his heart, and the transplant failed. They thought that the chances of being sued in those circumstances were very real.

To avoid this hazard they had decided they could only risk a transplant in a patient where, after routine heart surgery, the patient's heart did not take over. The choice was then either to switch off the heart-lung machine and let the patient die, or to take out the heart and do a transplant.

It was obvious that an operation could not be planned to coincide with a time when a suitable donor was available as it's impossible to predict in which cases the heart, after surgery, would not take over.

I therefore had the legal system of the United States to thank for the honour of being the first surgeon in the world to have done a heart transplant.

The meeting ended with all the members of the panel agreeing that heart transplantation should be continued.

Now I could get back to my problem with Louwtjie and hurried over to the elevator and went up to the 23rd floor. The door was locked and there were no replies to my pleas to be allowed in. Total, and terrifying, silence.

Jesus! What's happening? I went back down to the lobby again. No, the key had not been left with the concierge but the assistant manager had a pass key and could open the room. So he accompanied me back upstairs.

'Big crowd at your lecture, doctor – how did it go?' He was one of those chatty people.

'Oh, I think it went okay.' I wasn't in the mood for polite conversation. The only concern I had was what I would find behind those locked doors.

'Anything else I can do for you?' the assistant manager asked me as the door swung open.

'No thanks,' I replied, closing the door behind me.

The lounge was empty, and so was the open window. There was water running in the bathroom. My God, she's drowned herself!

I quickly opened the bathroom door – and there was Louwtjie lying with closed eyes in the bath with the water still running. My heart skipped a beat – and then began to race.

'Louwtjie!' I shouted in alarm.

She opened her eyes and I could see that she was calm and had come to terms with the situation. I closed the tap and she was the first to speak. 'What did I do to deserve this, Chris?'

I hesitated for a moment while I racked my brains for the right answer.

'It's not what you've done, Louwtjie. You've been a wonderful *wife* and you've sacrificed a lot to help me get where I am today, but what you have *not* done is you haven't tried to be a companion to me.'

She wanted to interrupt but I stopped her by raising my hand.

'You've been willing to share the bad times with me – why can't you share the good times too? Why must everything always be so miserable, why should we be wary of people – and unfriendly, why can't we just have fun?' I didn't think it was asking, or expecting, too much.

She raised herself out of the bath and I handed her a towel which she wrapped around her waist. 'Does that mean you can go to bed with every woman you meet? Is that the companionship you're missing?'

Louwtjie had always been a good lover. She was the first girl I had ever gone to bed with and I'm sure I was the first man in her life. There was nothing wrong with our sex life.

'No, it isn't that. Sex isn't everything.' Although I knew perfectly well what was driving me into other beds, I wasn't prepared to discuss it at that moment.

'I'll tell you what it is, Chris, you have a huge ego. You've proved to yourself and the rest of the world that there's no operation you cannot perform – now you want to show there's not a woman who won't open her legs for you. But I have news for you,' and she pointed to herself, 'here's one woman who won't satisfy your male ego any more.'

We had been married for 18 years so Louwtjie probably knew me better than anybody else. I just stared at her. So this was it. Was it what I secretly wanted, too?

'Please get out,' she said with a nasty edge to her voice, 'I want to get dressed in private and you can then take me to the dinner.'

I was relieved to get off so lightly, so I went into the lounge to search for the two missing slides.

She closed the door firmly as he left the bathroom and stood with her back against it and looked at herself in the mirror.

A short while ago, all she had wanted to do was kill herself. Now she just felt totally exhausted and wanted to sleep.

Were all men the same? Wasn't there at least one man in the world who could be a faithful and loving husband?

Sighing deeply she pushed herself away from the door and began the process of getting ready for the gala banquet scheduled for that evening.

But the evening was another disastrous event. No one took any notice of her – they only wanted to see, and be seen with, her famous husband – and, to make matters even worse, he was obviously enjoying every second.

He was taken from her side the moment they entered the banqueting hall and she was left in the company of strangers. Within moments she saw him laughing and joking with the VIPs, film stars and comedians at

109

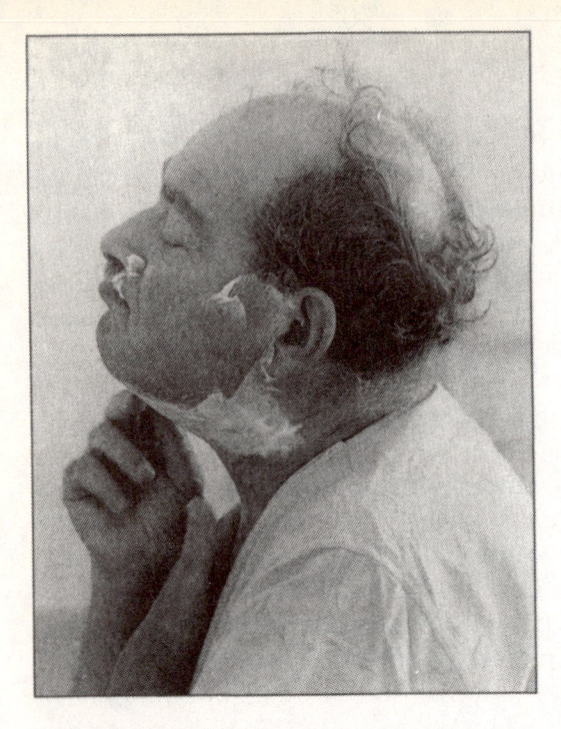

Philip Blaiberg shaving, 43 days after the heart transplant

the main table. Why was everything such a joke? She couldn't see anything funny.

How dare the organizers put her in this position – it was only right that she should have been given a place of honour alongside her famous husband – and, for that matter, why wasn't Chris himself doing something about it?

Even when the dinner and the speeches were over, her own personal anguish hadn't ended. Now there were queues of autograph hunters and photographers surrounding him. She was forgotten.

What about me! She'd wanted to scream.

Quietly she left the room, collected her room key, and went back to the room where, emotionally drained and unable to stay awake, she fell into a deep but troubled sleep.

3

As the plane landed and taxied towards the terminal building my thoughts went back to the 28th December 1955 when I first arrived in Minneapolis in sub-zero temperatures from the hot South African summer.

I'd never seen snow before, except on mountain peaks at a distance and couldn't make out what these walls of white stuff were on both sides of the runway. But when the door of the plane opened a blast of cold air soaked my clothes right through to the skin – as I had no overcoat in those days. 'We must be near the North Pole!' I shivered uncontrollably.

There was no one to meet me then – but I had the telephone number of a Mrs McKinley – and I phoned her after finding out what the instructions on the telephone meant by a 'nickel' and a 'dime'. She had a room for me and I stayed with her on the east side of the Mississippi River until Louwtjie, André and Deirdre arrived four months later.

Those were four months of the most unbearable loneliness I've ever endured. I usually stayed in the laboratory after the day's work until nearly midnight, just for the company of the people who came to clean it.

How different twelve years later!

There was a big, excited, crowd outside on the concourse and Professor Wangensteen – my old chief – and his wife Sally, were there too. Louwtjie and I were going to stay with them at their home.

The next day I went to the hospital where it had all started. It seemed like only yesterday that I'd first walked into the University of Minnesota Hospital on that bitterly cold December morning.

In this building, where I studied for two years, the foundation for the first human heart transplant had been laid. Now I had come back – for the first time since 1958 – to say 'thank you' and to share the victory of surgery over death.

There was hardly a corridor or a room that didn't hold memories for me – good ones and bad. I walked around a corner and there was the office of the hospital administrator who had reported me to the security staff for stealing a fan.

What happened is that we'd invited Professor Wangensteen and his wife to have dinner with us at our home. As it was a very humid, hot evening and I didn't have air conditioning, I asked Dr Perry, the chief resident in the lab, if I could borrow a fan for the occasion. He gave me permission so, that afternoon when I left hospital, I walked openly (with the fan in my hand) through the hospital, past the woman in the administrator's office, to the car park.

The next morning – thank God – I returned it because a few days later there was a phone call from hospital security.

'Hi, is that Dr Barnard?' a polite, but officious voice asked.

'Yes.'

'This is Security,' and the voice paused momentarily – probably to get the full effect – then added, 'Have you ever stolen anything?'

For a moment I was dumbstruck and then immediately realized what he meant. 'Are you referring to a fan?'

'Yes, Dr Barnard, the administrator's secretary reported it.'

He didn't sound very upset or too concerned, but I was shaking with anger. That bitch! 'I'll be with you in a minute,' I snapped.

I ran out of the laboratory, down the corridor and up the stairs four steps at a time, to the hospital security office. I didn't bother to knock and marched straight into the room.

'Sir, I'm here due to the generosity of this hospital,' I began, 'and I consider myself very, very fortunate to have been given the opportunity to study here. Do you think I would screw up everything for the sake of a miserable fan?'

The officer could see I was extremely upset and he shifted uncomfortably in his chair. 'Doctor, I'm only doing my duty. The secretary says she saw you taking an electric fan out of the hospital a fan belonging to the hospital.'

'But why didn't she call me and ask me what I was doing with it? Why did she have to report me to you? Now I'm on your records as a suspected thief!' I shouted.

After I'd calmed down I carefully explained what had actually happened. He listened carefully and, with a smile, he looked up and said, 'Okay Dr Barnard, your name won't appear on my records, there's obviously been a misunderstanding.'

I smiled myself now, as I recalled the incident – which had seemed so monumentally important at the time.

But, despite re-living the memories, I felt rather sad because there didn't seem to be much enthusiasm among my friends as I related my experiences with the first two transplants. They didn't appear to be interested and I thought I could even detect a little resentment.

My mood darkened even further as I strolled through the hospital after my lecture. The excitement of eight years ago was gone – so were many of the old, familiar, faces. I sadly remembered and murmured some lines of Wordsworth I remembered from my school days:

'Whither is fled the visionary gleam?
Where is it now, the glory and the dream?'

I was probably wrong to expect a sort of hero's welcome. To them I was still just the doctor from Africa, sitting alone in the lab at night.

Professor Wangensteen caught up with me. There had just been a message that the two of us were requested to give evidence at the sitting of a Senate Committee hearing, which was investigating the legal, moral, ethical and financial implications of heart transplantation.

His excitement was contagious and it lifted my mood very quickly. Even after all this time he was still a man who motivated me easily.

The next morning we left for Washington.

Since the drama in San Francisco, Louwtjie and I had been living like strangers – although we shared the same bed we were husband and wife in name only. I was sure that Professor Wangensteen and his wife noticed this strained relationship. I was quite a good actor but found it increasingly difficult to put on a bright front when it was so gloomy in my bedroom.

When we left I, again, reflected on how different it was from 1958 when I'd returned to Cape Town. Then I had to tear myself away from a girl I had fallen in love with. As a married man, I should have known better – but Sharon had been so close to me for more than a year and, when I told her I had to leave, she plead-

113

ed with tears in her big blue eyes for me not to go back to my wife and children.

I was an unfaithful bastard even then – so the 'fame' had changed me very little – it had just made it easier.

But, with a heavy heart, my deep sense of responsibility tore me away from her at that time. Away from the many dreams we'd had. The song, 'Memories are made of this' by Dean Martin, that we danced to – on those Saturday evenings when I could afford to take her out – haunted me now as I boarded the plane for Washington.

My evidence at the hearing turned into quite a lively discussion between the chairman, Mr Walter Mondale, and me. He seemed determined to give the medical profession in America a hard time and I was honoured that they'd asked for my opinion and suggestions.

Mondale's main concern was that in heart transplantation there were too many important considerations – and for that reason he believed he couldn't leave such decisions to the members of the medical profession to make independently.

I never quite understood who *else* should be considered to carry this responsibility. I certainly hoped it wouldn't be the politicians because their only concern would be the number of votes they could gain. High public interest in operations such as heart transplants was guaranteed to get good media exposure.

My standpoint was quite simple. Doctors are the only people capable of controlling procedures such as transplantation – just because the heart transplant had created such widespread interest was no reason to interfere with the systems already in place.

My argument was that the members of the medical profession were the *only* people trained and qualified to take the decisions required to select a patient, declare a patient dead – and also to do the operation. It definitely could *not* be a politician or, even worse, a committee of politicians – which would be unthinkable.

I cited the example of what would happen if a passenger plane developed mechanical trouble and the pilot had to make a forced landing. No one would expect him to ask the opinions of the passengers – or for their permission either. He, and he alone, was qualified to take the necessary steps because he was trained for it.

These arguments went backwards and forwards without any of us conceding any ground.

Mondale then decided to take a different approach and asked, 'Dr Barnard, who *pays* for these operations?'

This appeared to me to be totally irrelevant as I had never been in private practice, had never sent an account to a patient and was, at that time, earning the equivalent of $600 a month but I knew, instinctively, where this line of questioning was leading.

'I don't know who pays in this country but, in South Africa, these operations are only performed in provincial hospitals which are heavily subsidized by the government.'

I saw him smile shrewdly – as if he was thinking Aha! I've cornered this cunning little doctor! And, placing his fingertips together in steeple-like fashion he said triumphantly, 'So, Dr Barnard, the taxpayers foot the bill? If so, don't you think it's right that they should have some say in the matter?'

There were uncomfortable murmurs behind me but I knew that I now had Mr Mondale.

I met his gaze steadily and, being careful to speak slowly and in measured tones I asked, 'Sir, you are, at the moment, fighting a war in Vietnam? And who pays for that incredible waste of money? The taxpayers – am I correct?'

He still didn't see what I was driving at. 'Yes, that's correct,' he replied, still smiling craftily over his fingertips.

'Then tell me, Mr Mondale, every time the generals want to launch an attack do they first ask the taxpayers about the tactics and the weapons they should use?'

The press gallery burst out laughing and Walter Mondale looked around and, after the noise had subsided, sheepishly answered 'That is a good answer – no further questions, Dr Barnard – you may go.'

Professor Wangensteen slapped my back heartily and congratulated me on my performance, as we said goodbye to each other.

I never saw my old friend and master again. He died of a heart attack a few years later and I was told by his wife that his last words were, 'Where is Chris?'

Back in Cape Town, I called a meeting with the hospital authorities and told them that Bossie – who was the doctor supervising Philip Blaiberg's post-operative care – and I both agreed that there was no reason to keep our patient in hospital any longer and that we decided to discharge him on Saturday, 16 March 1968.

He was, at that stage, the only surviving heart transplant patient and would be the first to be discharged and go home to live a normal life.

'This news has to be kept totally confidential' I emphasized. 'I don't want any more accusations that we're after publicity – so I suggest that arrangements are made to increase security at the hospital exit. We'll also need to organize some kind of security at Blaiberg's home – otherwise his life will not only be made miserable by the press but they'll also expose him to a lot of bacteria.'

I also discussed these arrangements with Eileen Blaiberg. 'Tell absolutely no one – not your friends, not even your daughter – rather surprise everyone. It's critical that no one knows the date.'

She did exactly that and mentioned the date to no one. But the media guessed shrewdly that his discharge date must be close.

'My friends, the newspapers and television networks all over the world are phoning me day and night demanding to know when Phil will be coming home,' she complained.

'*And* they want to take pictures of the chair he's going to sit in *and* the bed he's going to sleep in – they'll drive me crazy!'

'Ignore them. Smile, and tell them you know as much as they do – probably less' I said, trying to give her some advice based on my own experiences with the media.

She agreed that this was the best plan and I told her to bring some clothes for him on the Friday afternoon.

And so, the day before we were to let Philip Blaiberg go home his wife arrived at Groote Schuur carrying a parcel for her husband who she'd thought would never leave hospital again – except perhaps in a coffin.

So the moment had finally arrived! Phil was coming home.

Dr Barnard had told her to bring some clothes for her husband to wear when being discharged.

With trembling fingers she packed an overnight bag with his Royal Dental Hospital blazer, shirt, slacks, shoes – and his favourite cravat. She still couldn't believe he was coming home – and yet, after all the trauma and tears, here she was actually packing for his return.

Katie, their maid, was furiously shining all the tables until they gleamed – everything had to be perfect, and perfectly clean, for Philip Blaiberg's homecoming.

When she arrived at the hospital she was sure there were more press men than normal – and, as usual, they asked her when the world's most famous patient was being released.

She wasn't a good fibber but said she really didn't know.
'What's in the bag, Mrs Blaiberg?' asked one astute reporter.
'Oh, it's just some clothes for Phil.' Which, of course, was the only confirming clue they needed.

Within hours media teams from all over the world arrived at the 'Big Barn' Hospital – Groote Schuur.

Later, she left her husband sleeping soundly – smiling as he snored gently into his last night in hospital.

Without hospital staff to look after her, Eileen – unlike her husband in hospital, managed only to get an hour or two's sleep – the telephone rang incessantly with calls from newspapers and television crews wanting the exact time of her husband's departure – she considered leaving it off the hook, but what if there was an emergency call from the hospital?

She kept up the 'top secret' pretence but she knew perfectly well that they all knew it would be the next day.

Her concern was more for her husband than for herself – after all, she'd run the gauntlet of newsmen so many times she hardly even noticed them now – but Phil was another matter altogether. Would his new heart cope with the strain and excitement? Will his new heart cope with me? she asked herself silently.

I walked down the tunnel from the old part of the building to the ear, nose and throat outpatients' department where our new transplant suite was situated. This was the same route that Washkansky's body had travelled to the waiting ambulance and the morgue. Now I was walking to the ward of a patient who was enjoying a new life with his transplanted heart, ready to be discharged from hospital.

The world was also waiting to see this man alive, with another person's heart beating inside his chest. They wanted to see whether he could walk out of the hospital as a fit man – or whether he would go out in a wheel chair as an invalid.

The question was what would his life be like. Would he be bedridden or would he be able to enjoy the things that everybody else can enjoy like walking on the glorious white beaches of Cape Town – along the Indian and Atlantic coastlines?

In the post-operative period, Louis Washkansky had been nursed in a single room on the same floor as the other patients who had undergone open-heart surgery. Opposite his door, the corridor used to be screened off for an area where the staff could wash and dress before entering his room. This arrangement was necessary to provide the precautions which would make cross-infection very unlikely.

For Dr Blaiberg the hospital authorities had, with unusual speed, transformed three rooms of the ENT outpatients' department into a transplant suite. It amazed me to notice how money was now rapidly available to proceed with the transplant programme. Where, before, it took months or even years to get new equipment, now I only had to make a casual suggestion and it was done.

I'm sure that if I'd requested Dom Perignon champagne and Beluga caviar for breakfast it would have been served the next morning.

I entered the 'dirty area' of the suite. The office was empty but I could hear laughter coming from Blaiberg's room, so I went into the change room, put on a scrub suit, overshoes, cap and mask and after scrubbing my hands, entered the 'clean' area.

Dr Blaiberg was out of bed, sitting in a chair with Sister De Villiers on his left and Sister Lindsay on his right. They both had their arms around him and hadn't heard me. The patient's face had become much rounder from the steroids – what we refer to as a 'moon face' – but he was otherwise the picture of health.

'So, are the two of you trying to get off with a married man?'

Both sisters jumped to their feet. 'Hello, Prof!' they said in unison.

'I'm glad you're back,' said Philip Blaiberg as he got out of his chair. 'There are a few things I want to ask you. First, when do I get out of this jail? Second, can I have sex?'

The two sisters screamed with laughter. This must have been the topic of their discussion before I'd arrived.

'The answer to your first question is tomorrow.'

'You see! I told you so – you've lost your bet!' Sister De Villiers interjected excitedly.

'And to the second question, of course you can make love – but you have to promise me that you won't put your heart into it.' I tried hard to look serious but we all burst out laughing.

'Now that we've sorted out your sex life let's see how your heart is doing,' I said, walking to the big chart pinned on the door. This showed his vital signs, lab results, electrocardiogram voltage and treatment from the time of the operation. I studied it for a few minutes, and the only aspect that worried me was that the ECG voltage remained low but there had been no change for the last four weeks.

'I see Bossie has reduced the cortisone to 30 milligrams a day,' I remarked, walking back to Dr Blaiberg. 'Can you get on the bed so I can listen to your heart?'

The two sisters helped him take off his gown and he jumped on the bed and lay back.

The wound had healed with no evidence of infection, the sternum was stable. All heart-sounds were clear with no evidence of systolic murmur.

I slipped the stethoscope out of my ears. 'Everything seems in order to me, Philip, but I'd like Professor Schrire to give the final okay.

'Tomorrow you will mix with the world again so I don't see the need for this anymore,' and took off my mask. 'The sisters can also show their faces to you so you can see who's been bullying you around for the past six weeks.'

Sister De Villiers and Sister Lindsay slowly took off their masks – and Dr Blaiberg watched this performance almost as a voyeur would watch a strip-tease artist. He'd never seen the faces of the nurses before, of course, and was smiling broadly in anticipation.

'My God, but you're beautiful!' Blaiberg exclaimed 'I don't think I want to go home any more!'

'Come on, your wife is much more beautiful,' they said, as I started to leave the room.

'Okay, see you tomorrow morning,' and I left the ward.

Sister De Villiers followed me to the office. 'We've missed you, Prof,' she remarked, looking into my eyes.

I knew what she meant. 'Well, I'm back now and we'll make up for it.' I moved closer to the long, slender, body and she opened her arms just as Dr Bosman walked into the office.

I spun around. 'You've done a good job Bossie, and I'm proud of the whole team' I said, recovering my composure quickly and trying to act as nonchalantly as I could.

'Thanks, Prof – do you think Philip can be discharged tomorrow?'

'Yes – but I'd like Vel to see him first.'

Bossie looked uncomfortable.

'I called him but he said the cardiologists didn't want to be further involved with the post-operative care of transplant patients. They have enough work to do.'

I had a notion things were going awry between Vel and myself. What a great pity. The success that the unit had since it started with open heart surgery in 1958 was due to the close cooperation between the cardiologists and the surgeons – but Vel had been my teacher and friend long before that – when I was preparing to write the M Med and MD degrees. Vel taught me cardiology – he was the best cardiologist I ever knew and also one of my best friends.

What was going on now? I knew that some of my colleagues were accusing me of stealing all the limelight – but surely not Vel? I had to go and speak to him.

'Well, Bossie, if that's the case we'll just have to look after the transplant patients ourselves. I want Dr Blaiberg to come back and see us once a week and he mustn't hesitate to phone us if something is worrying him. I'm going to change now and will be in my office for the next few hours if you need me.'

Bossie walked with me to the change room. 'If it's okay with you, Prof, I will see Dr Blaiberg every day at his house.'

'Of course Bossie – I don't mind.'

The nurses had already told me that Bossie Bosman had virtually adopted Dr Blaiberg and they'd become very close friends.

Back in my office, it was the usual shambles – hundreds of letters and invitations. Anne Levett hadn't been able to cope on her own so the provincial administration had seconded one of their secretaries, a Mr Stoffberg, just to take care of the invitations.

He was sitting at my desk as I entered.

'Morning, Stoffie, what's happening?'

He got up from the chair and pointed to the stacks of letters on the floor. 'Prof, I really don't know where to start – there are invitations and letters from all over the world.

'The city council has also decided to give you the Freedom of the City of Cape Town and the government has just told me that you've been awarded their highest honour – the Hendrik Verwoerd Medal.'

'Is that such an honour, Stoffie?'

'Well, only two people have been awarded it before you – there's also a fairly big cash award with it too – I think you should accept.'

But I still had my doubts. Dr Verwoerd, the previous prime minister, who had been stabbed to death in parliament, was the architect of apartheid that had caused so much misery to so many people.

As the son of a missionary who had seen the suffering of his coloured congregation under this inexplicable ideology, I felt uneasy about accepting a prize given under Verwoerd's name.

'Okay Stoffie, let me think about it.'

'There's also an invitation from Prince Rainier and Princess Grace to attend the Red Cross Ball in Monaco as their guest of honour.'

I turned around to face Stoffie. He had a twinkle in his eye and was smiling broadly.

'Are you serious?' I asked incredulously.

'Yes Prof, and I've already accepted – I hope you don't mind.'

'Hell no – that's fabulous!' I looked at my watch. 'Sorry, but I've got to run – Deirdre's arriving back from Australia this afternoon and I'd like to meet her at the airport.'

Stoffie was obviously disappointed that I had decided to leave so quickly but I had to get to the airport.

Deirdre and I had been very close over the past five years – in fact, until the transplant, I had focused most of my attention on her. Her achievements in water-skiing were major highlights in my life. She was not only my daughter but also my companion. Now she was coming back from Australia after having won the 'Moomba' and 'Australian Open' and I wanted to be at the airport to meet her.

My son, André (or 'Boetie' as we called him) was at school in Pretoria and was living with Martin and Kitty Franzot.

Martin was a patient of mine and I had already performed a mitral valve replacement and then, later, three by-passes on him. He had become like a second father to 'Boetie'; maybe he'd noticed the father neglecting his only son?

Driving to Zeekoevlei my thoughts kept wandering from those days of bliss with Deirdre gliding gracefully and expertly through the slalom course when the 'vlei' (lake) was smooth – to the Royal invitation. I wondered whether I would be able to dance with Grace Kelly. What would it be like to hold that beautiful woman in my arms? Would I have to bow?

The luxury of these thoughts was halted abruptly when I arrived at my house next to the lake – I couldn't call it 'home' any more. It had become a place where I ate and slept, especially now that I had no time to watch Deirdre on the water.

Louwtjie had become increasingly quiet and morose. Nothing made her smile or laugh. She was in the kitchen and had a blank look on her face, which was probably due to the Valium she was taking to help her cope.

'Blaiberg will be discharged tomorrow – what do you think of that? The first patient with a transplanted heart to leave hospital!'

'That's good.' But there was not a hint of enthusiasm in the monotone response. Then silence.

'Do you think, in your busy schedule, you can find time to go and see your mother again? You haven't been to see her since you've become famous,' she said wearily, busying herself at the sink.

The sarcasm made the truth even more painful. I had not been to see my mother at the old-age home for months. I wondered if she was even aware of the events of the past few weeks. Did she know her son had become a celebrity?

It was now six years since she'd suffered a massive brain haemorrhage but Maria Elizabeth Barnard's strong determination to survive had pulled her out of the coma – only to become a burden to her four sons.

She was virtually paralyzed on the right side and doomed for the rest of her life – or, rather, the rest of her 'existence' – to the bed and the wheel chair.

At the beginning, she was determined to get well and often, when I went to visit her, she would painfully massage her right hand – trying to bring life back into it – but the hand which had darned the socks of her sons and cooked the delicious bean soup for her family refused to obey the commands of her brain. Now she was a lonely old woman in an old-age home. Her life was brightened only by the infrequent visits of one of her sons.

Johannes, her eldest son, who actually lived in Cape Town, saw her maybe once a year. Dodsley, the second eldest, who lived in Vryburg (a small town in the far northern Cape over 1 000 kilometres from Cape Town) visited her once in the six years of her illness.

Marius and I saw her more frequently – but certainly not as often as she would have visited us had the circumstances been reversed.

This was the gratitude shown by her four sons for whom she had sacrificed her whole life. I think she had sensed she'd become a burden because she often asked me, 'When is God going to come and take me away?'

The plane arrived on schedule and Deirdre came running into

the reception hall with a big, cuddly, koala bear in her arms. She talked about everything except her achievements. I wanted to know about the competitions and how well she had done, but Deirdre only told us how wonderful Australia was and about the fascinating people she'd met there.

After collecting her skis and luggage she and Louwtjie left for Zeekoevlei in Louwtjie's car and I set off to see my mother in the old-age home.

All the residents were sitting on the stoep like little dassies (a South African wild rock-rabbit), dumped there by their loved ones on the pretext that they would enjoy it more than at home because they would be among people with whom they could identify. This is the most common explanation given to assuage the feelings of guilt in children. I know, because I gave my mother that same sweet talk.

As I arrived they all looked up and started clapping their hands – some because they recognized me and had heard about the transplant; others clapped simply to join in with everyone else.

My poor mother was bewildered because she didn't know what it was all about. She didn't know that her son had become one of the most famous doctors in the world.

She looked at me with an enquiring expression on her face. At the age of 85 she had hardly any recall. I sat down beside her and kissed her lightly on the cheek.

She smelt awful and her left hand was covered in faeces. She had become pathologically obsessed about her bowel actions and often scratched out the faecal matter with the finger-nails of her left hand.

I asked a nurse to bring a wet towel and cleaned her hand. Then I told her the story about the first heart transplant – and why her companions had cheered.

I don't think she grasped the significance or the importance of the events and immediately changed the subject to her own problems; the constipation and the burning sensation in her bladder when passing urine.

I looked at my watch every few minutes, to see if I had spent enough time visiting her and left as soon as I decently could.

I woke up uncomfortably on what was to be my day of triumph – a day of celebration for the first surgeon to be successful with a heart transplant and send his patient home from hospital.

But I felt miserable. Every movement was painful, from a flare-up in the arthritis – and I'd spent a miserable night trying to calm Louwtjie.

She was like an animal caged in her own insecurity and uncertainty. She considered me to be the only obstacle between her and happiness. Although I was desperately tired she gave me little chance to rest. She'd scared me half to death when, in the middle of the night, she'd clenched her hands tightly around my throat and screamed crazily. I'd woken immediately – only to look straight into her wild eyes.

Eventually I went to lie on the couch in the lounge. Fortunately I didn't have to operate that day.

I arrived in Philip Blaiberg's sterile suite as Eileen was being briefed on the finer details of home-care and medication procedure. She was obviously nervous – and shaking so much with excitement that I don't think she understood half of the instructions being given her by the nurses and Bossie Bosman.

My patient, in the meantime, was getting dressed – very jolly and cracking jokes with everyone.

And then Eileen walked into the sterile suite, for the first time in ten weeks not wearing her mask, took one look at her husband, and promptly burst into tears.

They clung to each other and I watched a couple – married to each other for a lifetime and still so much in love – blessed with, at least, *some* quality time together again.

How long they had didn't matter at that stage – the moment was enough. I felt pangs of jealousy that two people could be so emotionally close to each other.

After a flurry of awkward congratulations and good-luck wishes an orderly arrived with a wheel chair. Much against Philip's will, we insisted he sit in it and be pushed out of the hospital. I've often thought it was a ridiculous hospital rule – but it was taken very seriously – something to do with insurance I think.

But before he left, Bossie wanted to do one final electrocardiograph and, while the wheel chair waited, Sister Lindsay positioned the electrodes and the reading was taken.

'Perfectly normal,' Bossie announced with his schoolboy grin.

Then, 74 days after his world-famous operation Dr Philip Blaiberg was wheeled to the entrance of the hospital – accompanied by Sisters Lindsay and De Villiers and many others closely involved in his recovery – every one of them his friend – in fact I'd never seen a more popular patient.

The exit from the outpatients' block was surrounded by hundreds of people – television crews, photographers and journalists from every part of the globe.

I slipped past without being noticed and bumped into Don Mackenzie who had just taken a few final pictures of Philip Blaiberg getting ready to go home. He told me that the French singing star, Françoise Hardy, was waiting in the crowd to see Blaiberg leave and that she also wanted to meet me.

She had been booked to make three appearances in the Alhambra theatre in Cape Town for one day – the very day on which Philip Blaiberg was being discharged.

I watched as she walked towards me, and then we were face to face. She looked at me with those beautiful sloe eyes.

'Allo, Monsieur Barnard – excuse – Dr Barnard?'

'Hello,' I replied and, as she held my gaze for just a fraction longer than necessary, I suggested we watched the historic occasion together from a different angle.

So, we stood some distance away, and watched the seething mass of reporters and photographers descend on Philip Blaiberg. The car park was packed to total capacity with people – thousands upon thousands of journalists, hospital workers and well-wishers.

When he walked out of the main door the entire crowd erupted into one enormous roar – so loud that any soccer supporters' club would have been proud.

'I leave tonight – maybe you will phone me in Paris?' she suggested.

I told her I would definitely see her again – maybe that very evening – as I had tickets for her show.

When he reached the giant hospital doors, Philip Blaiberg decided he'd had enough of the wheel chair. Jumping up, he said to the group around him 'Look, there are hundreds of press and television teams waiting outside, as well as the public, who've been waiting for hours. They don't want to see an invalid so take this contraption away!'

He had no intention of allowing the world to see Barnard's patient leave the hospital in a wheel chair – he lifted himself out of the chair and walked steadily towards the door.

Outside, a feeling of elation swept over him as he faced a world that had expected him to die.

'I'm in the air and sunshine again!' He shouted and waved to the thousands of people gathered in the car park.

A young reporter grinned and called 'Hey Doc! What's it like to breathe contaminated air again?'

Blaiberg looked amazed for a moment. 'Contaminated?' Contaminated? This is heavenly!'

After final hugs with his two nurses and hand-shakes with hospital staff, he climbed into the waiting car with his wife.

Slowly, the big shiny Mercedes pulled out of the hospital grounds and along the freeway to the suburb where Dr and Mrs Blaiberg had an apartment – in a block called Highbury, which overlooked the beautiful Constantia valley long renowned for its fine wines, Napoleon himself having requested one last bottle before he died.

Philip Blaiberg couldn't wait to be home again to drink in the view once more – maybe even stroll around the vineyards?

When they arrived there were still more crowds, more reporters and photographers; he didn't mind.

I'm alive – really alive again he kept repeating over and over in his mind, as he was helped to flat 204 at the end of the corridor.

After all the excitement, their visitors left – leaving Philip and Eileen Blaiberg alone – in their own home again.

'You've got to be feeling tired by now Phil,' she said.

'A bit – but very excited – did you see all those people?'

'Yes,' she replied, 'I think I saw them – but I was really watching you!'

'Where was Professor Barnard? I don't think I said goodbye to him properly – today was more of a triumph for him than for me after all.'

'You got well again – I think that's all he wants – and you'll be seeing him again any way.'

'You know, Eileen, everyone reckons I was the brave one – but I wasn't really. I had no choice. I was dying. It was he who had the courage to transplant a new heart in me after Louis Washkansky died.

'They're making such a fuss of me and I can't help feeling a bit of a fraud. This is really Chris Barnard's day.'

He stretched out on his bed, feeling deliciously tired.

'Eileen,' he said. 'The world is marvellous. Just bloody marvellous.' And he fell asleep.

After waving goodbye to Philip Blaiberg, I went back to my office to meet Stoffie who had been busy arranging my next month's travel programme.

First to Rio where I was to be the guest of the Gama Filho University and receive an honorary doctorate, and then to Buenos Aires for an award from the Argentinian government. Then back to Cape Town for a week before Louwtjie and I would leave for Spain and France.

Before Stoffie had finished explaining the details, Ann Levett buzzed through on the intercom to tell me that a very sick patient had arrived from Romania and that the cardiac unit wanted me urgently. I ran down the corridors and up the stairs four at a time, white coat tails flapping behind me. I seldom used the lifts because I'm impatient to get where I'm going and they are interminably slow.

Marius was waiting for me in C2.

'What's the problem?' I asked, catching my breath.

'It's hard to tell actually. A distraught woman arrived here not long ago with her son. She can't speak English and I can't find anybody who can speak Romanian – the kid's very sick, though.'

We entered the single-bed ward. The boy was about 13 years old and as blue as a plum – even though he was breathing oxygen from a mask over his nose and mouth.

His mother looked up sharply at us. She was rubbing her son's feet in a vain attempt to improve his circulation and I could see the terror and deep concern in her eyes.

'It must have been a long journey,' Marius explained. 'When he arrived Vel Schrire insisted he be catheterized immediately, as there was little time to waste, in his opinion.'

As often happens with these blue children, his condition deteriorated further after our investigations. I smiled at the boy and felt his pulse. It was rapid and hardly palpable.

'What did they find?'

'They couldn't do a full study but Vel is sure it's a tetralogy.'

The mother suddenly seemed to recognize me and, grabbing hold of both my hands, began kissing them. Although I couldn't understand a word of what she was saying I knew exactly what she meant. She was wearing a simple, shapeless, black dress and had the hands of a hard-working woman – I couldn't even guess at how she had managed to get this far in her last-effort bid to preserve the life of her son.

The boy opened his eyes and gave a weak smile.

'She probably thinks you can perform miracles, Chris, so we'd better get going – I don't think this boy will live much longer. I've already organized the theatre and alerted Ozzie and the heart-lung technicians.'

There would be no Françoise Hardy concert for me that night.

Cardiac teams are used to working quickly and in emergency conditions so it was only a matter of minutes before the boy was prepped and being trundled towards the theatre – where we were already waiting.

The operation went off without a hitch and turned out to be a very straightforward and standard correction. All I had to do was patch the hole between the two ventricles (the lower chambers of the heart) and cut out the muscular and fibrous tissue that obstructed the free flow of blood into the lung.

'That was lucky,' said Marius when the operation was over. 'He should be okay now – his mother got her miracle.'

'Thank God we do get lucky sometimes,' I said, wearily taking off my gloves, 'but I wonder why she had to come all the way here – there must be dozens of clinics in Europe who could have done the same thing.'

Suddenly feeling exhausted, I added, 'Would you mind taking him back to the ward? I didn't get much sleep last night.'

My brother looked at me and nodded – I knew he understood.

The next morning Sister Geyer was in the office when I arrived for the ward round. She was a caring, motherly person, with kind twinkling eyes and rosy cheeks – the type of person you would want to tuck you up in bed all snug and warm – and she was one of the best nurses I've ever worked with.

Her patients came first and many times I'd seen her bustling around in the ward several hours after she was supposed to have finished duty. She always pretended to be strict and professional but, deep in her heart, I think she had a soft spot for me.

'How's last night's patient, Sister?'

She smiled. 'Good *morning*, Professor.'

I ignored the gentle reprimand for not going through the customary greetings. 'Have you managed to find someone who can speak Romanian?'

She walked passed me into the corridor. 'Yes, Dr Marius is with him in the ward.' And we walked briskly down the hall together.

I couldn't believe my eyes when we arrived in the ward. The boy who had been blue and dying only 12 hours before was now sitting up in bed – a healthy pink colour – and chatting animatedly with the interpreter.

As I walked in all the jabbering stopped and everyone turned their heads to the door. The mother fell on her knees as if God had entered. She clutched both her hands together over her heart, whispering a prayer as she stared at me adoringly with tears spilling onto her cheeks. I didn't know how to handle this embarrassing situation.

'Never mind, Chris, I had the same reception,' Marius said.

'But she has the most amazing story – the *sacrifices* this mother made for her son would make even the hospital superintendent weep!'

The miracle we'd joked about the day before certainly had happened – but it was the mother who'd made it happen – not really us.

It made me very heartsore because I could see my own mother sitting alone in a wheel chair on the stoep of the old-age home – maybe she was also thinking about the sacrifices she'd made for her own children?

Marius told me the story he'd heard from the interpreter.

Horia was born blue and, from birth, had been slow to develop physically although he was very bright. He was unable to play with his friends and his mother had devoted her entire life to him. She took him to the clinic in Romania but they all told her that nothing could be done for her son.

She then started saving money by doing extra work and, as soon as she had enough, she began taking him to other centres outside Romania. First to Germany, then to France, then to Russia, then to Poland. But she was always told the same sad news. Nothing could be done and her son would soon die. Still she refused to give up – mothers all over the world seem to have this tenacity about their children.

Then she heard the news about the heart transplant and was determined to bring her son to Cape Town. When she told the Romanian doctors of her decision, they told her it would be better to take him to England or France or Germany, because it would be less expensive to bring the body back after the operation – but she was not deterred by their blunt fatalism and was adamant that she would get Horia to South Africa and the Groote Schuur cardiac unit.

At that stage Romania was under communist rule and had no

diplomatic ties with South Africa. But she even overcame these hurdles and arrived in Johannesburg, flying via Frankfurt, without a visa or money. Just a note in English, 'For Dr Barnard.'

The immigration authorities cut through all the red tape and South African Airways decided to fly her to Cape Town without a ticket.

At Cape Town airport she was met by an ambulance that brought her and her son to Groote Schuur – where we took over.

Horia made an uneventful recovery and returned to Romania. Despite the communist-controlled press, he made headline news and from then on, we had a steady flow of Romanians coming to South Africa without visas or money. All of them received the same hospitality and treatment as South African citizens did and the operations were free. There were some weeks when I had more Romanians in my ward than South Africans.

Our unit built up a close relationship with the Romanian doctors and Marius went there twice with members of our team to help them start their own cardiac surgery unit.

Although I had travelled quite extensively I'd never been invited to any of the South American countries. This would be my first visit to Brazil. I'd heard and read so much about the Carnival and the beautiful hot-blooded mulatto women so it was with great anticipation that I stepped out of the South African Airways jet at Rio de Janeiro.

I was certainly not disappointed because, once I had passed through passport control and customs, it was exactly like the pictures I'd seen of the carnivals.

Outside the airport building there was a mass of colourfully dressed men and women singing and dancing to the rhythm of the samba bands – what a welcome! To me this didn't look like a country being run by an army which had seized power only four years earlier.

I was sure that my first visit to South America was going to be an exciting one and I was determined to have a good time.

The flight was a good start in itself. It was an eight-hour journey from Cape Town to Rio – but due to flying west the flight gained time. We took off at 5 pm and landed at 7 pm – it was the 'happy hour' all the way!

Although my invitation to Rio was from the Gama Filho

University, the minister of health was also at the airport to welcome me on behalf of the government of Brazil.

I really appreciated this gesture very much because, at that time, South Africa was being ostracized and isolated by most of the world for its racial policies and, as a South African, I was often snubbed or ignored by the politicians of the countries I visited.

In fact, the only press coverage my country was getting at that time was about Gary Player, me and apartheid. Gary Player, with his squeaky-clean and irreproachable lifestyle was getting 100% 'good' coverage. I was 50/50 good and bad (with no half-measures). Apartheid was justifiably 100% 'bad'.

Invariably the bad news makes bigger headlines – so South Africa continued to be the permanent whipping-boy of the world press.

I had many engagements – the most important being conferred with the honorary degree of Doctor of Science at the Gama Filho University, being made an honorary member of the Brazilian College of Surgeons, being given honorary membership of the research centre of Lagoa State Hospital, honorary citizenship of the state of Guanabara and the freedom of the city of São Paolo.

There were also engagements which were less glamorous – but more enjoyable. For the first time, on one of these trips, my security was in the hands of five plain-clothed and well-armed bodyguards. I felt rather foolish with these men around me wherever I went but, they also had their uses. When we went to night clubs, for example, they would ensure I had the most beautiful company – often for the whole night. Many of these girls were of heroic proportions and I really discovered the meaning of the word 'passion' in Rio.

It was an unbelievable experience for a barefoot Karoo boy – the son of a missionary – suddenly able to get virtually any girl he wanted. Many made written offers, like the letter I found recently in an old file: '...I am 19 years old with blue eyes and was a "Miss Brazil" finalist last year. I know you are busy but I would like to meet you. Maybe one night you will call me and I come to your hotel for some time and some fun?'

I have few regrets about what I've done in my life – and mostly, I only regret the things I *haven't* done. There were so many opportunities I didn't make use of – or simply didn't have the time for – but one man can only do so much. I can't even remember if I saw the Brazilian beauty queen or not.

The next stop was Argentina. In Buenos Aires I had no bodyguards – at least, none that I was aware of – and definitely no fun. After Rio, it was a boring experience.

The engagements were all very official and serious. I was told by the president of the Argentinian Medical Association that they were going to nominate me for the Nobel Prize, but I didn't take it seriously. Apart from the fact that the heart transplant was not a basic scientific discovery I was further disqualified for this prize by the fact that I was a South African – and a white one at that.

The lecture halls were full to capacity everywhere. I couldn't speak Spanish so I had to use an interpreter. I found this extremely difficult – especially if the translation was not simultaneous because I had to interrupt the lecture every few minutes and then wait for the translation. Stop-start talks can easily become tedious.

This had several disadvantages because the lecture took twice as long and I also found I could never make real contact with my audience. The one thing I did learn, however, is never to try to tell a funny story in these circumstances because you hardly raise a laugh. The punch line is invariably lost – humour doesn't travel well – what's funny in one country is far from funny in another.

A good lecture is one where you get excited and enthusiastic yourself and the audience soon picks this up – lecturing is, after all, a form of entertainment. But it was impossible to get into this mode when I had to stop talking every few minutes or so. Despite these restrictions, however, the audiences were enthusiastic and lively round-table discussions with many of their leading heart surgeons followed each one.

During one discussion, the indications for heart transplantation and the treatment of ischaemic heart disease (insufficient blood supply to the heart muscle due to blockage of the coronary arteries supplying the muscle) was raised.

We all agreed that when this had resulted in extensive death of the heart muscle the only option was a transplant.

I stressed that none of our patients selected so far had suffered from angina (which is ischaemic pain), because only *live* muscle can generate pain. The absence of angina is a clear indication of extensive and permanent heart-muscle damage – in which case the heart should be replaced.

One question was about what should be done if the patient still had considerable pain, indicating that there was still muscle which could be saved and that transplantation might not be indicated.

The moderator proudly pointed out that a young Argentinian surgeon by the name of Rene Favoloro, working at the Cleveland Clinic, had pioneered an operation where a vein is taken from the lower leg and the blocked area of the artery by-passed with the vein from the leg. This was made possible because a cardiologist, Mason Soanes, working at the same clinic, had developed a technique whereby a radiopaque dye was selectively injected into the coronary arteries and a cine picture taken during the injection.

This allowed him to demonstrate the position of the block and the potency of the artery's distal to the obstructed portion.

Favoloro, at that stage, had operated on sixteen patients, resulting in spectacular relief from pain. The question asked was whether this operation would make the transplant obsolete. I didn't think so and pointed out that it was no use watering a dead tree. The transplant would always be the correct treatment for dead muscle. Muscle that was still alive needed only an improvement in the blood supply – a by-pass.

Although the introduction of the by-pass operation did not create the publicity the heart transplant did (and the names of the surgeons who pioneered this operation would not be mentioned in the *Guinness Book of Records* as mine had been), the operation turned out to be of much greater value in the treatment of heart patients than that of the transplant.

In my opinion the by-pass has been one of the most important contributions in the field of cardiac surgery. The fact that it's one of the most common major surgical procedures in America, for example, proves what a fantastic surgical development it is.

Publicity and the media can so easily fashion history and distort our sense of values. Ask ten youngsters today who discovered penicillin* and I'm prepared to bet a lot of money that not one would know, but ask them who the Beatles were, and at least half of them will give you the correct answer.

---

* Two Britons, Australian-born pathologist Howard Florey and German-born biochemist Ernst Chain, developed an industrial process – after Gerhard Domagk's discovery of sulphanilamide – for the manufacture of penicillin, a mould whose anti-bacterial properties had been noted, but not exploited, by Alexander Fleming in 1928. Although Fleming, Florey and Chain shared the Nobel Prize for Medicine in 1945, it was Fleming who received all the popular acclaim.

Such is the fickleness of fame. It's the scientists and researchers who make the world a better place with their discoveries in medicine but, without fame, their efforts are much less likely to succeed because 'fame' tends to generate financial support through publicity.

My own fame – or notoriety (whichever you prefer) – did me and my family considerable harm. But it also did a great deal of good. The Chris Barnard Fund, for example, continues to assist major research into cardiac disease and people tend to listen when I speak. Fund-raisers are quick to recognize this phenomenon and use it whenever possible to help generate funds.

I was amused, a few years ago, when I had been invited to a dinner in Washington to raise funds for cancer research. Before the dinner started the guests were allowed to meet the specially invited celebrities – actors and actresses, boxers and pop singers. The organizers didn't consider that it was enough to meet *one* scientist and, in the excitement to shake the hand of Sugar Ray Leonard, the scientists – who were the real heroes of the day – were rudely shoved out of the way by the paying guests!

Favoloro, widely unrecognized for his brilliant surgical technique, eventually returned to Argentina and opened a cardiac surgery there. We became close friends and I often watched him operate.

He told me a very amusing story about how some American heart surgeons had reacted when I gave a lecture. He said they had planned to sit in the front row of the lecture theatre and, as soon as I started to talk, they would stand up and walk out.

The public may believe there is no professional envy between doctors. Unfortunately there is, in fact, fierce competition.

As far as these American surgeons were concerned, all I can say is they probably missed a very good lecture by walking out and I was very moved and greatly honoured when Favolora quoted some lines by Jonathan Swift for my benefit, 'When a true genius appears in the world, you may know him by this sign, that the dunces are all in confederacy against him…'

Doctors in other parts of the world, however, were kinder. When the South American chapter of the American College of Cardiology had their annual congress in Lima, Peru, for example, I was invited to relate our experiences with heart transplants up to that time.

Afterwards, the president of Peru awarded me the 'Member of

the Order Hipolito Unaneu' and I also received the 'Order del Sol'.

In Lima I travelled around in a big black limousine and was escorted by four traffic cops on big Harley-Davidson motorbikes, with sirens blaring to get the traffic out of the way.

It embarrassed me to see my friends waiting to be transported to the congress by bus when my special VIP transport arrived. I never asked for any of this special treatment – but I have to admit I enjoyed it when it was offered.

Louwtjie was at the airport in Cape Town, to meet me with a frosty welcome. After collecting my luggage, we left by car for Zeekoevlei. I was driving and tried to make some idle conversation when, out of the blue, she exploded and smacked me hard across the face. Whatever the reason was, I suppose I deserved it so I just kept on driving.

I realized that we had probably come to the end of the road.

He lined up all his pills with military precision. Twenty-two of them in a row. As he swallowed each one he ticked it off against a list he carried in his note book. It was a strict routine he followed religiously four times a day.

His wife called from the lounge and suggested a drive up to Rhodes Memorial – one of his favourite places – in the shadow of Table Mountain.

The entire estate once belonged to Cecil John Rhodes and on it, today, stands the official residence of the South African president as well as Groote Schuur Hospital and the University of Cape Town.

High up on the slope of Devil's Peak is the memorial, once the favourite spot of Rhodes himself – the man who'd made a fortune in diamonds and gold, who'd had a country named after him, who had directed the British ideal of enslaving a nation in its colonial quests, and a man who had destroyed his own political career when he was implicated in the disastrous 'Jameson Raid'. Jameson's forces of 470 men had been captured by the Afrikaners and Rhodes was forced to resign as premier of the Cape Colony. Ironically and typical of the British Colonialists' irrational politics, Jameson served a prison sentence in Britain – then returned to South Africa after the Boer War and, himself, became premier of the Cape Colony, later to be made a baronet.

Philip Blaiberg stood in front of the massive monument and re-read the inscribed words that Kipling had written on Rhodes' death, 'The immense and brooding spirit still shall quicken and control. Living he was the land and dead his soul shall be her soul.'

He turned to enjoy the spectacular view out over Cape Town and the distant mountains beyond, when he became aware of two men walking towards him – they were obviously medical people as they kept their distance – something he'd had difficulty in explaining to other people. Because his immune system was not strong he had to be extremely careful.

'Did you know you're a famous man in Britain?' one of them said to him. 'Name's Griffith, Kenneth Griffith – and this is Dr Richard Heald,' he continued, introducing his friend.

The three men sat on a low wall surrounding the Memorial and talked about Rhodes, the hospital, Christiaan Barnard and, of course, heart transplantation.

Kenneth Griffith was on a visit to South Africa for preliminary work on a film of Cecil Rhodes' life and Richard Heald was a young registrar at Guy's Hospital, London, then attending the biennial conference of the Association of Surgeons being held at Groote Schuur Hospital.

'I discussed your operation with Lord Russell Brock, one of Britain's leading heart specialists,' said Heald. 'He has great admiration for Professor Barnard and his achievements and is one of Britain's leading supporters of heart transplantation.'

They chatted casually about post-operative care, the drugs he was taking and the treatment he was still undergoing at the hospital. Philip Blaiberg didn't notice how critically, and professionally, the doctor had been watching and appraising him.

Their conversation lasted about half an hour.

A month later Eileen Blaiberg handed him a local edition of a Cape Town newspaper which reported on a letter the doctor had written to The Times of London which read: 'There have been a number of wild and varied reports about the quality of life being enjoyed by Dr Blaiberg since his heart transplant. I met him, and a brief description by an essentially unbiased observer, like myself, may be of interest.

'He walks and talks normally with the exception of a slight residual weakness of the legs. At no time did I observe him to be breathless.

"I have had a hundred days of good life on borrowed time," he told me, "and if I die next week from rejection, the operation on me will still have been a success."

'Having seen for myself that Dr Blaiberg is enjoying life, I can assure doubters that reports to the contrary are untrue.'

That should be of some relief to the hospital staff, Philip Blaiberg chuckled, as he began lining up his pills again.

When I arrived home, I phoned Bossie.

'How's Dr Blaiberg?' I asked.

'He's coming in for a routine check-up tomorrow morning. I think he's doing well.'

He didn't sound concerned at all and his tone of voice caused me no alarm but I always hated it when registrars told me what they 'thought'.

'You're not *sure*?' I asked, irritated by his uncertainty.

He was probably sensitive to my irritation and said 'No Prof, all the tests are within normal limits and he's enjoying life immensely.' But, when I think back on it, Bossie was probably very worried indeed.

'Bossie, I'm tired as hell. I've just come from the airport. I'll see you and Blaiberg tomorrow.'

The phone went dead immediately as he replaced the receiver without another word. There were none of the usual telephone formalities, just a hostile 'click'.

'What the hell's wrong?' I thought as I stared at the silent phone. Bossie had never behaved like this – I felt as if he, like Louwtjie, had also slapped me. I felt my nose again to make sure it wasn't broken.

Bossie had just finished doing the electrocardiogram when I arrived the following morning.

'Morning, Bossie. Hello, Philip – so what have you been up to since I saw you last, my celebrity patient?'

'I suppose the same as you, Professor', he said as a naughty smile lit up his round face.

'And what's that?' I asked curiously.

'Well, I suppose it's only proper to tell you everything isn't it?' He asked.

'Of course – why, is there something wrong?'

'No, in fact it couldn't be better, but maybe I should have told you before, that Eileen and I resumed our marital relations twenty days after I left hospital – on our wedding anniversary actually.'

Now, that would make a *great* story for some of the tabloid press and gossip magazines, I thought.

'I thought you should know – especially now that my medical history is being compiled for official records and textbooks on cardiology and cardiac surgery.'

'Quite right, Philip,' I smiled.

'Maybe,' he continued, 'I should tell others as well to avert any fears that some men might have, who believe their sex life will suffer after cardiac surgery?'

'I honestly think you should avoid making it public,' I replied, 'but I'm sure it will come as a great comfort to many who do have operations similar to yours in the future. Unfortunately, if you let that sort of thing become public knowledge, you'll have a major media headache on your hands – which could also be embarrassing for you and your family.'

The examination continued. It was 24 May 1968 and his 59th birthday.

'So, you're keeping well then?'

'Well, actually, I don't *always* feel so great,' he admitted reluctantly, 'and I often feel so terribly tired,' he added with a deep sigh.

There was something about Philip Blaiberg that was worrying me. All the tests appeared normal, but experience had taught me that studying the patient by simply watching him is as important as the special investigations. One eventually develops a sixth sense where one walks into a ward and, without feeling the pulse or taking the blood pressure, can see that things have changed. Maybe Bossie had also sensed this – which would have explained his curt manner the previous day.

My patient was not well.

I said earlier that I have no regrets about the things I've done but, looking back at those hectic days, I feel I made one mistake – and that was to accept too many invitations.

After all, I was primarily a surgeon and not a public relations officer for South Africa. Not that my patients were neglected because, fortunately, Marius was there to run the show when I gallivanted all over the world. But it wasn't the same – it was like the first mate being in charge of the ship while the captain was ashore.

So, despite the uneasy feeling I had about Blaiberg, I left with Louwtjie for Spain and Iran. Then I was to go alone to London to visit Dr Donald Ross, my old university friend.

We arrived early in the morning in the land of flamenco, the brave bulls and the most generous people I've ever met.

The minister of public works was at the airport to welcome us on behalf of the government and, after a short press conference, which Louwtjie refused to attend, we were taken to a suite in a five star hotel. There were beautiful flowers and a bottle of the best Tio Pepe. Although it was still early morning I decided to have a stiff drink. I needed some quick-fix immunity from Louwtjie's moodiness as the entire flight had been tense.

General Franco's only daughter, Carmen, was married to Martinus Bordeaux, head of the department of cardiac surgery at La Pas Hospital. With his marriage also came a title, the 'Marquis de Villaverde'.

There was a message for me at the hotel that I would be collected and taken to observe an open-procedure done by the marquis.

The department of cardiac surgery was equipped with the latest and best monitoring devices in an extremely modern intensive care unit and operating suites. There was obviously no shortage of medical funds.

I changed into operating clothes, cap and mask and entered the operating theatre where the marquis had already started a mitral valve replacement.

The patient's left atrium was small, making exposure difficult, and I sympathized with him as he struggled to see where to place his sutures.

As he'd been trained by Denton Cooley, speed was considered to be of utmost importance – which is the exact antithesis to my own approach. By nature I have never been a very dextrous surgeon and, to me, speed in ordinary circumstances is not an important factor. I would rather take ten minutes longer and make sure that every stitch was correctly placed and properly tied. I would probably have taken at least one and a quarter hours to replace this valve, but the marquis was finished in forty-five minutes.

He left the closure of the chest to his assistant. We showered and changed back into street clothes and left for lunch at the Jockey Club.

Fortunately I had the evening free to rest because the next day I was invited to another bloody event, a bullfight.

When we entered Las Ventas Plaza de Toros the atmosphere was electric. With a crowd of 24 000 spectators, the excitement and expectations lay heavy in the still air of the dusty, hot arena where it mixed with that unmistakable smell of death.

We took our seats in the *corrida*, antipodal to where the *cuadrilla* would make their grand entrance. To the right of the mid-line of the 50 metre wide arena, high up in the wooden shelters sat El

Presidente. He acted as the referee and would decide when the bull could be killed and also judge the performance of the matador.

Today, five bulls were to be killed. El Cordobés would fight three of them and two lesser-known bullfighters would slaughter one each.

Manuel Benítez, or El Cordobés, as he was known, was the most skilled, admired and highest paid fighter in Spain, having learned well from his peers, Juan Belmonte, Luis Dominguin and Manolete. He was now as immortal as they were – during the sixties, his posters were found in bedrooms and apartments all over the world.

It's rumoured that the evening before his first major encounter with the bulls, he'd said to his mother, 'Today I will dress you either in silk, or in mourning.' Fortunately for him he had dressed her in silk.

As we sat in the shade – which were the best seats as they were out of the sun's glare – I knew that he and his compatriots would be in the chapel, next to the small surgery, praying for bravery and honour.

Suddenly the chatter of the crowd was silenced by the fanfare of trumpets. The gates in the arena, opposite to where we sat, opened and the grand entrance began.

At the front of the procession were the mounted *alguaciles* who rode majestically up to El Presidente's box, saluted him by removing their plumed *monteras* – those three-cornered hats – and ceremoniously collected the key to the *toril* gate.

Next in the *paseo* were the matadors dressed in their sequined 'suits of light' (*traje de luces*) with bright-coloured tights and with their shiny black hair tied back in ponytails.

They were followed by *banderilleros* with their multi-coloured barbed sticks and the picadors with their padded horses and *vara* lances. At the rear came the members of the supporting cast – the *cuadrillas*.

The procession stopped in the middle of the arena. All of them turned to where the president sat and saluted him by bowing and removing their hats. Then they turned to where we sat with the marquis and acknowledged our presence as well.

The horses left and the others took up positions behind wooden shelters around the edge of the arena. A trumpet sounded and a gate – the *toril* – was flung open and a bull rushed into the arena. His huge muscles glistened and gleamed in the sun.

What a magnificent animal – all 450 kilograms of him! He stormed to the middle of the ring, stopped, lifted and shook his head as if to say, 'I'm not afraid of the lot of you.'

Each 'fight' lasts about twenty minutes and I watched three bulls literally bleed to death on the scorched red earth in front of me. I was also presented with two ears – an honour which would have been unthinkable to refuse.

I am a surgeon, so blood is nothing unusual to me – but this barbaric ritual was making me feel sick. As I was being bothered by people coming up to me all the time for autographs and photographs, I used this as an ideal excuse to leave early.

On the steps there was an American tourist, complete with camera on his shoulder and loud-patterned shirt, who had been watching this fussing around me. As I passed him he greeted me with great pride, 'Hi there, Dr De Bakey!'

Hemingway wrote, 'Bullfighting is the only art in which the artist is in danger of death and in which the degree of brilliance in the performance is left to the fighter's honour.'

But isn't this also true of boxing and maybe motor sports? Is it correct to call it an 'art'? When does blood-lust stop being barbaric and become a sport? There was a growing demand in Spanish society to ban bullfighting but, typically, no political party would endorse it – and risk losing votes. They can have my support any time.

I was filled with abject sadness when we drove away. The bull had entered the arena as a magnificent beast, the picture of strength and courage. He was then slowly worn down until he stood in front of the matador, head hanging and tongue protruding, pawing at the earth with his front hooves – which is a sign of wanting to make peace (not an act of aggression as many believe).

If he could talk I'm sure this bull would be saying, 'You've hurt me enough now, can't we please stop?' But the crowd yelled for more blood – they would show no mercy and only rarely is a bull spared.

All these bulls appeared to be exceptionally brave to me. None of them backed away when the picadors' lances plunged time and again into their hard back muscles until crimson with blood and the *banderilleros* stabbed the barbed sticks into their necks to make the beast's head droop.

We drove away without anyone saying a word. I turned to the

marquis, 'Martinus, thanks for bringing me to see the bullfight, but I never want to see one again.'

He looked at me in utter amazement. He couldn't believe what he'd just heard. In fact, as a full-blooded Spaniard, he was probably highly insulted.

'Why, Chris, what's wrong?'

'I don't know, I felt so sorry for the bulls – they were such magnificent animals and it was tragic to see them die. The whole event was very depressing.'

His face lit up. 'Chris, then the performance was a success!'

I couldn't understand.

Martinus continued, 'A bullfight *is* a tragedy – it's the death of a bull.'

'But the poor animals had no chance,' I argued – I still couldn't condone what I had just seen.

'Chris, look at it this way. If you were a bull and the farmer had given you the best grazing he had available for three years and now had to get rid of you. Which of the two would you prefer – to go to the slaughterhouse, or to fight for your life in the bull-ring?'

I decided I'd think about that.

The Spanish custom of having a siesta in the afternoon was greatly appreciated especially as Louwtjie and I would only be collected at 10 pm that evening for a dinner at the home of Eduardo Barreiros and Dori, his wife.

Señor Barreiros was a very wealthy industrialist and, among his many interests, he assembled automobiles in Spain. He was also one of the most generous human beings I've ever met and, from that evening on, took it upon himself to look after the Barnard family.

All the beautiful people of Madrid were invited and his magnificent home echoed to the sounds of Spanish guitarists and flamenco dancers. The marquis de Villaverde arrived late, with Audrey Hepburn and Doris (the ex-wife of Yul Brynner), who was Chilean and very hot-blooded as the Latin Americans usually are.

Audrey Hepburn has Dutch ancestry and could understand my Afrikaans so we chatted for a while. She was very beautiful – but sad. She'd just been through a divorce and those big brown plaintive eyes told me she wasn't much in the mood for a party. I would have loved the opportunity of bringing a smile back to that innocent face.

We left at 3 am the following morning and, at 10 am, there was a car to take Louwtjie and me to the studio of Juan d'Avalos, a famous Spanish sculptor. Eduardo Barreiros had commissioned him to make busts of the two of us. Mine is now in the Beaufort West Museum.

That afternoon we left for Majorca. Barreiros owned a lot of property on the island and he took us to show us a piece of land next to the ocean, where he said he was going to build a holiday home for his family – and also one for us!

They made a great fuss of Louwtjie and showered her with gifts. I was very pleased about this as it gave her back some of her old confidence – and I'm sure she felt less like second-fiddle, which had been making her so miserable and hostile recently.

Teheran airport is much like any other except that there was a visceral undercurrent of tension as we made our way through the buildings. There had been serious rioting a few years previously and the after-shocks hadn't been brought under control yet. I had been reading about a Muslim leader, the Ayatollah Khomeini who, although living in exile, was stirring up a lot of religious fervour and calling for violent mass action of the people.

Rampant inflation didn't help the plight of the shah either – and I felt very guilty when I first saw the turrets of his palace over the rooftops of the city – where I knew we'd be treated lavishly while the peasants drudged away outside its walls.

The meeting with the shah was a great disappointment. Louwtjie wasn't invited – but neither was the shah's wife. He appeared to be in a great hurry and our conversation lasted only about ten minutes. To be honest, I don't even remember what we talked about so it couldn't have been very important – or interesting.

Louwtjie joined me to look at the crown jewels. It was the first time in my life that I'd seen such treasures. The 'Peacock Throne' was absolutely incredible and the most valuable item in the collection was a dagger given to the shah's father by the sultan of Turkey. The handle of this magnificent weapon was studded with diamonds and rubies – some the size of walnuts. I couldn't even begin to imagine its value – but that's the paradox of the Middle-East, treasures beyond belief amid hunger, religious mania and war.

The members of the royal family and their friends treated

Louwtjie with great respect but, in the crowds at social events, she was shoved thoughtlessly out of the way and I often heard her cry in anguish, 'I am *Mrs* Barnard!'

To be fair, it was rather tough on Louwtjie – apart from the royal household, nobody took much notice of her – and, in a country where women are not held in high esteem, her presence was tolerated but with little, or no respect.

She sensed this and said as much. I agreed it was unfortunate but said that she should remember the culture of the country we were visiting and, in any case, they really wanted to hear me talk about heart operations.

Although I was being as gentle as I could she took that *very* badly and stormed away in a furious rage – shouting over her shoulder, 'You're so bloody full of yourself – it's always you! you! you!' She was right of course – but it wasn't entirely my fault.

I was deeply touched when the shah instructed the Pahlavi University of Shiraz to bestow an honorary doctorate of medicine on me. It was a great honour for someone of a different faith.

Shiraz was a most beautiful city, with streets lined with rose bushes which were in full bloom. The ceremony was just as colourful. I wore a special gown which was made specially for this occasion – a full-length, heavy robe in deep-coloured textures, lined with ermine, complete with gold clasps. When it was draped over me I was regally transformed and felt as important as a king when all the ceremonial pomp began.

After visiting the oil-centre, Basrah, and seeing the vast oil wells of Iran, Louwtjie returned to South Africa and I went on to London by myself.

When I registered at the Savoy Hotel I noticed with great pleasure and anticipation that Françoise Hardy was giving a concert in the hotel that evening. This meant she was probably also staying there. 'How very convenient,' I thought to myself with a smile.

After a quick breakfast I was collected for a visit to the National Heart Hospital where I met my old medical-school friend again, Donald Ross, who had just performed the first heart transplant in Britain. We chatted with the patient, Fred West, for a while and then I was asked to say a few words to a group of medical students.

There were always several questions which came up repeatedly – the cost was one of them, so I had the answer ready. I was sure the young student who'd asked this question was probably a radical, looking for an easy target for abuse or, at best, a member of the Labour Party which was fiercely anti-South Africa.

'I'm glad you asked that question because there is a misconception on the question of costs. However, I'm not sure I can answer you because, where I operate, the patient doesn't have to pay. I've never sent an account to any patient – white or black – since I've been practising open-heart surgery.'

A ripple of surprise ran through the audience and I could see the radical young man raising his eyebrows in contempt. I was sure he didn't believe me.

Looking straight at him I said, 'In case anyone misheard me, the government hospitals in South Africa are free to all – including foreign patients,' and I paused for a moment. 'Yes, *all* South Africans get free treatment and if you, young man,' and I pointed at him, 'were on holiday in Cape Town and suffered a major heart problem you might well end up under my knife – and it wouldn't cost you a penny.

'But let's say, for argument's sake, that it costs £30 000. I guess then, that the cost is very high but, from the nature of your question, you assume that *not* doing the transplant costs nothing?

'That is obviously incorrect – in fact it may cost more money by not doing the operation. Remember that the patient is in total heart failure and needs extensive medical treatment. Often he has to be re-admitted to hospital – that also costs money. Then he can never return to a productive life and never provide for his family again – unlike a patient who has had a successful transplant. How much does that cost? And, lastly, he's going to die within a few months, what value do you put on the death of a father, or mother, or brother?

'On a more personal note – if you came to me with your father or mother who could be saved by a transplant, how would you like it if I told you, "No, let him die – I'm not spending money on this, I prefer to spend the money on the starving children of Africa."

'The point is that there should be enough money *to do both* – to feed the children *and* to do the transplant. Yes, this *can* be done because, after all, there always appears to be enough money for politicians to buy expensive equipment to kill people in wars.'

The audience exploded in deafening applause – that was the kind of thing they loved to hear as the majority of students were totally opposed to war and armaments.

4

Jennifer was now 21 years old. I had met her for the first time two years before the transplant, when she and her mother came down from Pretoria with her father who had severe multi-valvular disease.

I had replaced both his aortic and his mitral valve and done an angioplasty on the tricuspid valve. She had been extremely grateful and had told me she was determined to show her gratitude whenever the opportunity arose – in a way that would be mutually enjoyable.

Jennifer was, then, working at the South African Embassy in London, so I phoned her just to hear how she was enjoying England.

'My professor!' She shouted gleefully. She always called me that although I had never taught her medicine. 'I'd *love* to see you while you're in London if you have the time.' And we arranged to meet that afternoon in my hotel room at 5.30.

We were still busy with thanksgiving when the phone in my room rang. It was MC Botha. He had just arrived from South Africa. 'Blaiberg is fine,' he said, 'but there is a nurse from Holland down here in the foyer. She used to work for you and she would like to see you and ask you a few questions.'

'MC, tell her I'll be down in about half an hour.'

He laughed and gave me his room number and I arranged to call him later.

Jennifer and I showered together at the end of our afternoon session and said goodbye.

I waited for twenty minutes and went down to the lobby. Gertrude saw me and flew into my arms and gave me a long, open-mouth kiss.

I knew she only wanted to ask me one question, but would I be able to reply? I was still a bit wobbly from being with Jennifer. But when I felt her naked body next to mine in bed the answer was there.

Gertrude left at about 8 pm and I was then so exhausted I decided not to contact Françoise Hardy after all.

But it's wonderful how sleep can recharge the batteries. I woke up at 10 pm fresh, and ready for the evening. I felt like phoning Jennifer again because I had grown quite fond of her but, instead, went down to see if Françoise Hardy's concert was still in progress.

She was busy with her last song. What a beautiful voice – sweet, melodic and haunting, made even more seductive by the French accent. I couldn't wait to see her after the show.

When we met she told me that she had no more performances to do so we went to the lounge for a drink and then up to her room for our own private performance.

Françoise had a beautiful face and a tall willowy figure – but she was very thin and with her small breasts certainly didn't match the reputation of the buxom and sexually uninhibited French mademoiselles.

I left her room in the early hours of the morning feeling rather disappointed but happy nevertheless as I sauntered down the thickly carpeted corridor to my own room where I fell into a deep sleep.

I met MC the next morning for breakfast. He slumped heavily into a chair and told me he'd just received very bad news from Groote Schuur Hospital. Philip Blaiberg had had a relapse and been readmitted to the intensive care unit. We decided to go back to Cape Town that evening.

The press also had the news by then and we spent the entire day dodging reporters and photographers.

The press annoyed me most of the time – but never more so than when there was bad news. The grief of others seemed to attract them like carrion to a corpse.

We were back in Cape Town within 24 hours and I went straight from the airport to see my patient. His condition had deteriorated considerably since I'd last seen him – and I blamed myself for going on the trip when I had sensed beforehand that something was going wrong.

The sparkle in his eyes had gone and, more seriously, he appeared to have lost the will to live. I hardly recognized the patient I had talked about in London – the man who had been enjoying life to the full and looking forward to celebrating the anniversary of his heart transplant.

I started examining him. He was definitely jaundiced – I could clearly see yellow discolouration of the whites of his eyes. His liver was enlarged and palpable below the rib margin. But what worried me the most was that he had all the signs of poor cardiac output.

I felt his feet – they were cold and the pulse was hardly palpable. His lips were blue and he was not interested in his surroundings – a sign of poor cerebral circulation. His chart showed that his urinary output was poor and the blood urea raised.

'How are you feeling, Philip?' I asked, hoping to get some kind of encouraging reply from my patient. He opened his eyes and managed a faint smile. I could see the great concern in Bossie's eyes.

'He's been going down the last three days,' he whispered. 'I asked the physicians to see him and they think it's all due to an infection.'

'Then why hasn't he got a temperature and why isn't his white cell count raised?' I asked sharply.

'They say it's due to the drugs – his immune system isn't able to respond.'

Bossie was paging through his notes to show me the physician's report and handed them to me. I read without comment. Professor Eales, after listing the symptoms and signs, had arrived at the conclusion that Philip Blaiberg was suffering from a severe infection. I looked at Bossie and put the notes down.

'Bossie, I don't think it's an infection. This is severe rejection. He's been rejecting since the transplant and that's why the voltage of the electrocardiogram never increased.'

I could see Bossie didn't agree, he was probably afraid we were going to make the same mistake as we made with Washkansky where our treatment for rejection had allowed fatal infection to occur.

'What about the jaundice, Prof?'

'Congestion of the liver,' I replied, 'and maybe, on top of that, the toxic effect of the Imuran.'

We wandered to a corner of the ward where we could talk without the patient hearing.

'Shall we increase the cortisone?' I asked.

Bossie looked nervously down at the floor as if he was going to find the answer there. 'Hell, Professor, I don't know, that's for you to decide.'

That was my problem. There was nobody in Cape Town who had any experience in this field whom I could consult. In fact, there was nobody in the world I could turn to. I felt totally alone.

'I see you've sent away several blood samples to the laboratory for culture.'

'Yes, – so far they're negative. The last time I phoned was this morning.'

There was no doubt that Bossie had done everything possible to give Blaiberg the best treatment while I had been away. He had virtually been living with the patient. I wondered whether that was good. Such close involvement could easily cloud a doctor's judgment.

The dilemma that faced me was that, if I treated him for rejection and his condition was due to an infection, I would virtually be signing his death certificate – because I would be suppressing his own body's defence mechanism. On the other hand, if it *was* rejection and I didn't treat it, his heart would be destroyed within the next day or so – to the extent that it would stop working.

I walked to the phone and called Vel at the cardiac clinic. Maybe he could help me to make the correct decision. There was no reply. I turned to Bossie as I replaced the receiver and said, 'I suppose Professor Schrire's doing his ward rounds and will probably pop in here later.'

Bossie shuffled uncomfortably and edged closer to me before saying, 'He doesn't come here unless we send an official referral to him.' His eyes wouldn't meet mine.

What the hell was going on with Vel? I was annoyed and astonished by such high-handed and callous behaviour, but made my decision anyway. 'Let's increase his cortisone to 60 milligrams a day – what do you have him on now – 20? Keep the Imuran at 200 milligrams.'

I left the ward. Alone.

She still visited Phil twice every day and she now saw him growing weaker and weaker each time. He could hardly speak and was dangerously underweight.

Then, on Thursday, 4 July, she was told that Phil had developed yet another complication – pneumonia – just as Louis Washkansky had.

She looked at him through the glass and tried speaking through the intercom – but the words wouldn't come. He seemed even worse than he ever had before. 'He's going – and there's nothing anyone can do,' she told herself as she left the hospital, 'it's over.'

Before reaching her car she saw Professor Barnard. Even from this distance she could see that his face was drawn and tired. She watched him silently.

He didn't see her as he walked with his shoulders hunched in resignation and defeat.

'Yes, it's over,' she repeated.

Philip Blaiberg was dying and there were two options available – so I asked to see Eileen Blaiberg.

It was a Saturday evening, 6 July 1968, when I found her in her husband's ward.

I spoke as gently as I could – but she was a strong woman who had faced all the previous dangers bravely – so I could talk directly and openly, 'Eileen, if you don't want to lose your husband, we'll have to consider giving him another heart transplant – and a lung as well.'

'Are you *serious*, Professor?' She asked me incredulously, her eyes wide with fright.

'Yes – very serious,' I said. 'We may try a serum first, although it's very risky – so I want your permission to go ahead with the arrangements for another transplant if it's necessary.'

She paled visibly – but agreed.

After she left I went to see Philip Blaiberg again. He was in a fitful sleep, but woke when he saw me. I explained the situation completely to him and he agreed with an air of finality. He'd always been a fighter but he looked, now, as if he was ready to throw in the towel.

When I had first prepared myself for the transplant programme I'd visited Dr Starzl in Denver – to learn how to prepare antilymphocytic serum (ALS), as he'd used it with good results in patients who had undergone liver transplants.

Human lymphocytes – isolated from the blood or lymph nodes – are injected into a horse. The animal's immune system then recognizes these cells as being foreign and begins producing antibodies to destroy them. Blood samples are taken regularly from the horse and the concentration of antibodies is determined. When this is high enough a few litres of blood are taken from the horse and the serum is separated out, producing horse antilymphocytic serum, or ALS.

We had never prepared the antilymphocytic serum ourselves but had received some from Professor Carras of the Pasteur Institute in Lyon and Professor Brendal of Munich.

The rationale behind treating rejection with this serum is that the patient's lymphocytes are the immunologically competent cells and are responsible for destroying the transplanted organ. If the antibodies made by the horse are injected they will kill these lymphocytes, reducing their numbers significantly and stopping the rejection. The only danger, however, is that the horse serum is a foreign protein and, when given to a human intravenously, can cause a fatal allergic reaction.

That evening I went to a hospital function – I don't remember what it was in aid of – it wouldn't have been a celebration as the news could not have been worse. The entire hospital was deeply concerned about Philip Blaiberg.

I had quite a few glasses of wine to help me escape from reality and was dancing with Sister Geyer when I was called to the phone. It was Bossie.

He told me that Blaiberg was not responding to the increased dose of cortisone and asked if he could try the antilymphocytic serum. We'd had no experience in using this drug but I knew the dangers. I also knew a decision had to be made one way or the other – and quickly. I remembered what Dr Perry once told me when I was a registrar in Minneapolis, 'Either get off the pot – or piss in it.'

I made a decision. 'Okay Bossie, work out the dose from the protein content of the serum, mix that with 250 millilitres of saline and give it intravenously – very slowly.'

It must have been the alcohol that dulled my reservations, but it turned out to be the turning point. The fruit of the vine helped save Blaiberg's life.

By now, of course, the press were driving everyone mad. And they were stuck between a rock and a hard place themselves – they wanted to condemn me for transplantation but, at the same time, didn't want to risk criticizing someone who was, after all, saving lives.

I still don't know who tipped them off about the possibility of a second transplant – but it seemed this was bigger news than the first operation.

Newspapers around the world carried this speculation as their front-page stories. Britain's *Daily Mirror*, in a statement of apparent paradox, attacked the publicity generated in a denouncement on their front page – while not committing themselves as being either in favour or opposed to the treatment of my patient – and pronounced didactically:

Everyone would like to cheer this courageous transplant survivor back to health. But no one can have an easy mind over the wave of publicity about his condition every time he has a relapse. Heart transplant operations themselves are still highly controversial.

They are made more controversial when they are associated, as in this particular case, with a constant bombardment of publicity, rumour and speculation.

There have been stories that Dr Blaiberg might be given a new heart and lungs. There have been reports that he refused a second transplant, reports denied by his wife and Professor Barnard.

The whole business is enough to make any heart patient think twice before going through the same ordeal.

Professor Barnard and Cape Town's Groote Schuur Hospital will always be under pressure to give out news, and they may not find it easy to achieve the right balance between candour and silence. But while the controversy about heart transplants continues, they should beware of the wrong kind of publicity and the harm it can do.

I wish I'd had the man who wrote that on my staff – he obviously knew how to avoid publicity and make our lives easier. I have to agree that what he said made perfect sense – for a newspaper to admit they were exacerbating a problem was an incredible confession.

Eileen Blaiberg was also reading the newspapers and was sick to death of the way her words were continually quoted out of context, misconstrued, distorted and sensationalized.

She was so very weary of the ceaseless hounding by journalists – each with a deadline to meet, who had to produce a story, any story, each and every day.

She was unspeakably angry with others who invaded her privacy, telephoned her in the middle of the night and gave her no time to rest or pray for her husband.

On Sunday, 7 July she met Dr Bossie Bosman who, taking her arm, said gently, 'Eileen, you had better go into Phil's suite and speak to him.'

She knew exactly what he meant by allowing her into the suite that had always been out of bounds to her – it was to be her last chance to say good-bye.

She didn't know for sure that Chris Barnard had decided to use anti-lymphocytic serum on Phil the previous day – in fact she thought he'd mentioned it only to be kind.

She put on her sterile outfit as usual and walked into her husband's room. Her legs felt weak and she was nauseous with fear.

Philip Blaiberg was deathly pale and perfectly still on his bed.

'Oh my God!' she cried. 'Phil...Phil!'

He opened his eyes and smiled weakly.

Then the tears began rolling down his face. He knew.

Keeping perfectly in control of herself she waited until he had drifted off to sleep again and then, quietly, left him for the last time.

When she got home she broke down completely with wracking sobs of grief. She cried – for the first time in weeks – uncontrollably.

She lay on the bed, close to hysteria, for what seemed like hours when suddenly the telephone rang.

'This is it then.' She braced herself as she picked up the phone. She couldn't speak.

She recognized Chris Barnard's voice – it was kind of him to call personally to break the bad news.

'Hello? Hello!' said the voice, 'are you there, Eileen?'

She tried to swallow a sob of grief.

'Eileen!' he said, 'I've got wonderful news for you – Philip's going to live. He's going to live!'

She didn't understand. In a hoarse whisper she asked, 'Have you found a donor then?'

'No!' he said excitedly. "We don't need a transplant – the serum worked! Your husband's recovering!'

The antilymphocytic serum had taken thirty-six hours to show its effects and we continued the treatment with highly satisfactory results.

We published the effects in the medical journals and many researchers around the world became extremely interested in, and heartened by, this remarkable drug.

Philip's recovery was now so normal, that bulletins were again issued only periodically and the press gradually eased the story off their front pages and then out of the news altogether.

The success we achieved with Blaiberg resulted in a spate of heart transplants all over the world.

I met Dr LAPA Munnik, the member of the executive council of the Cape Provincial Administration, responsible for hospital services, and suggested we should hold the world's first heart transplant conference in Cape Town. He immediately agreed and said that he would find the money to finance the whole show, including the delegates' air fares and accommodation.

So I personally invited the heads of 15 centres who had performed heart transplants at that stage. They all accepted except for Doctors Shumway and Lower who couldn't come personally but would send a member of their team in their place.

In the meantime, I had received the most generous invitation from Eduardo Barreiros. He'd offered to pay all the expenses for me, my family and some of our friends if I wished, to join his family for a holiday at Las Togas. Unfortunately, however, the dates overlapped with the time of the world congress. After some phone calls backwards and forwards it was agreed that Louwtjie and André would go with some of her friends, Tubby Farquhar and Maureen and Fritz Brink. I would join them later when Deirdre was skiing at Ruislip in London.

This arrangement suited me fine, as I was working long hours at the time and this would give me a chance to catch up. More and more foreign patients were being referred to my unit for treatment. The children with congenital lesions were, as a rule, the more complicated ones – like the severely blue babies with absence or underdevelopment of the arteries to the lungs, or children with three and two-chamber hearts and those with the main arteries coming off the wrong pumping chamber.

Because these defects were extremely difficult to correct and needed an experienced surgeon – either Marius or I operated on them.

I also still received a lot of mail which I wanted to attend to myself. This meant long hours in my office mostly after a full day in the operating room.

Although most of the letters were complimentary and flattering I was getting more and more poison-pen letters – most of them just rude and derogatory – but a few of them were full of anger and hate and made serious threats on my life.

My life, both private and professional, was attacked. Accusations ranged from being Satan to playing God, from being a dirty old man to being a playboy.

At the beginning I was naive enough to read these letters – and they hurt me very much. But I've since decided that, if the writer is too much of a coward to put his name and address on the letter, it goes straight into the wastepaper basket – without even a cursory glance at the contents.

I never took the death threats seriously – except one, when the time and place of my death had been clearly and carefully planned.

Louwtjie and I had been invited to the capital of the ostrich farming area, Oudtshoorn, in the Little Karoo. There would be an official dinner and also a visit to one of the great wonders of the world, the famous Cango Caves.

The caves had been discovered by the San – the original hunter gatherers of Southern Africa, who were systematically wiped out by marauding black tribes from the north and the white colonists from the south. The caves are in a kind of oasis in the hot and dusty semi-desert. The San had called this area 'Kango – place rich with water'.

Within this cave system is a fabulous display of speleotherms – stalactites, stalagmites and helictites, some of them absolutely enormous and thousands of years old.

Visitors are shown around these caves and, at one point during each tour, in order to get the full impact of the grandeur of this natural subterranean wonderland, the lights are turned off.

The writer of the letter I'd received knew that I was to visit these caves and said that, when the lights were turned off, I would be killed.

I tried not to worry about it but the South African police were more concerned and provided some bodyguards for me. Dutifully we all trooped into the caves and finally reached the spot where the lights were turned off. My bodyguards moved a little closer and I wondered if my paper assassin had already drawn a bead on me.

As the lights went out I couldn't help myself from shuffling a couple of spaces to the left but nobody attempted to kill me.

When we were all outside in the sun again one policeman said, 'There you are – I told you there was nothing to worry about.' But I couldn't help notice that he was sweating as much as I was and I detected a faint tremor in his hands as he lit a cigarette.

The following week Louwtjie, André and their friends left for Madrid to join Eduardo and his family.

Meanwhile, invited surgeons were arriving in Cape Town every day. Whenever possible I met them in person at the airport and with every arrival, of course, there was a press conference. Some answered the questions quite briefly – like Denton Cooley who, when asked what he had come for, joked, 'I've come here to save Blaiberg's life.'

'Too late,' quipped Bob Molloy, one of the few journalists I respected, 'he's already been saved.'

Dr Kantrowitz didn't joke and was most complimentary when facing the reporters as he arrived.

Adrian Kantrowitz, America's first heart transplant surgeon, faced the newspaper reporters on his arrival in South Africa with apparent ease and listened to their questions.

He gave his full attention to lighting his pipe before he spoke. Finally, after the third match, he said, 'Heart transplantation is still a clinical trial, except for one man Professor Chris Barnard.

'The man is relentlessly dedicated to his task and, as far as I'm concerned, Chris Barnard regards heart transplants as regular procedure – an achievement none of us can claim.

'Although heart transplant surgery is still in its infancy Chris Barnard has been doing better than all of us.'

Bob Molloy, a well-seasoned reporter from Cape Town, made precise notes and checked how much time he had before deadline to phone his story through to the Cape Times.

'Why should Chris Barnard be the only surgeon in the world to have been so successful?' he asked the professor.

'Why?' said Kantrowitz, removing his pipe and studying the glowing embers for a few moments, 'I'll tell you why – it's just that he's better than we are. All of us. He and his entire transplant team in Cape Town

are leading the field in this challenging and exciting branch of surgery – make no mistake about that.'

The conference was convened in one of the lecture halls of the University of Cape Town. There were two one-and-a-half hour sessions in the morning and two in the afternoon – for five days.

Each day was planned carefully and divided into major topics such as 'Patient Selection', 'Donor Selection', 'Surgical Technique', 'Rejection and its treatment' and, finally, 'Post-operative problems – results and the future'.

I was proud of the standard of the organization which had been handled mainly by Stoffie Stoffberg. All the finer details had been extremely well attended to and a lot of ground was covered over the five days.

The social side of the conference was also of the highest standard. The lunch at Leeuwenhof, the home of Dr Nico Malan, administrator of the Cape, was a memorable event. He gave a very inspiring short talk and recited a poem which both Denton Cooley and I have used since at lectures. It was written by an American poet named Sharp:

*Isn't it strange that princes and kings
and clowns that caper in sawdust rings
and common people like you and me
are builders for eternity.
Each is given a bag of tools,
a shapeless mass, a book of rules
and each must make 'ere time has flown
a stumbling block or a stepping stone.*

This poem has always been of great inspiration to me in later years.

One evening we had dinner with the prime minister at his official residence. John Vorster, with his dry humour, charmed all the guests.

Later that week, I gave a party at the house of my Italian friend, Emiliano Sandri. He was in Europe and had said I could use his home overlooking the sea, where the Atlantic rollers dashed against the rocky shore. He was a very successful restaurateur and his restaurant, La Perla, supplied the food and drinks.

Don Mackenzie, being a fashion photographer, also ensured that the most beautiful Cape Town models came to keep the surgeons happy and keep them up-to-date on female anatomy. Of all the cities and countries I've visited, I've yet to find one that boasts as many stunning women. The visitor to South Africa has only to stroll along Clifton Beach to understand what I mean.

When the surgeons finally left Cape Town, we gave each of them an ostrich egg signed by all of the doctors present. I've visited several of these surgeons since and the ostrich eggs take up a very prominent position in their offices.

Every day I received phone calls from Spain to ask when I would be arriving. According to Maureen Brink, Eduardo Barreiros had made the most extensive arrangements to please me. 'He's got a speed boat for skiing,' she said, 'there's trap shooting and, every night, the best dinners. We're just waiting for *you*.'

I realized that the correct thing to do was to pack my bags and join them all. But I didn't.

Then the news came that Deirdre had torn her medial ligament while jumping the ramps at Ruislip and she was to have an operation on her injured knee in London. Eduardo had arranged a private plane for Louwtjie and Fritz Brink to fly and see her. They would meet me in London and I could fly back with them.

I still didn't go.

Although it's painful to admit now, I realize that I'd lost interest in my family and old friends. The glitter of the new world I was living in had intoxicated me. I'd become addicted to all it had to offer and wanted more and more of it. My appetite for the good life seemed insatiable.

The final break with Louwtjie was looming fast.

I was determined to accept the invitation to go to the Red Cross Ball in Monaco, even though Louwtjie had made it very clear that, if I did, the marriage would be at an end.

I knew she was serious and, although I tried to rationalize the situation, I think I must have been feeling that if this trip did cause a break-up, then so be it. Maybe I actually *wanted* a divorce? Maybe that would be the best for all concerned?

I have, however, since changed my mind about divorce being the best for all concerned.

I had said to Louwtjie many times, 'How often will I get these chances? I've worked very hard in my life to get where I am and now I've got these great opportunities I'm going to take them – it can't last much longer, after all.'

But she remained adamant that this would be the end of us.

I still couldn't bring myself to refuse the invitation. What man in the world, on a government salary, suddenly finding himself in the limelight, and receiving a personal invitation from Royalty to be their guest of honour, would *not* go?

Fortunately, although the emphasis on my social and private life had shifted dramatically, the same didn't happen in my professional life. In fact, I was working harder than ever before – to show the world that what had happened wasn't a flash in the pan and, perhaps, to prove absolutely that I was one of the best cardiac surgeons in the world.

In the laboratory we were working with new ideas in the field of transplantation and clinically I was operating on more and more complicated defects – often in patients who were considered inoperable by their referring doctors.

As I've said before, maybe I travelled too much and perhaps I accepted too many invitations – because I was frequently away from the hospital and the laboratory. But I always tried to make my trips as short as possible and, when I returned to the country, I invariably went straight back to work.

I was also very fortunate, as I had extremely competent staff to care for the patients when I was away. And, of course, there was Marius.

Stern magazine asked me to address a meeting of high-school children in Frankfurt. The conference was known as the 'Jungen Forst' where budding scientists had an opportunity to exhibit their research projects.

I had an important operation to perform that week so I left Cape Town at 4 pm, flew 9 000 kilometres to Frankfurt during the night and arrived there the next morning. I attended the conference and gave a talk to a most excited and enthusiastic audience. I took the plane back that evening and was in the operating room the following afternoon.

This lifestyle was certainly not the best way to treat rheumatoid arthritis. I now had multiple-joint involvement and only found relief by taking excessive amounts of non-steroidal anti-inflammatory medication – often on an empty stomach.

One morning, getting out of bed, I felt unusually dizzy but thought it was due to the handful of aspirin I'd taken the previous night. Anyway, there was no way I could stay in bed, as the South African Medical Association Congress was in progress in Durban and I had agreed to read a paper at the cardiac session that afternoon.

In the toilet, I noticed my stool was black in colour but I thought that was due to some liquorice I'd eaten the previous day.

After a shower and shave I rushed to the hospital for a quick ward round before catching the plane. The dizziness persisted and, walking up the stairs to the ward, I felt extremely faint.

Sister Geyer was writing a ward-report in her office when I arrived. She stood up to greet me. 'Morning, Professor.' Then she looked more closely at me and added, 'What's the matter with you? You're as pale as a sheet!'

'Morning, Sister. I think I must have eaten something that didn't agree with me,' I replied wearily, slumping into a chair.

'Dr Marius is in the ward, why don't you let him have a look at you?'

I could see she was worried and I got up and walked to the doctor's office to look in the mirror – just as Marius came round the corner.

'What's up? Sister says you look terrible.' he said.

'I'm just dizzy,' I replied, sitting down again.

Marius moved closer and lowered my eyelid to see the colour of the mucous membrane.

'You've lost blood,' he announced immediately. 'Let me do your haemoglobin.'

He pricked my finger to get a drop of blood, put it on a slide and then peered into the haemoglobinometer. 'My God!' he exclaimed, 'your haemoglobin is 10!'

They called Dr Solly Marks, the head of the department of gastroenterology. I told him my symptoms briefly and he examined me, concluding that I was bleeding from a gastric or duodenal ulcer, probably caused by the medication.

'You'll have to stay in hospital for a while, my friend,' Solly pronounced. Then he added, 'How can an intelligent guy like you come to the conclusion that the melena (black stool) is due to liquorice!'

He prescribed two-hourly antacid and Tagamet, a revised, balanced diet – and lots of rest.

But it was serious and I actually collapsed before they could get me into bed. My friend, Don Mackenzie – always on hand with a camera – took a shot which he could probably have sold for a fortune but at my request, he never released it. I looked quite pathetic, being helped onto the bed by nurses and orderlies, in great pain and verging on unconsciousness.

The news hit the newspapers immediately and some kind things were said.

SUCCESS HAS TAKEN ITS TOLL OF BARNARD
Prof. Chris Barnard was admitted to Groote Schuur Hospital yesterday against a background of growing concern at the way he has been driving himself...

DOCTORS WARN BARNARD IT'S TIME TO SLOW DOWN
A long list of public appearances – including a Man- Of-The-Year award in London next month are now in the balance.

According to associates there is likely to be a battle of wills over his future activities.

His engagements are exhausting, and he has a natural diplomacy about not wanting to disappoint people but if he doesn't relax he will become a very sick man.

In the past nine months he has travelled 300 000 miles or an average of 1 000 miles a day. He has been to countless functions in scores of countries, has been grilled on television or by newsmen on an average of twice a week, and has made dozens of speeches.

There were also some nasty comments like the completely unnecessary: LOUWTJIE SAYS SHE'S NOT VERY WORRIED

And the most ridiculous report of them all – written by some lunatic in Italy: BARNARD HAS DEPRESSION OF SUCCESS

Professor Carlo Sirtori said Chris Barnard had a sudden success when he had made the first transplant and his magic moment cannot be surpassed whatever else he does in life.

'*He is trying to overcome his depression with his prodigious activity as a lecturer. The depression finally has affected that part of the brain called the diencephalon which contains all commands of the human body.*

'It is not excluded that Professor Barnard will undergo psychoanalytical treatment.'

Why they waste valuable newspaper space on crap like that I'll never know.

So I was now a patient in my own ward. The next day Phillip Blaiberg came to see me but he could only pronounce that there was nothing wrong with my heart and the newspapers carried a big story about the patient examining the surgeon.

I had many visitors but they only irritated me, because I resented having to admit to being sick myself. The one who annoyed me the most was the senior matron whose only remark, when she entered my ward, was, 'Oh! How the mighty have fallen.'

Spiteful bitch.

I was pleased with a get-well letter from Sophia Loren, but the flowers from Gina Lollobrigida were potential dynamite, so Stoffie pretended they were from his own wife – to avoid any unpleasant scenes with Louwtjie.

Fortunately, there was no further bleeding and the X-rays didn't show any stomach or duodenal ulcer, so I was out of hospital within five days and back in full operation – both in and out of hospital.

As it had been decided not to give me a blood transfusion, I was still anaemic and felt tired and listless. The trip to Monaco was within a week and, as I wanted to be in top form for this engagement, I decided to accept Martin Franzot's invitation to spend a few days in the Kruger National Park.

He had managed to reserve a private camp and suggested that the whole family should come up for a few days – to get away from the hustle and bustle of the city.

The Kruger Park is enormous by any standards and occupies nearly two million hectares between the Sabie and Crocodile rivers. Our camp was on the Lower Sabie river – which is in the best lion country within the park because of its large herds of antelope.

Although the park is majestic and tranquil – with the raw beauty of Africa at its very best on display – the holiday was not a happy one. In fact, I'd seen pallbearers having more fun. Louwtjie tried to dissuade me again from going to Monaco but, as adamant as she was that I should not go, as equally determined was I to go.

After a few miserable days, Martin drove me back to Johannesburg early one morning for my UTA daylight flight to France. Once in the air and being fussed over by the gorgeous stewardesses I quickly put the gloom behind me.

I arrived at Nice airport and was driven by limousine to the Hotel de Paris, next to the casino, where I had a beautiful suite overlooking the yacht basin – the parking-lot of the international jet-set.

The next day I had a press conference, visited local hospitals and then was shown around the famous casino, where millions are lost but rarely won. They pointed out tables where people had blown their brains out after losing their fortunes.

As I was leaving I met the son of Mussolini. He was a piano player in one of the bars. Meeting him reminded me of how time can change the apparently unchangeable and unthinkable. Not so many years before, his father, together with Hitler, had declared war on the world – now he was enjoying a certain celebrity status in Monte Carlo.

That afternoon I rested and prepared for the gala.

Angelo Litrico had made me a special 'smoking' suit (as he called it) for the event.

The ball was an open-air affair and all the special guests first gathered in a hall, where we were introduced to Prince Rainier and Princess Grace. She was even more beautiful than I'd imagined. After a glass of champagne we made our grand appearance and took our seats at the table reserved for the princess and her guests.

I was surprised that the prince didn't sit next to his wife. Prince Alfonso de Borbón y Dampiert, relative of the present king of Spain, Juan Carlos (since killed in an avalanche while skiing), sat on her right and I sat on her left. The next day the newspapers made a big thing of this – that I was not really the guest of honour; otherwise I should have been seated on the right of the princess. Also, Prince Alfonso had had the first dance with her.

I couldn't care less. It was a glittering occasion – there was a cabaret by Charles Aznavour, a spectacular fireworks display and, what I enjoyed most, a few dances with Princess Grace – extensively recorded by a horde of photographers.

She was bubbling over with laughter and chatting gaily but I had the feeling she was only acting. Was there something more that she wanted from life – something she was missing?

After the ball, a few of us were invited to the royal residence in the city – Prince Rainier excused himself and didn't join us – but we continued the party until the early hours of the morning.

Prince Alfonso de Borbón phoned me the next morning and said, 'Look, my yacht is down here in the harbour, why don't you take some time off and spend a few days cruising with us?'

I said that I couldn't because I had to go home; patients were depending on me and that sort of thing.

I say this only because it's true. People can speculate all they like about my private life-style but I retained a very strong sense of responsibility as far as the well-being of my patients was concerned. In fact I often said 'no' to extremely tempting offers, so that I could go back to South Africa and my patients (often to find, I might add, that I needn't have rushed back at all!).

So, I said I couldn't go and he suggested, 'Well, I'll fetch you tomorrow anyway and take you by yacht to Nice airport.'

The airport there is on the sea and he had all the necessary permits for mooring.

He came to fetch me and took me to the yacht and I could have torn my hair out for not accepting his invitation – there were such *beautiful* girls on the yacht, draped in their bronzed (and topless) glory all over the boat! It was like something out of a James Bond movie.

I was damned sorry to miss it. I should have taken Oscar Wilde's advice: the only way to get rid of a temptation is to yield to it.

Stoffie Stoffberg brought the big car to a standstill outside Chris and Louwtjie Barnard's home – 'The Moorings' in Zeekoevlei – and parked next to the silver GSM Dart that Louwtjie had been given as a gift from Eduardo Barreiros.

The press had been having a field day about Chris Barnard's current trip to Monaco – without his wife – and he knew, more or less, what to expect when he saw Louwtjie. The press thrived on sensation and rumours and she just couldn't deal with it.

As soon as he saw her he knew his suspicions were correct. 'I want everything out, Stoffie – everything!' she sobbed.

He saw the soaked Persian carpets – gifts from the shah of Iran – draped over the dustbin. It had been raining and he shook his head sadly.

'I'm sick to death of the whole thing, Stoffie,' she continued. 'All these stories in the newspapers – and I've been getting all kinds of sick phone calls from cranks. I just can't stand it any more!'

He knew about the rumours – Chris Barnard had, according to popu-

lar belief, been systematically sleeping his way through most of the attractive female staff at Groote Schuur Hospital – even before he hit the headlines.

Apart from the stories about Chris and Gina Lollobrigida there were also rumours about Sophia Loren who thought that her own husband was impotent at the time. As she wanted a baby, she had apparently discussed the problem with Chris – and now all kinds of stories were surfacing.

But he knew these weren't true – Chris himself had said so – and he told him most things.

'And I saw him dancing with that Grace Kelly – he even had his hand under her cloak!'

'Don't believe all the stories, Louwtjie,' he said.

'I don't care if they're true or not – I just want him out. Out!'

So Stoffie packed as many of the professor's belongings as he could into the boot of the car and set off for the airport to meet the plane.

He wondered absently as he drove, if the Persian carpets, worth thousands of dollars, had been permanently damaged.

In Nice – on board the playboy's yacht – I'd decided to go home. I think there was a large measure of guilt involved: How could I be here enjoying myself when Louwtjie was sitting miserably at home? So, reluctantly, I flew back to South Africa where Stoffberg came to fetch me at the airport.

As we were driving away, he said, 'By the way, all your belongings are in the boot of the car. Louwtjie has thrown them – and you – out of the house and she says she doesn't want you back. I packed as much as I could in the time.'

'It's been a long time coming, Stoffie,' I said with a sigh. 'Has she filed for divorce?'

'I don't think so – yet – but she says she's going to.'

He drove me to Clifton, a beautiful suburb on the Atlantic coast of Cape Town where the beaches are white and the homes are extremely expensive. In summer the four sandy coves are littered with gorgeous bikini-clad (and some topless) girls, all in lemming-like pursuit of skin cancer and preparing their bodies for future wrinkles.

A very kind lady, Mrs Krugel, had two apartments in a block called La Corniche, and she said I could use the empty one until I found a place to stay.

So Louwtjie and I were to be divorced. This was to have a profound effect on several lives, especially those of my children. At

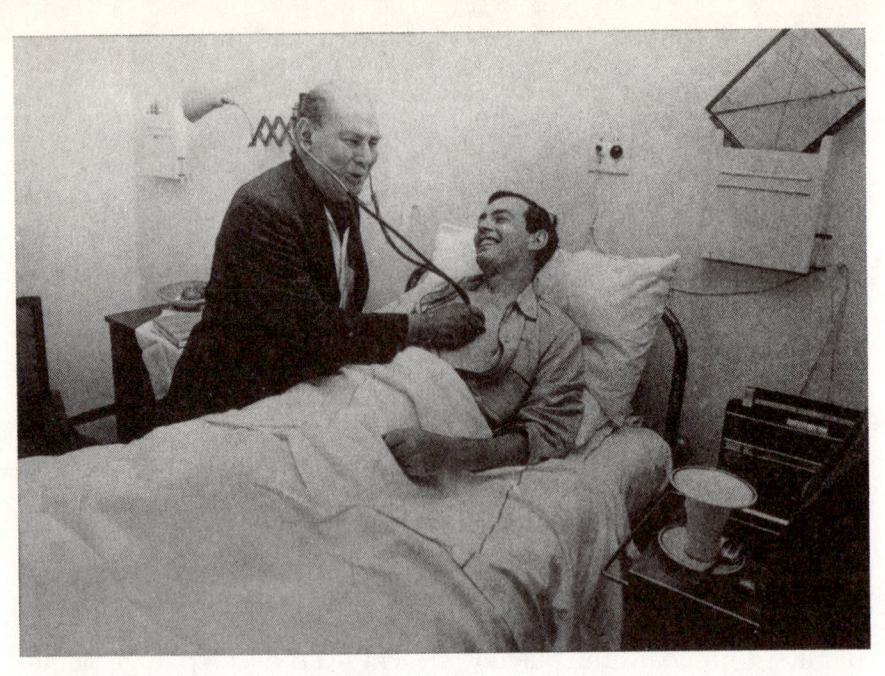

Patient Philip Blaiberg as the doctor

that time André, in his last year of school, was about to join the navy for his national service and Deirdre was at university – and a divorce like the one we were headed for is very tough on the children.

Our children found out about the probable divorce through the newspapers – *before* the two of us had even discussed it properly and before we'd had a chance to tell them personally.

André told me that he heard about it for the first time when he was coming out of his school in Pretoria one afternoon. He read about his parent's separation on the newspaper posters in big bold print. Who can ever quantify the effects of such shocking news to a boy that age?

He'd wandered the streets aimlessly and alone until late that night, in a torment of anger and bewilderment. The one thing about a divorce, and there's no doubt about it, is that it's the children who *really* suffer. I believe that for a child to grow up normally, he should have the mother and the father and, as far as possible, a stable home.

The children of divorce are frightened and frequently depressed orphans of quite a different kind. Even though the parents may be concerned they are seldom able to provide sufficient help and moral or emotional support – so the children live through periods of great stress – confused, helpless and lonely.

In our children's case it was made much worse by Louwtjie's bitterness and animosity and the wide publicity the proceedings attracted. Personally, I would have preferred a quiet and dignified divorce, but that proved to be impossible.

There was nothing we could do to prevent the publicity, so both our children suffered great anguish – probably more than we did ourselves. They read about their own family's unfolding tragedy every Sunday in the South African yellow-press.

I decided the best therapy was to throw myself into my work – and keep a low profile as far as other women were concerned.

I had done two further transplants and we had, at that stage, three out of four transplant patients alive and there was an increasing amount of routine surgery to do.

Patients were now coming from all over the world because they thought we were the only surgeons who could do these operations. They came especially from countries like Italy, Portugal, Romania, African countries and even from Britain.

Diane was an English girl who worked as a freelance journalist in America. She phoned my secretary and asked whether she could interview me for an article she was preparing for a magazine.

Louwtjie, being uncharacteristically cooperative, had allowed her to come to 'The Moorings' and not only helped her with the interview, but also given her lunch and allowed her to rest for a few hours.

I was about to leave for Johannesburg but, to help her, I agreed that, if she could get a seat next to me on the same plane, we could talk during the flight.

When I boarded the plane I made my way to my seat and found Diane already there. We talked for about an hour and as she walked down the aisle to the toilet I noticed she had a fabulous body – not that there was anything I could do about it then.

During our conversation, I mentioned that I would be in Amsterdam in a few days' time. When she suggested we could meet again there I agreed enthusiastically and gave her the name of my hotel.

In Johannesburg she took a plane back to Cape Town and I left for Europe – not thinking I would see her again, as she probably had all the information she wanted. But I was wrong. She was waiting for me as I booked into the hotel in Amsterdam a week later.

I was sure, now, that she was after more than just a story so I told her that I needed a bath and if she wanted to interview me further she would have to do so while I was in the bath.

So we continued our talk – with me lying in the bath and Diane sitting next to me on a stool.

She was asking me about people I'd met and, heaven only knows why I did this – probably to impress her – but I said, 'Diane, if I tell you a story about something quite sensational that happened to me, will you promise that you'll never write about it or tell it to anyone else?'

She promised on her word of honour.

Like a stupid fool I took her at her word – and told her all about my affair with Gina Lollobrigida.

Then she left the room and went back into the suite while I finished my bath. When I got back into the bedroom my journalist was waiting for me under the bedcovers. Maybe it was the story that turned her on or maybe, as Graham Greene once wrote, 'fame is a powerful aphrodisiac'. I don't really know but I slid in under the sheets next to her – and it wasn't to finish the interview.

Some girls are good in bed and some are bad. As far as I was concerned, Diane was really awful. It wasn't making love – we were just having intercourse. It was mechanical, unimaginative and unfulfilling.

When we were finished I lay back in bed and noticed there was a guy outside cleaning the window of the bedroom. I don't know how much he saw but I'm sure he was even more bored than I was.

Lying back in the rumpled sheets I was reminded of a story which made me chuckle. It was about a little French boy who was playing in the garden of his father's *pension*. He came running back to tell his father that there were two people making love on the lawn.

'My son,' said the father, 'it's Paris and it's spring – it's only natural.'

'Yes Papa,' said the boy, 'but the lady is dead!'

This was serious, so the father went outside to see for himself, and what his son had told him was true, so he ran back inside and phoned the police.

'Constable! There are two people making love on my lawn,' he said breathlessly.

'Monsieur,' he said, 'it's Paris and it's spring – it's only natural.'

'Yes, I know that, but the woman is dead!'

So the large gendarme, complete with waxed moustache, cape and stick came to the house and the father showed him the way to the garden.

After a minute he returned smiling broadly – he had solved the case. 'Monsieur, the lady is not dead – she's English.'

I had agreed, with some reluctance, that we should have dinner together that evening and Diane finally left for her own hotel.

I was enjoying the warmth of the bed and idly watching the window cleaner when my phone rang. It was MC Botha. He was in Amsterdam and told me we'd been invited to what promised to be a fabulous party at a friend's country house. Jan de Hoop was a bachelor who knew all the beautiful girls of Amsterdam. We agreed we would go together.

I immediately phoned Diane and told her I couldn't make dinner that evening as my immunologist had arrived and that we had important matters to discuss.

The party was everything that MC had promised. There was a whole troupe of the most beautiful women I'd ever seen – a huge harem, a wondrous assortment of shapes, colours and sizes. I felt like a schoolboy being given the freedom of a sweet shop – and I couldn't make up my mind which of the goodies to grab first. But then I met Monique Pell who was absolutely stunning. She wore the shortest mini-skirt imaginable – not much wider than a leather belt – the crowning glory of the most shapely legs I'd ever seen. Her halter top fitted like a second skin and her spectacular breasts strained against the silky material.

She'd arrived with a friend of ours – an immunologist called Hans Balner – but that didn't stop me from giving her all my attention. I really turned on the charm as I tactfully steered her away from the rest of the group and into a quiet corner, where I did my very best to persuade her to travel with me.

Stern magazine had arranged for me to go to Heidelberg the next day by train to lecture at the university. I asked Monique to join us and she said she wasn't absolutely sure, but promised to meet me at the station if she could change her plans.

The following morning I was waiting on the platform with my colleagues for the train – anxiously searching for Monique and hoping that she would make it – when fate dealt a cruel blow – because Diane came tripping through the station.

She swooped down on us like a hawk and started chatting excitedly about coincidences – while I silently prayed that Monique *wouldn't* show up now.

Of course, a few minutes later she came running down the platform towards us, struggling with her suitcase. While trying to avoid gaping at her deliciously long legs and the promises they carried I introduced her and pretended she was Hans Balner's friend.

But Monique turned to me and laughed, 'So, I kept the promise I made last night at the party to come to Heidelberg with you!'

Diane looked at me and I could see the venom in her narrow eyes. I'm sure she would have loved to have screamed, 'You bastard!' but, instead, she picked up her bag and said, 'Well, I mustn't keep you, Professor, I can see you have things to do.' She turned sharply about-face and marched off down the platform.

Oh well, she was a lousy lay anyhow. Although I knew this could be trouble, I didn't realize just how much.

Heidelberg, on the River Neckar, has the oldest university in Germany and is famous for its 12th century castle. I had been warned before the lecture that there might be demonstrations by the students against South Africa. I decided to use the technique that General Smuts had used when addressing a group of striking Welsh miners. When he'd begun to talk he had said, 'Gentlemen, I've heard so much about the Welsh and how beautifully they can sing, I would appreciate it so much if you would sing me a few songs before we start.' They'd sung with great enthusiasm and, after that, were eating out of his hand.

The hall was packed with students when I walked up to the podium. 'Ladies and Gentlemen,' I began, 'I believe there's a song called "I lost my heart in Heidelberg" – do you know it?'

'Yes! Yes!' they shouted.

'Would you mind singing the song for me? But first I need a conductor.' So I chose a very pretty girl in the front row and invited her on to the platform.

The students sang enthusiastically and she conducted them vigorously. There was no demonstration and I made many friends among the students. I think they admired me as much for my taste in women as they did for my work, because many of them looked enviously at Monique.

After the lecture a journalist said to me, 'You will never be accepted as a professor.'

'Why not?' I asked.

'Because you don't behave like a professor.' He was probably referring to my informality.

I turned to the journalist and said calmly, 'I would much rather be remembered as Chris Barnard the human being, not Chris Barnard the professor.'

During my career I've never lied about my results and I've never pretended to be what I'm not. My honesty, I'm told, is usually so blunt, it borders on being rude. Maybe that was responsible for a lot of my troubles.

'Heaven has no rage like love to hatred turned, nor hell a fury like a woman scorned'. I was painfully reminded of that truth when Bill Pepper phoned me from Rome two weeks later.

'Chris, you'd better come to Rome and make amends to Gina because she's going to tear you to pieces – she's as mad as hell!'

'Why? What have I done?' Not understanding the problem.

'There's an article in a German magazine this week. Don't you remember an interview you gave to an English journalist in Amsterdam?'

Oh my God. How could I have been so stupid as to trust such a bitch? I said, 'I can't come to Rome now.' I wanted more time to think.

'Chris, I think it's vital that you come as soon as possible – your whole future's at stake.'

'Okay, I'll be there tomorrow night,' I reluctantly agreed.

Bill fetched me from the airport and took me to his apartment in Trastavere. When I walked into the lounge, Gina was sitting in an armchair and I think she'd had a few drinks. As soon as she saw me her eyes flashed and she greeted me, 'You fucking bastard!' This, I sadly reflected, was rather different from the endearments we'd exchanged the last time we were together.

I said, 'Darling, please don't be like that – I'm as angry as you are and very sorry too.'

'Don't call me "darling" – look what you told these people,' she screeched, waving a newspaper wildly in front of my face. 'How *could* you!'

I lied like crazy and, with fingers crossed behind my back, pleaded, 'I never told them Gina – I don't know how they got the story.'

She was still as mad as all hell and demanded 'Here's a piece of paper – now you write down what a fantastic woman I am and you apologize to me and say how sorry you are!'

Well, I didn't have any option, so I wrote what she wanted me to say and that seemed to calm her down.

When she finally left the apartment with a few choice Italian phrases which I guessed weren't meant to be complimentary, Bill said, 'Look, here's the letter!' She'd obviously dropped it on her way out so I quickly picked it up and the evening ended there – for me at least – because I believe Gina crashed her car into a wall, or a pole, on her way home.

But the *trouble* didn't end there because, a few weeks later, she sued me and the magazine for an enormous amount of money. I almost passed out when I saw her lawyer's letter. Where was I going to raise that sort of money? But my lawyer, and old friend, Noel Tunbridge, somehow got me out of it without my having to pay a cent.

That was the last time I had anything to do with Gina Lollobrigida until quite recently when I saw her sitting with a gentleman in the bar of the Pierre Hotel in New York. I decided to say hello to her so I wandered up to where she was sitting and said, 'Hi, remember me?' She looked up with a withering sneer and snapped, 'Unfortunately, yes – go away.'

The man later phoned me and apologized for her behaviour.

Gina, if you read this book, I want you to know that I deeply regret what happened. You are a very special lady and I'll always treasure the wonderful time we spent together. The media are really the reason our relationship didn't succeed.

The transplant programme was slowing right down because of the lack of donors. Several of the patients referred by the cardiologists were excellent candidates but they died before suitable donors could be found.

There were several reasons for the shortage of donors. In those early days, we had not yet perfected the technique where the heart could be preserved for several hours before transplantation. This meant the donor had to be in the adjoining operating room so that the heart could be connected to the patient's circulation as soon as possible after removal. It was therefore only possible to use donors who were pronounced dead in our hospital or in a nearby hospital and could be transferred to our unit very quickly.

Today, with the technique of paralyzing the heart while cooling it down – known as cardioplegic hypothermia – and then keeping it on ice, one can safely transplant a heart up to four hours after removal. This makes it possible to remove hearts from donors in hospitals several hundred kilometres from the transplant unit and then even fly the heart by jet to the recipient if necessary.

The second reason for the shortage of hearts was the publicity that donors and their families were subjected to. Soon after every transplant, the reason for the donor's death and every intimate detail about his or her life were extensively exploited by the press, often causing acute embarrassment.

I remember being presented with a young girl of 18 who was a very suitable donor. We had a patient who was very close to death and waiting in the transplant unit for news of a new heart.

When I approached the father for permission to use his daughter's heart, he said, 'Professor, I have no objection against my daughter's organs being used for transplants – you can have her kidneys and her eyes – but not her heart. You see, she committed suicide by taking an overdose of barbiturates. If I donate her heart the details of her suicide will be in the press and I cannot allow that to happen.'

As a result of this refusal the recipient – my patient who was waiting for transplant – died before we could get another donor. I suppose one could say the press were ultimately responsible for this death – but it's an academic argument.

Last, but not least important, was the lack of cooperation from the neurosurgeons. Their approach was 'why should we bother when Chris Barnard is the only one who benefits from our hard work'.

They became petulant about the heart transplant programme and, whenever the opportunity presented itself, expressed their 'moral indignation' about it. But, moral indignation is, in reality, only 2% moral, 48% indignation and 50% pure envy. They conveniently forgot the dying patients – and that only they could prevent these deaths by helping us with donors.

I was told a story by a doctor working in the multiple injury unit at Groote Schuur who'd called in a neurosurgeon to declare a patient brain-dead. After the surgeon had examined the patient and agreed there was no evidence of brain activity he suddenly decided he wanted another blood test, for reasons nobody could understand. It was late that afternoon and he said he would come the next morning to look at the results.

The young doctor, realizing that during the night the patient's circulation could deteriorate so drastically that the heart could never be used by my team for a transplant, suggested that he deliver the results to the neurosurgeon's house as soon as they were ready.

The neurosurgeon turned on the doctor and snapped, 'If you come to my house and disturb me I'll put my dogs on you!' And he stormed out of the hospital, determined to be as uncooperative as possible.

Because of these problems, I decided to explore the possibility of using animal hearts – xenografts. The baboon is a primate readily available in South Africa where they are considered as vermin and often killed by the farmers – so we gave serious consideration to using them as donors.

The virologists, however, warned us that there was a virus endemic in the baboon that caused only mild illness in the animal due to its naturally acquired resistance – or immunity – but in humans, who had no natural resistance, it could cause a fatal infection. It was therefore necessary to test every baboon and isolate those which showed they had not yet contracted the infection. Eventually we had about a dozen of these virus-free baboons of various blood groups.

We realized that control of rejection would be a major problem and decided we would resort to transplanting a baboon heart only in extreme emergencies.

The possibility presented itself when a young Italian boy, Paolo Fiocca, arrived at our unit. The newspapers said he had been referred to me by Sophia Loren although I had no way of knowing this, as she'd never personally spoken to me about him.

I could see the suffering in this little boy's pale blue face. He had never known what it was like to be normal, what it was like to breathe without struggling for breath. He'd never experienced the excitement of being able to play and keep up with his friends. How unfair, I thought, when I examined him for the first time. What sin had this little fellow committed to be punished like this?

Paolo was a brave kid, mentally advanced beyond his age and willing to cooperate, although he often objected loudly – in his broken English – to the treatment that he had to receive.

On investigation we found that his heart was extremely deformed. He had been born with only one lower pumping chamber, the right one being functionally absent. The only reason he survived at all after birth was that there were large holes between the two upper and two lower chambers. This allowed right-sided and left-sided blood to mix freely and also made it possible for the left lower chamber to pump blood both to the body and to the lungs.

The major problem, however, was that because of the reduced resistance of the lung – being much lower than in the body – it received about three-quarters of the blood with every contraction of the pumping chamber. Consequently the lungs were being persistently flooded and were extremely wet most of the time, leading to severe breathlessness and repeated attacks of pneumonia.

This brave boy was dying without ever having had the opportunity to enjoy life.

I'd never operated on this type of abnormality. We usually considered them, in those days, to be uncorrectable and sent them home to die.

But now we could replace the heart. If successful, it would be the answer. We decided that the only way to save Paolo was a heart transplant.

There was only one snag – we couldn't use the heart of an adult donor as it wouldn't fit into his little chest. Donor hearts usually came from people who had been assaulted or had been involved in motor car accidents. Children were infrequently available as donors.

We waited and waited and, before our eyes, Paolo deteriorated until it was essential for us to act without further delay. 'We have to operate today, Marius,' I decided one morning after visiting Paolo.

'But what about a donor Chris?'

'We'll use a baboon,' I tried to sound as confident as possible.

'Are you *serious*?' Marius stopped dead in his tracks.

'Yes, do you have a better suggestion?'

I phoned Bossie at the medical school laboratory and told him to get one of the baboons in isolation, with a compatible blood group, ready. He would have him shaved, anaesthetized and draped and, when I gave him the signal, he would remove the heart and rush it to the Red Cross Hospital about 5 kilometres from Groote Schuur, where I was to perform the operation.

When I opened the sac in which the deformed organ was hidden it seemed to want to burst out of the chest. It was severely enlarged, due to the seven years of labour under an increased burden, and the arteries to the lungs were at least three times the normal size – dilated to cope with the excessive amount of blood being carried.

'Tell Bossie to start taking out the baboon's heart,' I said – to no one in particular.

There was one other option. I could band the pulmonary artery and, in that way, increase the resistance to the flow in this vessel thus reducing the quantity of blood flooding into the lungs from the heart. Should I risk that first and do the transplant if it failed?

The problem is easy to understand, as I've explained many times. If you imagine a pump pumping water into two pipes; one pipe leads to a patch of grass slightly uphill and the other to a patch of grass slightly downhill. You'll find that due to the decrease in the resistance in the pipe running downhill, more water will flow to the patch it supplies and it will soon become flooded. Due to the increased resistance in the pipe running uphill there will be less water on that patch of grass.

To correct, or balance, the situation, one can partially close the tap on that pipe running downhill, thus decreasing the quantity of water-flow.

In cardiac surgery this is done by snaring the pulmonary artery (the artery that leads to the lung) with a cotton tape and then slowly tightening the snare, until the resistance it creates is about equal to the resistance imposed by the artery leading to the body. There is, however, a very small margin for error because, if you tighten the snare too much, the heart will fail acutely and the patient will become very blue – and die.

I placed the tape around this enormous pulmonary artery and monitored the pressures in the artery distal to the tape and also the pressure in the aorta.

I started tightening the snare – no change. A little tighter – still nothing. Tighter still. Then Ozzie called excitedly, 'Chris, it's working! The pulmonary artery pressure's dropping as well as the venous pressure – the circulation has improved too.'

'Okay Ozzie, I'm going to tighten it some more – keep telling me.' I started tightening the snare even further, little by little. Suddenly the heart slowed down.

'The arterial pressure's dropping and the venous is rising!'

'I'll loosen the tape slightly.' Immediately the heart picked up again. I looked at Marius, 'This seems to be as tight as we should make it – let's fix it in this position.'

'The baboon heart is here, Prof.' It was Bossie putting his head around the operating room door.

'Fortunately we won't need it, Bossie.'

The baboon had given his life in vain and Bossie, a great animal lover, drooped his head as he turned and left.

Paolo did well and went back to Italy – not to return to his usual life but, to a life of significantly improved quality.

When I discussed the operation with Vel Schrire the next day, he said he was glad we hadn't used the baboon heart, because it would be interpreted by the press that we were experimenting on children and the public wouldn't take kindly to that.

I didn't see it the same way. If I'd had to use an animal heart, I would have offered the child the only treatment that was available. That was my duty as a doctor. But, then, I've always been less diplomatic than most surgeons and certainly not as cautious.

Although Louwtjie and I were not yet divorced, she and her lawyer had drafted a document outlining the conditions for the settlement and served it on Noel Tunbridge, who was acting on my behalf.

In the final analysis it meant I would become as impoverished as they could make me. All I would be allowed to take from my house in Zeekoevlei were my clothes. Louwtjie would continue to live there until she died, or got married again. I would pay for the rates, taxes, insurance and maintenance of the property. She also asked for an allowance of R500 a month – and I had to pay for the education of our two children as well.

This placed an awesome financial burden on someone like me. At that stage, I was earning only R1 200 a month – before tax (at a time when the rand was worth about $3). But, as I didn't want the divorce to become a protracted legal wrangle, I was totally compliant and instructed Noel – against advice given me from many quarters – to agree to everything.

I was now leading a bachelor's life in the two-roomed flat on Clifton beach so generously offered to me by Mrs Krugel. She lived with her boyfriend and daughter, Mercedes, at San Michele – a block of flats next to La Corniche. Giela Krugel was an exceptionally good cook and I was often invited to have dinner with her, her boyfriend and her ex-husband – who had an apartment in the same block. They had such an amicable arrangement and I fervently hoped this would be the case after my divorce too. But I knew it was highly improbable.

I had resolved not to get married again but I found it unbearable to come home at night to an empty and silent flat. There were none of the usual domestic noises, nor the earthy smell of a woman around.

This wasn't difficult to remedy. But I decided to be very discreet as I was attracting constant attention from the press. I made sure I was hardly ever seen publicly in the company of women. When I arranged to meet a girl it was always at the flat. Some were friends and just came round for a social drink. Some were more than just friends and would sometimes stay the night.

Because of my reputation people assumed that every woman I met ended up in my bed, but most of the stories were wildly exaggerated.

Some time ago I was even listed by *Paris Match* as one of the four greatest lovers in the world – along with Princess Astrid of Belgium, Björn Borg and Christina Onassis.

As Louwtjie correctly said in the hotel in San Francisco, I just wanted to satisfy myself that I could get any woman I wanted – but she was only partly right because, although I loved female company, I often found the chase far more enjoyable than the conquest.

I think, generally, that women enjoyed being in bed with me because, when it came to making love my own satisfaction was not as important as feeling their excitement and climax. I truly enjoy anticipating a woman's desires and fantasies – and making them happen – hopefully with a bang.

There was one girl, however, who carried this a bit too far because every time she had an orgasm she would lose all bladder control and wet the bed, which wasn't romantic. I suppose I could say I got pissed off.

5

Due to the resistance we encountered in the hospital, it was now nearly 9 months since our last transplant. This wasn't good for the morale of the team, or for the programme as a whole, as the experience gained by the previous operation became vague with time.

The requirements for a successful heart transplant are a patient with terminal heart failure as determined by the cardiologists and a patient whom the neurosurgeons have declared brain-dead.

We'd had a few referrals from the cardiologists during this time, but they all died because donors couldn't be found.

Then 32 year old Pieter Smith, who had reached the terminal stages of a heart muscle disease of unknown cause, called idiopathic cardiac myopathy, was admitted. As the deterioration of his heart was very rapid his general physical condition hadn't suffered very much. Patients in long-standing heart failure often become cachectic – like a patient suffering from cancer. Experience has shown that they do not do well on high doses of cortisone. So Pieter Smith was an ideal candidate for transplantation – we could save his life.

The team was alerted and we were all geared for the operation. Meanwhile, however, he was so desperate and in such pain, that he actually attempted to commit suicide to relieve himself of the suffering. That's how bad it was.

The evening after he tried to end his life, the neurosurgeons finally, and I suspect reluctantly, phoned to say they had a black woman whom they had declared dead and whom we could consider as a potential donor.

All the tests indicated that she would be an excellent donor. The only problem was that it was about midnight and we couldn't find any relatives to give permission for the removal of her heart. We sent the police to look for the relatives but in those days, in the height of the apartheid regime there was no question of locating anyone in the black residential areas at that time of night.

In extreme circumstances such as this, the law does allow permission to be given by the district surgeon and medical superintendent. But they both hesitated, because it involved a black donor and they were terrified it could lead to a scandal. Their recalcitrance would prove to be much more harmful in the end.

When I realized they were still agonizing over the problem and nowhere near a decision – while the donor heart was deteriorating and another man's life was in the balance – I phoned the attorney general in desperation and explained the dilemma I was in, asking if he could give permission.

'Professor Barnard,' he replied, 'I don't have the power to give that permission, but I do understand your position. There is only one way in which I can help, I will undertake not to prosecute you.'

That was enough permission for me and we performed a very successful transplant that night.

The next morning the local papers started sniffing around and guessed there might be a 'good' story. They sent out reporters and, after several hours the following day, found the relatives of the donor. We, on the other hand, hadn't had the luxury of time and daylight.

Of course, the relatives, when encouraged by reporters, were 'against' the transplant and would 'never' have given permission. A well-posed picture was published of a black man and some children huddled forlornly together, bemoaning the lack of respect I had for their feelings.

Then one of the newspapers decided to give these people the legal assistance to sue me. It would be scurrilous for me to suggest that the story was 'created' rather than 'reported', but there *was* a proliferation of 'cheque-book journalism' in the sixties.

We had not released the name of the donor because, after consultation with me, Dr LAPA Munnik and the hospital superintendent had decided that it would be hospital policy from then on not to announce the name of donors. So I was prevented from confirming (or denying) that the woman in question was, in fact, the donor.

Unfortunately this event received wide publicity – not only in South Africa, but also from the international press.

I didn't feel guilty at all because I had followed the legal procedure – to the letter. But, because the superintendent and district surgeon were timid beyond belief and wanted to avoid confrontation, they actually exacerbated the situation and made the whole thing much worse. All the fuss would have been avoided had they simply done their jobs.

Meanwhile, Pieter Smith made a remarkable recovery and was discharged from hospital six weeks after the operation. He did a lot for the heart transplant programme, as he was the first patient with a new heart to play on a tennis court and prove that transplant patients could fully participate in competitive sports.

He unfortunately died – not from his heart – but from a carcinoma of his stomach, two years after his transplant.

Everybody warned me to refuse the invitation by David Frost to appear live on his show in London. Several previous guests had been brought close to tears by his vicious interview techniques but, to me, this was a challenge – after all he couldn't know more about heart transplantation or, for that matter, about medicine generally than I did – so how could he embarrass me?

When I arrived at the studio one afternoon I briefly met David and he was very charming and friendly. Being a doctor, I closely scrutinized him and my eyes finally rested on his hands. I noticed that his fingernails were very dirty – which I thought might be useful retaliatory information if he became nasty during the interview.

My white shirt wasn't suitable for TV so I changed into a blue one and we took our seats in front of the cameras and the live audience.

After the opening credits of the *David Frost Show – live from London* Frost turned to me and asked, 'Professor Barnard, you removed the heart of Evelyn Jacobs without the permission of her relatives – how could you be so insensitive? Or is it that, as an Afrikaner, you have no respect for the feelings of black people?'

I was caught completely unawares. I had no idea that his questions were going to be in that direction. But, I recovered quickly enough to hide my surprise.

'Mr Frost, where did you get the name from? Because we aren't allowed to name the donors.'

'It was in all the newspapers!' he exclaimed, waving a paper with the family picture in my face.

'Mr Frost I'm surprised that an experienced journalist like you would believe everything you read in the newspapers.' I could see, with some gratification, that he was getting annoyed.

'But was she the donor?' he demanded.

I sat back in my chair – now completely relaxed – and replied, 'I just told you, we aren't allowed to identify the donor.'

We argued backwards and forwards on this point and then, in desperation, he asked, 'Have you ever removed a heart from a donor, without getting permission from the relatives?'

He's got me now, I thought. I could not lie but, as a heart surgeon, I had learned to think quickly. Looking as innocent as possible I replied, 'Mr Frost the law of my country clearly states that I have to get permission before removing any organ.'

I was praying that he wouldn't ask the obvious, such as whether I'd ever disobeyed the law – but he didn't.

We then went on to other aspects of transplantation and eventually I had him so confused, that the audience was laughing at him openly.

Frost was furious and continued the programme for fifteen minutes longer than its allotted time, but he couldn't get the better of me because anger only amplifies stupidity.

It was exhilarating to see a favourable report about me in the newspapers the following morning for a change, and I was delighted to read the main story of the day:

FROST NO MATCH FOR
QUICKSILVER BARNARD
David Frost clearly met his vocal match during his interview with Professor Barnard.

The brilliant Frost, who has handled a cardinal, the Prime Minister and countless other celebrities with equilibrium, was noticeably out of his depth with the quicksilver Prof Chris Barnard...

When I left he wished me a pleasant journey home and, as soon as I'd gone, he arranged for one of his researchers to visit Cape Town a few weeks later to gather information on my activities.

Two months later I was invited back on his show but decided that the better part of valour was to turn down the invitation.

T.V. STAR FROST, BEATEN BY BARNARD, WANTS A RETURN MATCH.

Smarting under the defeat he suffered at the hands of Professor Chris Barnard in a television debate three weeks ago, Mr David Frost has been trying to get Barnard on his programme again to even the score.

Professor Barnard was not available for comment this weekend but it is believed to be highly unlikely that one of the busiest surgeons in the world will drop everything and fly to London to satisfy Frost's vanity.

Frost couldn't swallow the defeat and did a show about me anyway – without my being there – saying how I'd deceived the public.

Little did I know that our paths would cross again in time.

Meanwhile, Giorgi Mondadori was unhappy about progress on the biography. As I had promised all the royalties from the book to the Chris Barnard Fund, Lionel Murray, chairman of the fund, suggested to them that they should send Bill Pepper to Cape Town for a few months.

I liked the suggestion because, in the brief period that we were together, I became very fond of Bill. It was a great pleasure to work with such a wise and sensitive man. He eventually arrived in Cape Town and stayed at the Clifton Hotel – next to La Corniche.

During the following weeks we worked together whenever possible together on *One Life*. We decided that the book would deal with my childhood, my student days, my days as a young doctor and culminate with the first heart transplant.

I showed Bill the medical school where I'd studied, the laboratories where I did my research and the hospital. He watched several heart operations so that he could experience the smells, the sounds and the exciting atmosphere of the operating room.

We visited Ceres, the town where I'd settled as a young married man in family practice for two years. We travelled 450 kilometres to Beaufort West where I was born and went to school. It is a little farming town in the Karoo where my father was a missionary for nearly 50 years. I hadn't been back there since my father retired in 1950.

The scars of apartheid were everywhere in the area – but nowhere more painful for me than when I walked into my father's church. It was no longer being used as a church, because it had been built 75 years previously in an area of the town that had since been declared for whites only. My father's congregation had been mostly coloured people and they loved him.

The pews had been removed and the organ sold. The pulpit, in front of which I was baptized 45 years previously, had been torn down. The empty shell had now been converted into a badminton court.

As I stood before this sacrilegious destruction, I swore vehemently that I would never return to the town until my father's church was restored.

Since then, both the church and the house next door, where I was born, have been restored and converted into a museum. The organ has been re-purchased and re-installed, the pulpit replaced and the baptismal font returned.

Bill left for Rome after about two months. I was sad to say farewell to him, as he had become my adviser and given me moral support. But he'd collected all the material necessary to complete the book.

When one makes a friend like that it is inconceivable, at the time, that such a friendship could ever fade away. Unfortunately, after the book was published our paths just drifted in different directions – for no specific reason – rather like the song, 'And remember that the best of friends must part...'

When I look back over my life it's quite uncanny how my destiny has been fashioned by casual meetings and irrational or unimportant decisions. I had never heard of Minneapolis, nor did I have the vaguest notion of studying there until one day, purely by chance, I bumped into my professor of medicine – Dr Brock – in the parking lot of the medical school. At that stage I was a registrar in general surgery. (A registrar is a hospital doctor, senior to a houseman but junior to a consultant, specializing in either surgery or medicine.)

'Chris, how would you like to go to Minneapolis?'

'Minneapolis?' I asked, completely dumbfounded by the suggestion.

'Yes, I think I can get you a bursary to study with Professor Wangensteen.'

So I went to the University Hospital of Minnesota and studied general surgery. But it just so happened, unknown to me then, that in those days one of the leading cardiac surgery teams in the world was very active developing the heart-lung machine, so that surgery could be performed for an extended time inside the heart. This made it possible to perform a wide range of open-heart surgical procedures – including, ultimately, the heart transplant.

About eight months after arriving there I was working in the dog lab one day on a new technique to join the gullet. Just by chance I walked past another laboratory – where Dr Vince Gott was experimenting with a heart-lung machine.

'Chris, would you mind scrubbing up and giving me a hand? My assistant is sick today.'

That was my first encounter with the heart-lung machine and it was responsible for my changing from the general surgery programme to cardiac surgery.

Another change in destiny happened back in Cape Town about three months before I performed the first heart transplant. Professor Kench, for no apparent reason, accused me of being selfish and riding roughshod over my colleagues. That's just the way I am – I expect perfection from myself and from those around me. Often I'm brutally honest, as many theatre nurses and sisters will testify. I've never changed.

Anyway, I left the meeting feeling deeply hurt and, when I sat down in my office, I started idly paging through the latest *British Medical Journal*. I saw an advertisement for a surgical post at the National Heart Hospital in London. I thought, to hell with these people in Cape Town, and applied for the job.

Fate stepped in again in the form of a postal strike and my application arrived in London too late. I did not get the job. It's certain that if I'd uprooted myself and gone to London, I would never have done the first heart transplant.

And another casual meeting, which would *dramatically* change my life, happened after I'd taken Bill Pepper to the airport on his way back to Rome. As I parked my car at the hospital I met Solly Marks, who'd treated my ulcer several months previously.

'Chris, I believe you're a bachelor now,' he smiled.

'Yes, can you find a wife for me?' I joked.

Solly thought for a moment and said, 'You know, I'm going to give a party at my home tonight and I've invited a few friends – one of them is a patient of mine from Johannesburg and he has a fabulous-looking daughter. I think she's just the girl for you – why don't you come?

As it happened I was working that evening and couldn't go to the party but, for some unknown reason, the idea of meeting that 'fabulous-looking' girl haunted me.

A few days later I was invited to the unveiling of some spectacular wood carvings at a synagogue in Johannesburg. I remembered what Solly had said and phoned him. 'Listen Solly, I'm sorry I couldn't make your party the other night but I'm going to Johannesburg tomorrow. Do you think you can arrange for me to meet that girl you told me about?'

There was a long pause and I added, 'Solly, are you still there?'

'Yes Chris, I was just thinking about it. She's barely 18 and the only child of a very wealthy German industrialist. They're quite austere but, what the hell, I'll phone them anyway.'

Fifteen minutes later Solly phoned back, 'You lucky bastard! It so happens that they're having a black-tie dinner at their home the night after your function and they say you're very welcome.'

I booked into the Sunnyside Hotel and went to the function at the synagogue that night. The next evening, I put on Litrico's smoking jacket – the same outfit I'd worn at the Monaco Ball – and went down to the lounge.

There was an old couple having a drink there and I started chatting to them. They must have thought I'd seen a ghost, because I suddenly stopped talking and my mouth fell open as I stared across the room. One of the most incredibly beautiful women I'd ever seen had just walked in and had paused in the doorway, her gaze sweeping the lounge – obviously looking for someone. I prayed this was the girl that Solly had talked about.

Suddenly she recognized me and, without any change in her cool expression, walked towards me.

I'd seen many beauty queens but they all looked the same: long blonde curls, round face, big eyes and lots of teeth. This girl was in a different class altogether. Dressed in a flowing black gown she moved gracefully across the lounge taking long, elegantly slow, strides – the sort of movement to make a poet throw away his pen.

She had brown hair and blue eyes, but her face was so different from the chocolate-box beauties. Her eyes were small, her nose pert and slightly turned up and she had a deep-bronze suntan. Maybe each feature, alone, was not exceptional, but the combination was electrifying.

She stopped in front of me and extended her long, delicate, arm offering me her hand – I glanced down at her perfectly manicured nails as she introduced herself.

'I'm Barbara.'

'Oh yes, yes,' I spluttered. 'I'm Professor – I mean I'm Barnard – I mean – sorry, I'm Chris.' I finished lamely.

Her expression didn't change. 'My father's waiting outside in the car, shall we go?'

I was introduced to Fred Zoellner and we drove in a big black Cadillac to their home, 'Three Fountains' in Inanda, a suburb of the very wealthy.

There were some guests already standing around drinking Moët et Chandon from fluted, crystal glasses. The house was exquisitely furnished. Dr Zoellner had an impressive jade collection and, on the walls, were original old masters. I was completely ignorant about art – although the name 'Brueghel' did ring a bell.

Barbara introduced me to a beautiful blonde German divorcee who would be my partner for dinner. I also noticed an Italian-looking young man by the name of Philip, who was obviously Barbara's boyfriend.

I've often thought I must have been stupid even to have entertained the notion that I had the remotest chance with this beautiful girl – 27 years younger than I was – and the only daughter of very wealthy parents. I couldn't possibly fit in with these people, who talked about art and classical music, but I was determined to try.

The dinner was quite unremarkable, but the wines were of the very best French cultivars and vintages.

One thing I really dislike about dinner parties is sitting around the table afterwards making small talk – so, when the evening reached that stage, I said, 'How about some music and dancing?'

The suggestion was met by some surprised looks. My continued presence was, I think, only tolerated because of who I was and not what I was. They all probably thought I was an uncultured boer, but there was an element of ingenuity in my strategy. I'd realized that my only chance of getting close to Barbara was to dance with her.

Couples began dancing. Philip watched Barbara very closely. After a polite interval I asked Barbara to dance. Fortunately, it was a slow, romantic tune.

She had fantastic rhythm and, what really surprised me, was

that she danced more closely than I ever expected. I well remember the surge of passion that raced through my body as she moved gently against me.

During the dance I casually asked, 'What would you say if I asked you to marry me?'

She looked at me without speaking for a few moments and, with her head tilted quizzically to one side, held my gaze with her smiling eyes and murmured, 'Well, that's an interesting question.'

I didn't know what to say, so I concentrated on dancing but deep down, I had a feeling at that very moment that this young girl in my arms was, one day, going to be my second wife.

When I arrived back in Cape Town I decided to take a break and visit my old friends, Rita and Hentie van Rooyen, in Buffelsbaai (Buffalo Bay) where I'd spent holidays with my wife, and two children, at Christmas for the past four years.

This holiday resort, on the Indian Ocean shores of the Eastern Cape, had several kilometres of spectacular white beaches and I found it very relaxing to go for a long stroll in the early morning and contemplate my life and my lifestyle.

One day, my retrospection was interrupted when I met a mother with her little girl of 6. She stopped me and asked if she could take a photograph of her daughter and me.

'Of course,' I said, and asked the little girl, who had beautiful blue eyes, to come and sit on my lap.

Little did I know that I'd just had a picture taken with my third wife.

Refreshed by my brief holiday, I was looking forward to getting back into the operating theatre and the children who had been admitted to the Red Cross Hospital while I had been away.

On account of my heavy work load and my frequent absences, I decided to move Terry O'Donovan to the Red Cross Hospital virtually full-time. It was essential to have a more senior surgeon on call there. Marius was fulfilling the same duty at Groote Schuur Hospital. These two members of the team were of invaluable help to me in those days and contributed immensely to the successes we were enjoying with very sick patients, who had extreme complications.

Normally, I'd spend the whole of Monday in surgery at Groote Schuur hospital and later, do pre-operative ward rounds at the

Red Cross Hospital. Tuesday was the day I operated on children. Although they were admitted a few days before surgery for tests and studies, I had a rule not to see them until Monday afternoon. I carefully examined the tests and studies beforehand but visited the children themselves only once before the operation. This was because frequent visits could lead to emotional attachments with these little creatures, which might affect my judgment at a critical moment during surgery.

After the operation was finished it was different, and I would make frequent visits to see them in the intensive care wards.

One Monday I was late for the Red Cross Hospital ward rounds and Terry was waiting for me, looking at his watch as I arrived.

'Yes, I'm sorry I'm late, but one of the patients started bleeding and I had to re-open him. Anyway, what do we have?'

'Prof, there's a little girl here from Ireland – she only has a single atrium.'

'Yes, I remember seeing the catheter findings on Saturday,' I said as we walked into the first room.

There, in the ward, and sitting upright, was the most beautiful little girl staring at me with her wide, blue eyes.

'Hello, darling. And what's your name?' I smiled.

'Aileen Brassil – and what's your own?' she asked in her delightful Irish accent.

'Mine is Chris Barnard. But tell me, what's wrong with you, honey?' I asked, taking her hand in mine.

Those blue eyes looked straight into mine as she said, 'Doctor, I have a broken heart.'

Tears suddenly filled my eyes and I started paging through her notes to give me some time to regain my composure. It had probably been the best way her mother could explain what was wrong with her.

I couldn't sleep that night and went over and over in my mind what I had to do. I had to put the superior vena cava catheter in as high as possible and the inferior vena cava catheter as low as possible, so that I would have room and they wouldn't be in my way when I partitioned the common atrium into right and left halves with a plastic patch.

I was confident that I could successfully mend her broken heart without much problem.

Everything went well. Terry already had the heart exposed when I entered the operating room. I inserted the two catheters as planned and went onto by-pass. I made a large incision in the atrial wall and Terry retracted the two edges.

I put the sucker in to empty the heart of the remaining blood and then stared into the cavity in complete disbelief. There were portions of the two valves separating the upper and lower chambers just hanging limply and unattached – with the cordate dangling in the atrium.

'What the hell is this, Terry!' I asked, completely confused. I'd never seen anything like it.

'It looks like a single-chamber heart. I can't see any ventricular septum either,' he replied incredulously.

The division between the upper and lower chambers had not occurred during development of her heart; neither was there a division between the lower chambers. She most certainly did have a broken heart.

I didn't know where to begin correcting this mess. With dissecting forceps, I pulled the unattached portions of the mitral biscupid valve around aimlessly – it looked totally hopeless.

Suddenly it all became very clear to me – an instant revelation – and I knew exactly what I had to do.

It reminded me of a remark Giacomo Manzù, a very famous Italian sculptor, once made. He was doing a bust of me and I went for sittings at his studio several times. One day, walking up the path to his studio I noticed several big blocks of marble just lying around and asked, 'Why haven't you done anything with these?'

He replied, 'Professor, I cannot yet see what's inside them.' I thought that was a very beautiful thing to say. He wasn't, of course, the only sculptor to think this way because I remember seeing the slaves by Michaelangelo, where he didn't quite complete the sculpture, but left the figures emerging from the block of marble.

It was the same with Aileen Brassil's heart – I could now see exactly how I would repair it.

I divided the lower chambers by stitching a plastic patch between them, then I attached the loose leaflets of the mitral and tricuspid valves to the top of this patch – and tested them to see that they wouldn't leak, by filling the lower chambers with water. I divided the upper chamber by stitching a second patch in position.

In order to give me adequate exposure and room to manoeuvre –

so that I could put the stitches in exactly the correct position – I stopped the heart by cooling it down to a low temperature. When I'd finished all the stitching we had to re-start it and then we could also test the efficiency of the reconstruction.

There were two dangers. The first was that because the heart wasn't beating when I placed and tied the stitches, I had no way of knowing whether or not I had damaged the conducting bundle. This could result in heart-block and Aileen's heart would have to be driven by a pacemaker – maybe for the rest of her life.

The second danger was that if I had not attached the loose leaflets of the mitral and tricuspid correctly, it would result in leaking valves. If the leakage was slight it wouldn't matter very much, but if severe, then the heart would fail immediately.

'Start re-warming, Johan,' I ordered the heart-lung technician.

'Warming on, Prof.' The reply came immediately and the tension was running very high. Everyone in the room knew this was the moment of truth. Would this little girl live?

We waited.

I watched the second hand of the theatre clock slowly tick by.

We waited.

Tick-tock, tick-tock. 'Oh aching time, Oh moments big as years.'

Then, very slowly, the miracle we call life began coming back into the heart. The first sign was that it changed colour from a sick blue to a healthy pink. Then, the flabby feeling of the relaxed fibres changed to the firmness of contracted fibres.

'There's ventricular fibrillation!' somebody called out and I could see the uncoordinated contractions of millions of muscle fibres.

'The atria are beating!' another shocked voice said.

To my absolute horror I saw that the upper chambers were contracting, but that the lower chambers were not responding. Oh dear, sweet Jesus – after all this struggle – we've ended up with severe heart-block!

'Give some isoprenaline, Ozzie!' This drug would increase the receptiveness of the ventricles.

'The ventricles are beating, Prof.' Dene's voice sounded far away in the operating room, and only the persistent rhythmic hum of the heart-lung machine pumps could be heard.

Yes! Yes! There was an occasional ventricular contraction. 'Come on, baby!' I whispered urgently, trying to urge life back into the reluctant heart muscles – and, slowly, the heart rate picked up.

'Let's see an ECG strip,' I asked.

Ozzie gave me a printout of the electrical activity so I could study it. It was a 2-1 block – that is, when the ventricle only responds to the second atrial beat.

'She's going to come out of block,' I heard myself say and it was as if Aileen's heart actually heard me. Her heart rate doubled immediately.

'She's out of block!' It was the first time that Terry had spoken.

'But I still think we should put in a temporary pacemaker – these patients can easily go back into block later.'

I stitched some electrodes onto the right ventricle muscle, connected them to a lead and handed the other end out to Ozzie.

'Ozzie, set it so that the pacemaker will kick in when the heart rate drops below 100 – I'll feel much safer that way.'

We closed the atrial incision and stopped the heart-lung machine.

The pressures in the left and right atrium felt low, indicating that there was not a serious leak of the valve.

'Terry, put your hand in and see whether you can feel a thrill.'

He first felt behind the heart over the left atrium and then, in front, over the right. 'No, Prof, I think they're competent.' I could hear the relief in his voice.

The first few days of post-operative care were rough. Aileen went in and out of heart-block a few times but, fortunately, the pacemaker took over every time.

After about three weeks in hospital, she had recovered enough for me to discharge her and she went back to Ireland a few weeks later.

There were all kinds of press reports going on at the time – and a few politicians and rankled doctors also used the opportunity to get some coverage for themselves.

The world can think what it likes about whether I seek publicity or not, but I will always remain absolutely adamant that, where my patients are concerned, I have never had any desire to profit from their illnesses – either financially or in terms of publicity.

It may be true that I am a playboy – it may be true that I am a philanderer and an adulterer. But it's also true that I am, first and foremost, a doctor. That, and that alone, has been my motivation.

BARNARD IN BIG DEMAND
South African heart surgeon, Prof Chris Barnard arrived in Rome today in answer to an appeal by Sophia Loren to examine a group of ailing Italian children.

The fanfare of publicity which preceded Professor Barnard's arrival has led to about 100 Italian mothers asking him to see their children.

Prof Barnard said he didn't know how many children were now awaiting him but added 'I will see them all if they want me to…'

Professor Barnard is expected to communicate with Sophia Loren about Paolo Fiocco and a four year old girl, Silvana Cavallini.

Where they got all these reports and quotes from me, I'll never know. I don't even know if Sophia Loren had anything to do with these patients in the first place – she certainly never wrote to me about them. And it wasn't just happening in Italy either.

BARNARD GIVES HOPE TO ENGLISH PARENTS
A two-year old English child, condemned to death within five years because of his critical heart condition, has been offered a chance of normal life by Prof. Chris Barnard.

Little Philip Camfield's parents of Reading were told by surgeons that there were no facilities in Britain to deal with their son's hole-in-the-heart complication and that he would die any time within the next five years.

The only chance of curing him was to send him to South Africa.

Townspeople of Reading started a collection to send Philip there when they received a letter from Dr Barnard's secretary saying that the treatment in South Africa is free.

Mrs Camfield said the news was 'absolutely wonderful – now there is real hope for Philip'.

As it happened we were able to cure Philip Camfield but then we started getting criticism from different quarters. I myself, or my department, was accused of seeking publicity. Each time a child came to us, the media used every conceivable angle to write controversial headlines.

HEART BOYS IN S.A. CRITICIZED
Italian Minister of Health, Mr Georgio Bonadies said the transfer of Paolo Fiocco and Fabio de Fabris – after an appeal by Sophia Loren – could have been avoided since some heart damage can be treated with surgery in Italy.

BARNARD FACES MEDICAL ROW
Doctors are becoming increasingly annoyed at the way patients are contemplating visiting Professor Barnard for surgery which could just as well be done in Britain.

Dr Derek Stevenson, Secretary of the British Medical Association, told the Daily Express yesterday, 'It is widely recognized that facilities for research into and the treatment of heart cases in Britain are second to none.

'Individual patients would be well advised to consult their own doctor here before making the long and expensive trip to South Africa.'

When I spoke to Mr and Mrs Camfield about the sort of coverage the press was giving the controversial treatment they'd decided upon for their son, they just shrugged and said, 'They told us Philip would die – you said he would live.'
   To them it was as simple as that.
   Then there was Suzanne Jones, a blonde and blue-eyed minx with a lilting Welsh voice who was a heart-stopper for every male who spoke to her – especially me. She was five years old and had the tell-tale blue tinge around her lips – a sure sign of heart disease.
   There had been all manner of criticism about this operation. William Breckon, writing in Britain's *Daily Mail*, said that the operation 'could just as well be carried out by surgeons in Britain' and went on to report how doctors at Cardiff's Sully Hospital were 'angry at the way Professor Barnard's staff have handled this case'.
   Sometimes these reports made me so damned angry I'd kick my desk in frustration. I just couldn't believe these accusations. We weren't canvassing for patients as our case-loads were too heavy

as it was, but if a new patient came to us we simply went about our business of curing them. I didn't give a damn if my patients came from Timbuktu, whether they were black, white, English or Russian. I was a doctor and when patients with diseased hearts came to me I did my best to make them well again.

Breckon went on to say, 'It's heart-warming that well-wishers have contributed generously to the fund to send Suzanne to South Africa – but does it make sense? The fact is that the money will go on a trip that is not necessary...'

Whether it was necessary or not I leave the reader to decide – what did happen is that Suzanne Jones from Glamorgan, Wales, came to Cape Town for a heart operation – *after* the British surgeons had been reluctant to operate.

When I saw her, I dismissed the media hype surrounding her visit – I just wanted to save this fragile little beautiful life. I wanted to see her eyes laughing and hear her beautiful Welsh voice singing a lullaby again – without gasping for air like a fish out of water.

I knew from her records that she had multiple heart defects and after her tests at Groote Schuur Hospital, it was obvious that the defects were severe.

Just how severe only became clear in the operating theatre. It was like a knee to the groin when I realized how slender was the thread upon which her life hung.

How *dare* Breckon say 'gradually we would be able to build up her strength and eventually, possibly with the help of a series of correcting operations, give her hope of some semblance of normal life.' She had *no* hope whatsoever! If she'd stayed in England and nothing was done, they would have buried her before Breckon could write his next article.

The fact that she was alive at that very moment was a miracle in itself. The anger I felt was so intense that I had to take a few moments to calm down before I carried on.

All I knew was that there was a very minimal chance of her survival and – I say this with all due modesty – she could not have been in a better place. She was now lying on a table surrounded by the best medical facilities in the world, the best technicians, the best surgical and nursing team ever assembled in one operating theatre and as a bonus we also had luck on our side.

But she lay there, her chest cut open and cranked apart from neck to navel, with her pathetic little heart beating weakly and sporadically. I was amazed that it could move enough blood through her body at all, with its valves and chambers hopelessly grown awry from some strange mischance in her genes.

I put her sweet face and her enchanting personality out of my mind entirely and looked at the body as a surgical problem – as coldly and unemotionally as I could.

We succeeded – and I could almost hear the entire little Welsh mining valley rejoicing. Her village sent me a genuine miners' lamp as a gift later – one of the proudest awards I've ever received.

I left the theatre and went to the waiting room where I knew her grannie was anxiously pacing up and down.

I have always cried easily and, taking one look at this lady, I didn't dare speak – I grabbed her around the waist and we polka'd around the room like two crazy people, laughing wildly and ecstatically happy.

Later, in the changing room, I sat on the bench and cried. Uncontrollable sobs of pure joy. 'Thank you, God, for allowing me to be a part of these miracles – I can take all the ridicule and the false accusations – just please allow me to continue doing what I do now.'

Although newspapers and their reporters have always been my pet aversion, an article from The Argus London Bureau in December 1970, pleased us all very much:

BARNARD'S BABIES
Throughout Europe and Britain there are at least 15 children who, with serious heart defects, made the trip to Prof. Chris Barnard and his team in Groote Schuur Hospital, Cape Town, and who are today leading normal lives.

And, wherever these children and their families live, there are heartfelt thanks, admiration and respect for the man who 'gave the children new life'.

In Rome and other parts of Italy there are no fewer than 12 such young people:

Fabio de Fabris, who had his operation in September 1968, now, according to his father, 'runs about like a demon'. Before, his heart condition made it difficult for him to move about at all. Today his passion is football which 'he plays from morning to night'.

Domizia D'Agostino, who was operated on in February 1967, is now seven. Her parents recall that she was unable to go to school and had to have a teacher at home before the operation. 'She is back in full swing,' says her mother, 'she is always on the run and sometimes we have to warn her to slow down. She still cannot believe it is really true that Professor Barnard has made her into a normal child.'

Walter Gaggioli had his operation in November 1968. Earlier, when he was three years old he had been operated on by noted Italian surgeons. 'Before Walter had his operation in Cape Town he could not move' says his mother. 'Now he is so vivacious we have to discipline him and he has put on weight.'

Thirteen year old Pier Luigi Buttone was operated on just over three months ago and, according to his mother, is perfectly normal 'although he is still taking things slowly'.

Giovanna Bon was operated on in August 1969 when Professor Barnard replaced an artery, deformed since birth, linking her heart and her lungs. Her widowed mother says, 'Giovanna is the happiest child on earth and she owes it all to Dr Chris.'

The Italian parents warmly praised the doctors and hospital staff at Groote Schuur who, they said, were at all times understanding and helpful.

'We weren't made to feel like strangers,' said one mother, 'nor were we made to feel that doctors, nurses and the rest were doing us a favour...'

'But for Professor Barnard she would be dead today,' said the mother of now 20 year old Maria Margarida Lopes Barros of Lisbon who had suffered from faulty heart valves and for 12 years had been unable to live a normal life.

Aileen Brassil's parents have a deep conviction that Christiaan Barnard was the answer to their prayers. 'She is now a normal healthy girl – who even goes swimming in the sea, and anyone who has experienced the temperature of the water around this part of the Irish coast will know how sturdy she must be to do that!'

When Suzanne Jones was recently in South Africa one of her first 'get well' cards was from Aileen.

Philip Camfield's mother says her son's recovery was 'a miracle' as she recalled that before his operation British doctors had given him not more than five years to live. 'Some of the best doctors in Britain told us that the necessary operation could not be performed in this country.' Before he flew out to South Africa Philip was in hospital and doctors gave him 48 hours to live. His mother went to the hospital, dressed him and drove him to London Airport. 'My own doctor told me afterwards that he did not expect to see Philip again. In fact he said he did not think he would reach South Africa.'

Whenever I was in Johannesburg I tried to see Barbara and had dinner with her and her parents several times at their home. At one of these dinners, I again made an ass of myself when they served artichokes.

I'd never had them before and thought you had to eat the whole thing. Hell! I thought, this isn't properly cooked! But I kept chewing until eventually I gagged down the woody fibres. Then I noticed that the others only ate the soft end and put the remainder back on their plates. I was very relieved, as I could never have finished them the way I'd started. I'm still not very fond of artichokes.

Barbara's mother, Ulli, told me they were leaving for Ischia – an island about 20 kilometres off the Italian mainland from Naples – in a few days' time as Fred went to the health spa at the Regina Isabella Hotel every year. They said I was welcome to join them as their guest for a week.

We really had a great time there and I was 'unofficially' dating Barbara – although there was nothing serious or permanent. Every night the four of us went dancing in night clubs and I thoroughly enjoyed their company – especially Barbara's.

One night we were all invited to a party by Ernst Sachs, the brother of Gunther Sachs, who had a beautiful house on the island.

When we arrived the party was in full swing and, typical of the international jet-set, dozens of beautiful women were there. I really fancied one blonde German girl very much, so during the evening I said, 'I'm going to go home with the people I came with, but I'm going to come back.' And she said, 'Sure, come back and we'll get down to some serious partying!'

So, just after midnight I left with the Zoellners, said good night to them at the hotel and went up to my room. After a few minutes I went downstairs again and took a taxi back to the Sachs' house.

The party had broken up by the time I arrived and there was nobody left except the blonde German girl who was dancing with a tall Egyptian girl – it looked like a set from a Bertolucci film with these two girls lazily moving in time to some haunting music amid the debris of a finished party.

I found a bottle, opened it and joined them. It was the first, and last time, I was ever part of a *ménage à trois*. I didn't enjoy it – it was too much like wrestling, with arms and legs everywhere. I did quite enjoy the bath we took together afterwards, though.

The next morning at about 5 am, the girls drove me back to the hotel. The front door was locked so I went around the building and found the kitchen door. Then I went to bed – this time to sleep.

The doorman must have told the Zoellners that I had gone out again and only come back early that morning because they wanted to know all the details. I just told them I'd decided to sneak back to the party, where I had a couple of drinks with these girls. I was cautious in case they were offended in some way, but they thought it was a huge joke and I was so pleased that Barbara wasn't jealous. I was to find out later just how terribly wrong I could be.

The remainder of my stay on Ischia was idyllic. Barbara and I were enjoying each other's company very much, but I still felt slightly nervous around her and couldn't find the courage to attempt making any serious advances.

I had to attend medical conferences in Berlin, Toronto and Budapest during the following two weeks, but Barbara agreed to have dinner with me in Rome when I returned.

While I was away more rumours began about me re-marrying. Even Gina Lollobrigida told the newspapers I'd asked her to marry me and that she'd said 'no'. (I never did ask her.) I also met Françoise Hardy once more in Berlin.

Now, back in Rome, they found me having dinner in a quiet restaurant with Barbara, Bill Pepper and his wife.

A photographer sneaked in and took pictures by poking his camera lens through the leaves of some pot plants. Bill spotted him and politely asked for the film to be removed – which, surprisingly, was done. Of course, the newspapers carried a slightly different story:

BARNARD RIPS OUT FILM AS MAN TRIES TO GET PHOTO
A press photographer who took pictures of Prof. Barnard dining in a Rome restaurant with an attractive girl, had his camera seized and the film ripped out.

Professor Barnard was eating with Barbara Zoellner and Italian magazines have romantically linked him with the tall, blonde Miss Zoellner, daughter of a South African industrialist.

Professor Barnard, who left Rome for Cape Town last night, has denied any romantic links with her.

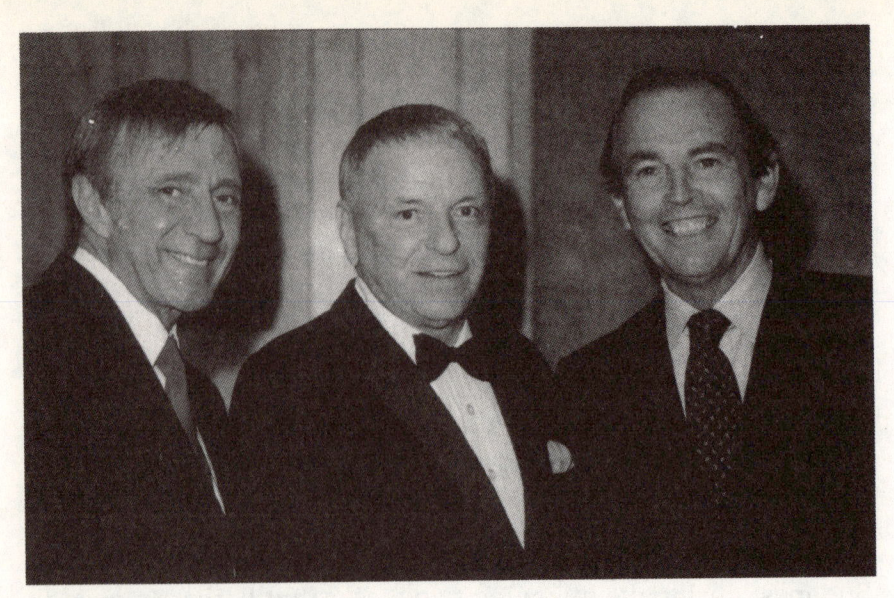

Nazih Zuhdi, Frank Sinatra and I

It's amazing how a few exaggerated adjectives can put a totally different slant on a report – of course some newspapermen are extremely good at doing just that.

I was in Majorca when my divorce from Louwtjie was finalized in the Cape Town Supreme Court. It was a sad day. They say that when you drown, just before you lose consciousness, your whole life flashes through your mind. This day turned out to be a kaleidoscope of the twenty years I'd spent with the woman I was about to be legally and irreversibly parted from.

I re-lived the day when I first saw her as a patient in Ward C2, the same ward where Washkansky died. In those days it was for sick nurses.

Those wonderful few minutes when we kissed and cuddled and said goodbye in the shadow of the hospital chapel, before the doors of the nurses' home were closed at 10 pm.

That dreadful and awkward speech I'd made at the reception after my wedding to Louwtjie at the Groote Kerk ('Big Church' of the Dutch Reformed denomination).

Our honeymoon along South Africa's Garden Route and how it had been spoiled by my getting severely sunburnt.

Memories. The words of that miserable Irish poet, Thomas Moore, seemed appropriate then:

'... Fond memory brings the light,
Of other days around me;
The smiles, the tears,
The words of love then spoken;
The eyes that shone,
Now dimmed and gone,
The cheerful hearts now broken.'

We'd settled in Ceres, and our first child, Deirdre, was born at the Booth Memorial Hospital where our second child, André, also came into the world. This was the same hospital where, many years later, my mother left the world.

And so, the whole day, I re-lived my life with Louwtjie. How sad that it all had to end like this. And it was even worse, because Louwtjie and I would never become friends again.

But memories are hunting horns whose sound dies on the wind and, after all, life has to go on.

6

I returned home and saw Barbara often. Her mother was happy with our relationship, but I think Fred wanted to see it end – and he decided that Barbara should study art at the Louvre. So she and her mother left to go and live in Paris.

We stayed in touch by phone but I also dated some other girls. The fact is that I wasn't sure I wanted to get married again – although I knew, deep down in that part of the heart which the surgeon can never reach, that I was slowly falling in love with Barbara.

In the meantime the press linked me romantically with women all over the world. There was Johanna in Spain, Princess Pinatelli in Rome, Doris Brynner in Paris and Janice in Cape Town.

Of course Barbara read all this and, as a result, I'm sure she didn't take our relationship very seriously.

The Marquis de Villaverde hosted a transplant congress in Madrid and invited Marius and me. He also asked me to bring Pieter Smith, who at that stage was the only patient to illustrate what an active life could be led by a patient who had had a cardiac transplant.

At the congress there were surgeons and immunologists from all over the world – including Denton Cooley and his wife, and also Carras (who'd supplied ALS). Carras' wife was a sexy little number and certainly knew how to make the best of her raw sensuality, especially on the dance floor. I'd had some volatile experiences with her myself when I'd been invited to Lyon a few months earlier.

One evening we all went to an open air dance. When the party was in full swing I thought I'd have some fun and pointed her out to Denton and said she was very keen to dance with him. The unfortunate and gullible Cooley fell for this line and asked her for a dance. He was about 6'2" and she about 5'3". As the dance progressed, I could see him getting that all-too-familiar vague and glazed look in his eyes. At that stage she was just about dancing between his legs and I could see he was excited to the point of frenzy, as she rubbed herself against him. I was bent double with laughter and tears rolled down my face.

When the music ended he came back to the table and with his Texas drawl, said, 'That's the first time I've ever done it with my clothes on – I should have worn your aluminium underwear.'

The meeting in Madrid didn't focus too much on medicine. The Marquis de Villaverde made sure his guests enjoyed themselves.

At a ceremony one night I was honoured by General Franco with the Blue Cross, which impressed me enormously – but not as much as the blonde American girl I met at the disco later in the evening.

Sean Rayan was the daughter of an American couple who had a summer house in Madrid. She was not as pretty as Barbara but I hadn't seen Barbara for several months, and my memory of her had faded a little. I was immediately knocked off my feet by this vivacious American and saw her virtually every night – and most days when we'd play tennis or just sunbathe.

What fascinated me most about Sean was that I couldn't work out how she felt about me and she played very hard to get. But, as I've said before, I enjoy the chase.

I left with Denton Cooley and his wife for the US but I promised Sean I would join her in St Tropez a few weeks later.

From America I went to Copenhagen to spend a few days with Deirdre who was preparing to take part in the European water-skiing championships.

My heart went out to my daughter. She was not with her father any more, she wasn't skiing well and, worst of all, she was considerably overweight. I realized then how a physical defect visible to others caused much more suffering than one that was hidden from view. I would never again criticize people who resorted to plastic surgery.

I took Deirdre shopping and bought her some clothes that would hide the bulges. She pleaded with me to stay on because she needed some security. But I was drawn like a magnet to St Tropez.

Sean came to fetch me at the airport. She was very tired and slept all the way back in the car. I could see immediately that she was burning the candle at both ends.

That evening at about 10 pm a few of us went disco-crawling until 5 o'clock the next morning.

At one of the clubs I saw Odette – an old friend of mine – and wife of the late Rubirosa, the famous playboy who had been killed in an automobile accident.

I met her several times, at parties given in my honour at the house of Paul-Louis Wellier, an elderly Frenchman who knew everyone of note in the world. He entertained lavishly – from presidents to kings.

He was a *commandeur* and had been awarded the *Légion d'honneur* – an order of distinction instituted by Napoleon in 1802 – a five-branched cross with a medallion, bearing a symbolic figure of the *République Française* which he wore with great pride. We became very good friends and every time I visited Paris I stayed with him.

That evening, while I was dancing with Odette, she told me that Paul-Louis was at his home, 'Reine Jeanne', about 40 kilometres from St Tropez. I asked for his phone number, just in case I wanted to call and say hello.

These parties with Sean went on one night after the other until they merged into one long, hedonistic blur. One evening we were invited to an all-night party on a luxury yacht. I arrived there and, as they were about to set sail, I decided that I'd had enough of this kind of life and stumbled back down the gang-plank.

I went back to my hotel, sat down on the bed, and said to myself, 'Chris, you are losing your grip – you're floating around aimlessly and you'd better get yourself back to some solid reality.'

I decided to phone Paul-Louis.

It seemed ages before anyone answered the phone and, as I was just about to replace the receiver, a voice said, 'Bonsoir, la residence de Commandeur Paul-Louis Wellier, que puis-je pour vous?'

I didn't understand what he said but I did recognize Paul-Louis' name so I must have had the right number.

'I'm sorry, I don't speak French!' and as I was afraid he would hang up on me I tried, 'Non-parlez Francais – praat Engels asseblief' (starting in French and ending with Afrikaans).

In perfect English the bastard replied, 'I beg your pardon, Sir, to whom would you like to speak?'

I was so relieved. 'I would like to speak to Mr Wellier, *please*.'

'I'm sorry, Sir, but Commandeur Wellier is dining at present, could you telephone later?' I knew this man had been instructed to discourage callers.

'No, no, tell him it's Professor Barnard.'

Immediately his tone changed and I was absolutely delighted that my name had an effect on his high-handed attitude.

'Oh, certainly Professor, please hold the line for a moment.' After about two minutes, I recognized the voice of Paul-Louis.

He greeted me warmly and when I told him I was in St Tropez, he immediately invited me to spend a few days with him at 'Reine Jeanne'.

He said he had some interesting guests he would like me to meet. Then, as an afterthought, he added, 'By the way Barbara's also here.'

I was absolutely dumbstruck! How the hell did she get there? When I'd phoned to ask her to meet me in Madrid, she'd said she couldn't make it. Something must be wrong. Panic seized me – she must have another man.

'Can I speak to her, please?' I asked, trying to keep the desperation out of my voice.

After another few minutes Barbara's voice came over the phone. 'Yes?'

I was even more furious with this casual response, when she knew perfectly well who was on the phone.

'What the hell are *you* doing there!' I demanded. 'Have you become just another French tart?' I knew this remark was totally uncalled for but I couldn't help myself.

Barbara, like her father, was strong-willed and her voice had a definite edge to it, 'How *dare* you say that when your name has been splashed all over the newspapers with a new girl every time! Well, I've decided I'm not just going to sit in Paris while you're having a good time – I'm having a holiday too.'

We argued backwards and forwards for a while and then, slowly, my anger subsided.

'But tell me, Barbara, what *are* you doing there?' I asked more reasonably and politely.

She'd also had enough and said tenderly, 'I don't really know myself – why don't you come and see?'

Paul-Louis sent his chauffeur to collect me and when I arrived at 'Reine Jeanne' he and his guests were having after-dinner drinks in the lounge. Barbara was standing with a goblet of cognac held in her right hand and a cigarette between the delicate fingers of her left hand. She looked at me and smiled when I entered the room, and I could see the previous aggression had evaporated.

Paul-Louis greeted me and introduced me to his friends. I can't remember them all but I do recall Merle Oberon with her husband, the Russian prince. A member of the Norwegian royal family was also there but the one guest who did fascinate me was Paul Getty Senior – then one of the richest men in the world. Subsequently I learned he was also one of the meanest men in the world. There was a story that he'd installed a public phone box in his English manor house so that guests could not charge calls on his account.

As I'd been going to bed at sunrise for the past week I asked to be excused and Paul-Louis showed me to my room. He also casually mentioned that Barbara's room was right next door to mine.

I undressed and lay down on the bed. The party was still in full swing downstairs and I could hear all the laughter. I was also under the impression that her companion was the Norwegian prince. My brain was full of irrational thoughts and I was so confused that I couldn't settle. I drifted into a half-sleep and images of women kept floating past me ... Barbara ... Sean ... Odette ... Barbara again ... Monique ... Barbara ... always Barbara. What did I really want?

After another hour I heard Barbara entering her room. I wasn't sure whether to go next door and talk to her, or just forget about the whole thing.

Eventually I summoned up the courage and, in my pyjamas, I quietly tip-toed to her door and knocked softly.

There was no reply.

I tried the door handle. The door was unlocked and, hardly trusting myself to breathe, I opened it fully and Barbara was waiting for me...

The standard of reporting of medical events in the South African lay press was very poor. The reason was that they didn't have reporters who specialized in this field– unlike those I'd encountered in the United States and Britain.

I often encountered reporters who would pester me for an interview and, after reluctantly agreeing, would find myself sitting opposite a dumb-looking or disinterested journalist whose first question would be something like, 'So, Professor Barnard, what's new in your field?' This inevitably meant they knew very little about the subject nor had they attempted to prepare for the meeting.

In these circumstances, I would patiently explain that I was very excited about a new surgical approach to coronary artery disease, for example, and invariably the reply would be, 'What's coronary artery disease?' They'd eventually admit that they usually covered women's fashion or football – but that they'd been asked by the editor to 'get an interview with me'.

As a result of their incompetence, the articles that appeared were perfunctory. The Sunday newspapers, especially, focused more on the sensational aspects of our work rather than those of real scientific significance. The social problems of the donors, for example, were easier to grasp by these so-called science writers, than the progress we were making in overcoming the difficulties with which our patients confronted us.

Gradually, a bad relationship developed between the medical profession and the media and the South African Medical Association convened a meeting between the two groups to see if a compromise could be reached.

The meeting was held in Johannesburg and I went there well prepared, because I felt very strongly about the harm that this sensationalism was doing to our work.

There was a lively discussion on how much information the doctors should give the media without making inroads on the privacy that the patient was entitled to.

The question of paying for information at hospitals – chequebook journalism – was also raised and vehemently denied, but everyone in the room knew that information – even disinformation – was being paid for all the time.

When my turn came, I said I had no objection to the media having access to medical information and events and that we would cooperate but that what upset me was the irresponsible way in which information was used. The goal of the reporting appeared to show little concern with facts but seemed, rather, to be to sell more newspapers.

Freedom of the press was essential but so was the responsible use of this freedom. 'You are the first to cry "unfair!" when the censor prevents you publishing – yet you ignore the appeals of those who suffer from the lies you write. You take no notice when we say "unfair!" – in my book that's hypocrisy.'

To illustrate what I meant I showed some slides of front page headlines I'd had photographed where, in the one issue there was a sensational story about the donor whose heart was used and, the very next day, the headlines said that this was *not* the donor.

The editor of *Die Burger* (a leading right-wing Afrikaans newspaper), Mr Piet Cillié, was absolutely outraged and after attacking me about my unfair comments, concluded by saying, 'Professor Barnard, you must realize that, in your profession you get good doctors and bad doctors, and in our profession you get good journalists and bad journalists.'

'Yes, I know that,' I interjected, 'but the only difference is that you can choose the doctor you'd like to treat *you*, but I can't choose the journalist to write about *me*.'

I don't think the meeting solved anything at all. It didn't change reporting techniques, nor did it prevent dishonest journalism. In many parts of the world, events and the lives of certain members of the medical profession became very profitable merchandise for the media.

Medical meetings continued to be turned into shambles by reporters, photographers and TV crews. I found nothing more distracting than a photographer popping up and flashing his camera in my face during a lecture. And nothing more annoying than TV lights illuminating the screen and overpowering the slide I'd just asked to be projected.

In my own case interviews concentrated more on my private life than on the contents of the papers I came to present. And sensational media reporting wasn't only confined to newspapers either.

One day I arrived at Bulawayo airport, on my way to a meeting of the Rhodesian Medical Association (as it was known then). I was invited to a TV studio for a short interview before going to my hotel. This was a very popular chat show they told me, and they'd very much like to talk to some of the doctors attending the conference.

When I arrived at the studio they were busy talking to Dr Hansen, a paediatrician from the Red Cross Children's Hospital in Cape Town. He sat with a young boy on his lap discussing kwashiorkor – a condition resulting from malnutrition in infancy which is, unfortunately, very common in Southern Africa.

I thought I had nothing to worry about as Dr Hansen left the studio with a smile and I settled down in front of the camera.

'Professor Barnard, we've heard a lot about your work tonight, do you mind if we now talk about you, the man?' the interviewer smiled.

'Of course,' I agreed – still expecting nothing out of the ordinary.

'Professor Barnard, there have been many pictures of you dancing with beautiful women – what does your wife say about that?'

I gripped the armrest of my chair tightly. I hadn't imagined the 'personal' interview was going to take this direction. I'd thought he would talk about my youth in the Karoo as the son of a missionary or something like that.

'Like any other woman, my wife doesn't like these pictures but, then, would you prefer to see me dancing with a man?' I replied, trying to pass it off as a joke.

He didn't smile or waver but continued the 'in-depth' interview – which was more like a character assassination. I answered his questions and innuendo unruffled and smiling as best I could.

Then he made a mistake.

'Professor Barnard, stories about your operations and patients are in the newspapers and magazines all the time – isn't this tantamount to advertising? Something that the medical profession frowns upon?'

You clever little bastard, I thought – now it's *my* turn to make *you* uncomfortable.

'Tell me, Sir,' I said. 'We are now appearing live on this show, viewed by 300 000 Rhodesians?'

'Yes,' he agreed proudly.

'So, one could say I'm advertising here tonight?'

'Yes, you could say that,' he admitted, looking slightly uncomfortable, but still not seeing where I was headed.

'Now, did an agent or did I, personally, request this appearance or am I here because you asked me?'

'Well, no, we asked you seeing as how you are in the country for the conference.'

'Just two more questions then: are you paying me a fee for this appearance?'

'No, no.'

'Are *you* being paid to interview me?'

'Yes, of course, that's my job.'

'In other words, you are making money out of advertising me?'

'Well, I wouldn't put it quite that way,' he stammered.

'How *would* you put it then?' I asked innocently. The interview ended abruptly.

The 2nd January 1969 was the anniversary of Dr Blaiberg's transplant. He was the first man to have lived one year with the heart of another man beating inside his chest.

I was on holiday in Knysna but *Stern* magazine had come out for this event and had sent a private plane up the coast to bring me back to Cape Town for an interview and a photo session.

They had a cake with one candle and there were a lot of well-wishers, photographers and reporters in the room when I arrived.

Bossie was fussing around like a mother hen with her chicks – to protect his favourite patient from the crowd.

'We hear you're writing a book, Philip,' one reporter shouted. 'What are you going to call it?'

'*Looking at my Heart*,' came the immediate reply.

'Why the unusual title?' another wanted to know.

'Because I am the first man to have held, in his own hands, the heart that kept him alive for 59 years.'

All the reporters looked confused.

'What Dr Blaiberg is referring to,' explained Bossie, 'is that after his own heart was removed it was preserved by the pathologist in a specimen jar and one day Professor Barnard show him the specimen.'

'And how did you feel about looking at your heart, Doctor?' a young girl wanted to know.

'When Professor Barnard pointed out to me the things that were wrong with it, I was glad it was in the bottle and not in my chest any more!' And they all laughed.

'I think Philip has had enough questions,' Bossie said, trying to get rid of all the people.

'One more question,' somebody from the back insisted.

'Okay then, just one more and then you must please leave,' Bossie implored.

'Dr Blaiberg, you've had a big operation, you've been in and out of hospital and you're still taking handfuls of pills. Do you think it was worthwhile?'

Philip Blaiberg looked up from his cup in amazement and said, 'Of course it was worth it!'

'Dr Blaiberg, when did you realize it was worth it – is it today after having survived one year?'

I was extremely interested to hear my patient's response.

'No, not at all, I knew it was worth the risk and the trouble as soon as I came round from the anaesthetic and I realized I could breathe again. Before that moment I had been gasping for breath day and night. Do you know what it's like not to be able to get enough air into your lungs?' He paused for a while, but nobody spoke. Then he continued, 'As soon as I gained consciousness after the surgery I immediately recognized that life was different – it was more enjoyable. I could breathe freely again.'

Flying back to Knysna in the little plane across the Hottentots Holland mountains and along the southernmost coast of Africa, I was thinking about what Philip Blaiberg had told the reporter.

For the first time I fully understood that the goal of medicine was not to prolong life – the real goal should be to improve the *quality* of life. If, by improving the quality of life, we also prolonged it, which we often did, then that was a bonus. I had long held this opinion but it was Philip Blaiberg who confirmed its importance.

This lesson stood me in good stead in the next few years – and for the rest of my career – especially when the poor results of cardiac transplantation discouraged many surgeons, and one unit after another stopped doing the operation, preferring to leave their patients with the misery of total heart failure.

I always remember those words of Dr Blaiberg, 'As soon as I recovered from the anaesthetic I knew the operation was worthwhile.'

In April 1969 I performed two cardiac transplants. The first was on a 63 year old male who was in very bad condition as a result of long-standing heart failure due to coronary artery disease.

Ten days later I did the first transplant on a female patient – 38 year old Dorothy Fisher – who was in terminal heart failure from rheumatic disease of the heart muscle. So, when I was invited to the second International Heart Congress, organized by Dr Grondin in Montreal, we had four patients alive out of the five we'd operated on so far. At that stage it was the best result reported by any unit in the world. Norman Shumway had done another 12 transplants of whom 3 were still alive.

However, some of the Americans were, in my opinion, doing too many transplants too quickly and this 'race' induced other less-prepared units in other countries to perform transplants – often with extremely poor results. At that time 133 operations had been performed in the world with only 13 surviving patients. This did almost irreparable harm to the transplant programme and some of the more conservative medical associations, like the British, placed a moratorium on heart transplantation for a number of years.

I now had a home whenever I was in Johannesburg as Barbara insisted I should always stay at 'Three Fountains'. Her parents seemed happy with this arrangement and Ulli was still keen on our relationship. I was never really sure about Fred though. There was something worrying him.

There was something bothering me too – the 28 year age difference. Would I be able to enjoy and cope with the social life of an 18 year old? And, as time went by, and the novelty wore off, would I be able to remain sexually active enough to satisfy her? Sex, after all, is a vital aspect of any relationship between two people who love each other. This was a very real concern – especially as Barbara, quite normally, was proud of being a woman and enjoyed being a full partner in the intimacy between lovers.

I used to lie awake at night pondering about what the future would hold for us if we were married. When I consulted my close friends they would simply say, 'Well, do you *love* Barbara? If so then there's no problem.'

My dilemma was, and still is however, that I don't quite know what is meant by 'love' between two totally unrelated individuals.

The only love as far as I could see was the love of a parent for his child – because this is the only totally unselfish love. A father loves his son and a mother loves her daughter without expecting anything in return.

In the case of lovers, there are other aspects of love – like sex, security and companionship.

It's these issues which cloud or distort the truly divine nature of love. 'Love gives naught but itself and takes naught but from itself. Love possesses not nor would it be possessed; for love is sufficient unto love' – as Kahlil Gibran reminds us.

So why, then, would Barbara – a beautiful, wealthy, young girl fall in love with a man more than twice her age and of different social and economic background?

At the beginning I couldn't fathom this out but, with time, I realized that the one thing in life Barbara really craved was security. During her childhood I think she often felt extremely insecure so she needed to surround herself with a family of her own – with a man whom she could both love and trust.

She saw me as a man who was mature, had achieved something

in life, was respected and gentle. I was the man who could give her stability and, unfortunately, in her pursuit of this dubious security, she tended to make our love into a bond, and left no space in our relationship for any independence. There was no room to grow and, as an indirect consequence, like two flowers growing closely together in the same pot, we eventually suffocated and wilted.

Three days after the transplant on Dorothy Fisher, I left on a UTA flight to Gabon with Jack Penn who at that stage was one of the leading plastic surgeons in the world. In Libreville I met President Bongo and at his request, examined his heart. We also visited Lambarene where Albert Schweitzer had devoted most of his life to combating leprosy and sleeping sickness among these unfortunate people. His daughter, Rhena Eckert, gave me a copy of her father's biography and showed me around Lambarene.

Dr Schweitzer is mostly remembered as a great humanitarian and medical hero and, of course, he won the Nobel Peace Prize. But the obviously unsophisticated and ill-equipped clinic reminded me of his reluctance to accept modernization. When he said, 'Progress is the suicide of civilization,' was he right? I think not. I think he was wrong, but I did agree with him when he said, 'Treat not only the sickness – treat also the man.'

There can be no doubt that this brilliant man worked wonders in Africa but the evident lack of facilities and suspect hygiene made one wonder how he achieved so much in a place such as that.

In Gabon, I also witnessed the suffering that refugee children were subjected to as a result of the Biafran war – a war that divided an entire country and its people, at the whims and complicity of two major powers. There were no winners, only losers. Africa is a violent continent, raped and pillaged by the early colonists, who having shown the people the Western form of barbarism, simply turned over the running of the countries back to them, heedless of the consequences.

Barely six months before I'd performed the first heart transplant, Colonel Ojukwu proclaimed a large area of Eastern Nigeria – populated mainly by the Ibo tribe – as the independent republic of Biafra. General Gowan, the Nigerian president, immediately sent in his troops and a merciless intertribal war erupted. The British supported the Nigerian federal forces while the French supported the Biafrans – like a chess game using human beings in a nightmare of suffering. The conflict was still in progress when I was there, with the last Biafran resistance defiantly struggling until the end, while their leader fled to the Ivory Coast.

During and after the war, the biggest casualties were not the fighters, but defenceless and helpless children – orphaned, diseased, homeless and without a soul in the world to care for them.

Up to that point I had never seen children who were starving to death. They were past tears and cries – they had enough energy only for pathetic and lethargic mute appeal. I realized that starvation was more than just a pain in the belly. It's the terrible and disgusting agony of the body literally cannibalizing its own tissues in its futile struggle to fight off inevitable death.

Reality can never be captured on film. There is a stink to starvation that cannot be seen on the TV screen. It assaults the nostrils and revolts the stomach – a smell I can never forget – a stench of obscenity.

I have been trained – as all doctors are – to face human suffering with as little emotion as possible. But the sight of these swollen-bellied children surrounded by filth and flies and the certainty of death reduced me to wracking sobs of sorrow. Never before had I felt so helpless and so utterly appalled, in this place that God appeared to have deserted.

I was severely depressed at having to leave this suffering without being of any help but thankful to be away from the squalor and misery.

My engagements took me to Paris, London and Naples. In Rome Princess Luciana Pinatelli gave a dinner party for me at her home. Among her guests was Audrey Hepburn, whom I hadn't seen since we'd met in Madrid. I was delighted to meet her again. The ex-king and queen of Greece were also there.

Luciana Pinatelli was a very special woman in my life, although I did not see much of her. She was very mature, honest and wise – with a razor-sharp sense of humour. She helped me tremendously in sorting myself out – both then and later. She was a true friend to me and I've known many who use the word 'friendship' as a means to a totally different end. She just liked me for myself – a feeling which was always mutually reciprocated.

The following day she took me on a guided tour of all the various boutiques in Rome to help me buy a dress for Barbara – a dress which Barbara liked so much, she wore it at our engagement party.

Our fourth heart transplant patient, Mr Killops, had not done very well after his operation and died 64 days later.

Our own experience, and that of other surgeons, indicated that we were wrong in assuming that a patient was never 'too sick' to be helped by a transplant. We realized that we should accept that there are certain contra-indications – these had nothing to do with the patient's inability to tolerate the surgery – even a terminally ill patient could survive the operation and enjoy immediate benefit from the improvement in the circulation. What they didn't tolerate were the high dosages of steroids that were prescribed, especially when there was evidence of acute rejection.

Not only do the steroids suppress the immune system but they are also what are known as an-anabolic agents – the drug prevents constructive metabolism, where simple nutritional substances are synthesized into complex materials of living tissue – the synthesis of proteins from amino acids for example.

For this reason, the patient who was already in a malnourished state from long-standing heart failure, literally fell apart under the high steroid doses. This was especially true when they were elderly.

In retrospect I now realize that four of the five patients we operated on for heart transplantation did not qualify under the new criteria – only Dorothy Fisher, our fifth patient did.

The fact that two of the four lived for more than fifteen months and, during this bonus time, enjoyed tremendous improvement in the quality of their lives, was testimony to the dedication and skill of the Groote Schuur transplant team.

Dr Blaiberg died two months after Mr Killops.

During the three months before his death there was a gradual deterioration of his circulation, with electrocardiographic changes which seemed to indicate ischaemia (a starvation of blood to the heart muscle) rather than rejection.

As Philip hadn't responded to the increase in anti-rejection treatment, I suggested that we should transplant another heart into him, but Vel Schrire didn't want to hear about that – and I think he also persuaded Mrs Blaiberg against taking my advice.

We were all sad to see this courageous, likeable man, slowly slide downhill towards the inevitable. He had done so much for cardiac transplantation throughout the world but he'd had at least 18 full months of very enjoyable life and, in that time, wrote a book (*Looking at my Heart*) and was able to provide financial security for his family.

Bossie, who had cared for Blaiberg with total and absolute dedication, was especially shattered and I don't think he ever fully recovered. He deeply mourned the loss of Philip Blaiberg.

He committed suicide a few years later.

'I don't believe it!' was Professor Thomson's comment when he cleared the pericardium from Dr Blaiberg's heart. We were all gathered in the morgue again, just as we had when Louis Washkansky died. 'The coronary arteries are extensively diseased. The new heart developed the same pathology for which you had removed his *own* heart!'

He turned briefly to me. 'Chris, how old was the donor?'

'Clive Haupt was about 35 when he died of a brain haemorrhage.'

'Are you sure he had no arterial sclerosis when you removed his heart?' asked the pathologist.

'No, not that I could detect on clinical evidence and I saw nothing during surgery but, of course, we didn't do a coronary angiogram.'

'No, there would have been no reason to do one,' he agreed as he lifted the heart of Clive Haupt out of Blaiberg's chest.

With small scissors he opened the main coronary artery and its branches. 'It's only twenty months since this heart was transplanted,' he observed speaking in a monotone.

For the first time in a human, we were witnessing the pathological changes caused by chronic rejection – an accelerated atherosclerosis of the coronary arteries. This proved to be – and still is – a major clinical problem. Ischaemia doesn't manifest itself with pain or angina pectoris – because the heart has no nerves. Extensive narrowing of the coronary arteries can occur even though the patient shows none of the symptoms – the surgeon's first warning is sudden death due to ventricular fibrillation.

Yearly coronary arteriograms are the only method by which the progress of the disease can be followed.

Experience has shown us that the treatment for this disease is to re-transplant. My recommendation to Vel Schrire and Eileen Blaiberg was the correct one. Philip Blaiberg could have lived longer.

That afternoon, all the members of the transplant team gathered in a small lecture room at the medical school. There was an ominous cloud hanging over the gathering and the main question was whether we, like so many other teams, should abandon the programme.

I was infuriated beyond belief at this line of thought. We still had two patients doing very well – both out of hospital – and Philip Blaiberg had really enjoyed the months that his life had been prolonged.

'If he was here today,' I said, 'I'm sure he would be the first to encourage us to go on.'

After some further discussion, and with reluctance, the team agreed to continue with heart transplantation.

To make matters worse, an interview with Philip Blaiberg's daughter, Jill, appeared in one of the local newspapers in which she claimed that her father's life, after the transplantation, was only one of suffering and that he regretted ever having the operation.

I knew this wasn't true but didn't have an opportunity to discuss it with her before she returned to Israel, where she'd lived for many years – even during her father's post-operative period.

Previously she had been enthusiastic when talking to the press but subsequently we learned that she had been paid by a reporter for the interview and that the contents of the article were mainly the impressions of the reporter – not the views of Jill Blaiberg herself.

All these events resulted in not a single transplant being performed in 1970 – but we continued with our various research projects.

The early diagnosis of rejection and the treatment of this complication still remained the most pressing problem and we concentrated on this aspect.

Our research findings had substantiated our clinical impressions that the methods available for diagnosing rejection at that stage, were unreliable and that often severe rejection was present long before it was evident clinically. This resulted in the clinical manifestation of rejection, often being acute and terminal. We could never be aware of it until it might be too late – so we developed a new anti-rejection protocol where, during the first three months after surgery, we gave our patients a bonus of one gram of cortisone intravenously every one or two weeks.

The rationale behind this approach was that, if rejection *was* present and we couldn't detect it clinically, this treatment might stop the progression of the complications.

Although it didn't receive wide acceptance by researchers in other parts of the world, we obtained the best results at the time with this shot-in-the-dark approach. In fact, the longest survivor in the world today – 22 years after his transplantation – was treated in this manner and he never received cyclosporine – an immunosuppressive drug, developed in 1976, which has transformed transplantation. This drug is isolated from the fermentation broth of a soil fungus found close to a stream running into Hardanger Fjord in Norway. Rejection hasn't been abolished, but it's not as severe and doesn't occur as frequently. Infections are not as frequent because lower dosages of other immunosuppressants can be used.

And in 1974 Dr Caves, working with Norman Shumway, made what I consider to be one the most significant contributions in the field of cardiac transplantation. He suggested that serial biopsies be performed on the transplanted heart. These specimens of heart muscle, obtained by biopsy, could then be examined under the microscope for evidence of rejection. So we had a way to detect rejection long before it became clinically evident.

The biopsy is a minor procedure that can be performed without the patient being admitted to hospital. Using local anaesthetic, a catheter is introduced through a vein in the neck, and guided under X-ray screening into the right pumping chamber of the donor heart. Small biopsy forceps are then introduced through the catheter and two or three small pieces of heart muscle are snipped off and extracted.

The muscle samples taken in this way are then examined by the pathologist, who reports his findings to the surgeon the next day.

This valuable contribution made a huge difference to the management of patients who'd had heart transplants. It has certainly saved a great number of lives – and is further proof that scientists should cooperate fully and work together to increase the efficacy of their research and the value of their discoveries.

During a visit to Miami I was invited to the home of an amateur jeweller where I saw a very beautiful ring. It wasn't a diamond ring but had several stones. It looked like Barbara's style so I bought it as a present for her.

When I came back to South Africa, I visited the Zoellners. Barbara, Ulli and I were sitting at the dining-room table when I remembered the ring and said, 'I've got a present for you,' and I went up to my room and fetched it. It was to be our engagement ring – although that wasn't my intention at the time.

Barbara and I were seeing one another frequently so she and her mother suggested I speak to her father and sort of pop the question.

One evening after dinner, the four of us were having coffee in the family room when, after a lot of hand signs, Barbara and her mother left the room and closed the door. I don't think Fred fully realized what was happening, but I knew exactly what was expected of me.

It wasn't going to be very easy – he was a tough man with a strong Germanic disposition and an iron constitution. He'd been told to slow down his lifestyle because he had high cholesterol but that didn't stop him enjoying a big fried breakfast every day, often washed down with an Amstel lager – he was that sort of guy. He epitomized the expression 'Nothing succeeds like excess' and he's still alive today, despite all the grave warnings.

After testing the mood of the man who I hoped would be my future father-in-law, by discussing the steel industry and his steel mills, I began.

'Fred, you must have noticed that Barbara and I are very fond of each other.'

After taking a puff of his cigar, he nodded. His expression told me nothing. He carefully examined the ash at the end of the Havana.

Clearing my throat I continued, 'Would you have any objection to our getting married?'

Fred took a sip of the coffee and paused. 'Chris, do you think you can both be happy? Let's face it, you're much older than Barbara. Now maybe, and for the next few years, it'll work out – but what then?'

This also troubled me and I had thought about it a lot. 'Fred, the way I see it is like this: now is life, not tomorrow or next year, or the year after that. If we can be happy, if only for a few years, then it's worth the risk. I'm sure you'll agree that there are great advantages to Barbara marrying someone my age and being happy, if only for a relatively short time, than marrying someone younger and being unhappy for longer.'

Fred reflected for a while and then put his hand out and said, 'Chris, if that's the way you feel, and you honestly believe you can make Barbara happy, then you have my full support.'

Barbara and Ulli burst into the room – I don't know how they knew that Fred and I had agreed. We kissed and laughed and opened a bottle of Moët et Chandon. It was a very happy moment, one of those moments in life that are never forgotten.

Barbara and I announced our engagement to a small group of friends at a private party at the Zoellners' house.

It was a memorable Friday. The evening was a perfect Transvaal summer night. The stars had never looked as beautiful as they did then – the only things sparkling more brightly were Barbara's eyes as she stood next to me, while we held hands for most of the evening. She radiated happiness and my heart ached with love and tenderness as she stood by my side. I'd never been so proud.

It was a very quiet and private affair – and we'd managed to keep it that way because it had all been arranged on the spur of the moment. I was to leave for New York after the weekend, on my way to a convention of the American College of Cardiology in San Francisco.

We had decided not to tell the press but, of course, they soon found out. What amazed all of us was the sheer volume of newspaper space devoted to it. We were so much in love we didn't give much thought to the publicity and, looking back now, it was probably the press and their sensational reporting that hammered the final nail in the coffin of our marriage – but that was to come much later.

In the meantime, after a quiet weekend at 'Three Fountains', where we refused to take calls from reporters, Barbara drove me to the airport and I left for New York. Barbara was wearing the ring I'd brought back from Miami and the photographers spotted it immediately.

Although we'd decided on 'no comment', it soon became obvious that we'd have to make some kind of statement – especially since Barbara's picture was on front pages the world over: Cape Town, London, New York.

When I phoned her from America we decided to confirm we were getting married, and she agreed to see a reporter and tell him the story.

Nervously, she showed the journalist into her parents' lounge and, sitting down with more confidence and poise than she felt, she smoothed out her cream linen skirt and began answering his questions.

'Miss Zoellner, you're 19 and have been described as a Johannesburg socialite. Would you agree with that description?'

'Well, I am 19,' she admitted, 'but I'm not a socialite. I just haven't started working yet, that's all.'

'And is it true that you are engaged to marry Professor Chris Barnard?'

'Yes.'

'And he's, let's see,' the reporter thumbed through his notes, 'he's in his late forties?'

'No, he's 46.'

'Yes, does the difference in age bother you?'

'Not at all.'

'Even though he's only two years younger than your mother and has a daughter almost your own age?'

She frowned slightly at the persistence. 'It doesn't matter – it makes no difference to us at all.'

'Why did you decide to get married?'

'I'm not sure what you mean – why does anyone decide to marry?'

'Is it because he's famous?'

'Absolutely not! And I hope no one thinks so. Of course, when I met him I was aware of who he was, but the only thing that impressed me was his charm.'

'What about his reputation of being a playboy?'

'I don't think he deserves that description at all and I'm sure the publicity he's received hasn't altered him – he's still the same man.'

'So what about the stories of him with other women?'

'I have no problem with Chris being photographed in different parts of the world with different women – what man, given the opportunity, wouldn't enjoy the attentions of beautiful women?'

He wasn't getting much of an angle here – she was too controlled – so he changed tactics.

'Where did you meet?'

'At a dinner party – in this house actually.' And she waved her hand around the room. 'After that we met again at various places but it was only when we met again on the island of Ischia that I realized I regarded him as so much more than a friend.

'From then on, things just kind of happened and last Wednesday he proposed and I accepted.' She added simply.

'Why did you and Chris deny the romance then?'

'Well, at first the stories were ridiculously premature – the newspapers were saying we were in love long before that actually happened – and, when it did, Chris was simply trying to protect me.'

'Protect you from what?'

'From persistent hounding by your colleagues and interviews like this one – I don't like them very much, I feel awkward.'

He decided he could probably get away with one last question, *'When do you plan to marry, Miss Zoellner?'*

'It's all in the air at the moment. I've only known Chris for 8 months but I don't believe in long engagements so we'll probably be married within a year.'

It hadn't been a great interview he thought – but a headline like *'CHRIS IS NO PLAYBOY – says Barbara'* might work well.

I wearily climbed out of bed one morning. We'd had a heavy schedule the previous day at the Red Cross Hospital and a long day in the operating room often caused my arthritis to flare up.

I felt as if I had been in a rugby match – not as a player but as the ball. Struggling to the bathroom I thought to myself as I looked in the mirror, Maybe you *are* older than you think and the time's come to slow down. But I was still deeply committed to my work, and was looking forward to seeing how the children on whom we'd operated the previous day were doing.

I filled the basin with hot water and immersed my hands as I flexed my fingers. Then I did the same using cold water. Somebody had told me that the sudden change in temperature would help.

I'd received hundreds of 'cures' from thoughtful people all over the world. These included the popular copper bracelets, copper pennies taped above the right ankle and a nickel coin on the left ankle, gin, oil of rosemary, green tomato juice, raspberry tea, parsley, celery, transcendental meditation, scientology, vitamin pills for dogs, brake-fluid, Brasso, rust remover, boiled guava leaves, burial in hot sand, Malaysian seaweed, stinging nettles, a potato in each pocket, Spanish fly, peanut oil, green plastic hair-curlers, blood from umbilical cords, various roots and acupuncture.

I haven't tried many of them but, 30 years after the initial diagnosis, I still keep it under control. The agony is sometimes unbearable, even though I have a high pain threshold.

So I shaved with difficulty that morning and dressed – although I struggled to get my left arm into my jacket sleeve. Curiously, after I married Barbara, the arthritis went into almost total remission and I often joked that the best cure was a young wife.

Outside it was a beautiful, cloudless day. The beaches were deserted, except for a few fitness fanatics jogging on the pure white sand of Clifton beach. I watched some boats out at sea and a cormorant diving for its breakfast. Then I turned to look up at Lion's Head and thought, What a beautiful country I live in – how can we allow politics to make it ugly?'

Dismissing the painful arthritis, I left for work.

Driving to the hospital, I thought about the little black boy Marius had operated on the previous day. He was only six years old, but rheumatic fever had destroyed his heart valves to a such an extent that one of them had to be replaced with a prosthetic valve.

There was a big campaign at that time being launched against heart disease. They meant disease of the coronary arteries. In bold black letters it was claimed to be the number one killer in the Western world. Also, in South Africa, emphasis had been placed on the high incidence among Afrikaners. Everybody, by then, knew the risk factors such as high blood pressure, high cholesterol, lack of exercise and smoking, but very little was ever said about rheumatic heart disease which is, without a doubt, the most common form of heart disease in South Africa.

Was this because 'heart attacks' occurred mainly among whites and the well-to-do, whereas rheumatic heart disease more frequently affected the non-white population and those socially deprived?

The irony of the situation is that we have very little knowledge about why people get heart attacks at all, and we certainly don't know how to prevent them. On the other hand, it is quite clear how people get rheumatic fever – and we also know how to prevent it.

In the Scandanavian countries today, rheumatic fever is virtually unknown. But in South Africa it's reached epidemic proportions.

The authorities seem to prefer spending millions on managing the complication, rather than spending the same amount of money to prevent the disease by giving the sufferers better houses, more food and better medical facilities – especially in the rural areas.

It was with a feeling of hopelessness that I sighed and walked into the intensive care unit of the Red Cross Children's Hospital.

Over the years, experience had taught me to sum up the clinical condition of a patient in a few minutes. I immediately recognized that 'Johnny' (we called him that because we couldn't pronounce his Xhosa name) was very sick. In fact he was dying.

The cardiologist had recognized that he still had acute rheumatic inflammation of the heart muscle and that we should really wait until this had subsided but, due to the severity of the valve lesions, we had had to operate immediately.

On examination he had hardly any blood pressure and was gasping with each breath.

I turned to Sister Meyer. She had been in charge of the intensive care unit for a year and was a wonderfully caring and devoted nurse who celebrated joyously with every child who recovered and grieved deeply for every one that died.

'What's going on, Sister?' I asked, knowing exactly what the problem was.

'Dr Marius has been in and he says it's myocarditis (inflammation of the heart muscle).' She tried to disguise her distress with a curt, professional, no-nonsense nursing attitude. She wasn't being very successful.

'Did he have any suggestions?' I wanted to know what treatment he'd prescribed.

'He suggested that we increase the steroids but that we should check with you first.'

'I agree with that. Is there anything else?' I asked, knowing there was little further we could do.

'Yes, he asked Johnny what he would like to have.' And her brave attempt at being emotionally detached began disintegrating as big tears welled up in her eyes.

'What *does* he want?' I asked softly.

I could hardly hear her answer and her voice broke completely. 'A piece of bread,' she choked, her chest heaving with deep, uncontrollable sobbing, as she turned her face to the wall.

The room was too small for me and I hurried to the men's room where I wept. I wept because we couldn't save this little boy's life. I wept because of the evil society which had deprived him of so much and allowed the disease to strike. I wept because we were able to give Johnny all the modern medical treatment and insert an expensive heart valve bought in America, but what we did not give him in time was a piece of bread – that's all he really wanted – something to eat.

Johnny died two hours later.

There was a phone call from Dr Watermeyer, the superintendent of Red Cross Hospital. He wanted to see me urgently.

I walked heavily down the steps to his office on the ground floor, each step leaden with bible-black sorrow.

'Come in,' came the reply after my knock at the door.

Dr Watermeyer sat behind his desk with a worried look on his face. He'd probably heard about Johnny's death I, thought. I was wrong – he had other 'more important' issues to deal with.

'Professor Barnard, you have to stop mixing the races.' He announced bluntly.

'What?' I was sure I hadn't heard him correctly.

'I'm sorry, but we've had instructions from head office that it is against the government's policy to have white and black children in the same ward.'

I could feel the fury rising in me like a volcano. My blood ran icy cold, as my face flushed hotly. My eyes narrowed and I gripped the back of the chair until my knuckles were white. I couldn't trust myself to speak.

'I'm sorry, Professor Barnard, I'm only doing my duty.' He could clearly see my anger and my guess is that he wanted to avoid the inevitable confrontation.

'Dr Watermeyer,' I said carefully, regaining as much composure as I could, 'let me tell you what your duty is, as head of this hospital. Your duty is to tell those bigoted shits in head office to go to HELL! In fact, if you don't want the message to appear to have come from *you*, then you tell them that *my* answer is that they should go and get fucked!'

I turned to leave the room.

'Professor Barnard, please don't get upset.' I could see he was very uncomfortable and, maybe, he was just protecting his own job. But I could still feel Johnny's pulse-less wrists in my hands.

'What do they want me to do?' I asked resignedly – suddenly feeling very, very tired.

'Well, the problem is the intensive care unit. I've been turning a blind eye to it, but a parent has complained that his child has to lie next to a kaffir.'

'Tell him to take his child to another hospital if he's unhappy here.' I sighed.

'But they want *you* to operate on their children.'

The secretary brought in two cups of tea and I decided to have mine black, without sugar.

'If they want that, then they'll have to get used to my ideas.' I raised my hand and stopped Dr Watermeyer from interrupting me.

'Let me explain to you the problems that face me. Even if I

wanted to make those insufferable bureaucrats happy – as well as those misguided and spiteful bigots which some unfortunate white children have as parents – it's impossible.

'We have only one post-operative intensive care unit. There's no way that I can operate one week on whites only and the next week on blacks only, it just doesn't work that way. Illness doesn't distinguish between white and black and neither can I.'

'So what do you suggest?' he asked, beginning to understand what I was talking about.

'I suggest we just go on the way we are now. I'll give those parents who object the choice: either they go to another hospital or I will nurse their children, after surgery, in the general ward where, of course, they will not get intensive care.'

Dr Watermeyer started fidgeting with his pen and paper on his desk. I could see the anguish in his eyes when he looked up at me. 'There's something else.'

"For the love of God – what now?" I thought.

'There have also been complaints that you are using coloured nurses to look after white children.'

What disease had infected my country? I should have accepted one of the many jobs offered me after the transplant and left this God-forsaken and forgotten corner of the planet. I was so offended by this repulsive remark that I could only say, 'Dr Watermeyer, if there's anybody who can run my unit better than I can, I'm happy to step down immediately.'

I took a sip of the black tea but it was bitter – like South African politics – so I returned the cup to its saucer.

'In the meantime,' I continued, 'I will do everything that I feel is in the best interests of my patients. Do you even *begin* to appreciate how good our coloured nurses are? Ask Dr Van Riet in charge of the burn unit – ask *any* doctor working here. We should go on our knees and thank God for them. What amazes me is that they are still willing to nurse the offspring of our "superior race" after the way we've treated them!'

I couldn't face talking to him any more – this man whose job it was to enforce the disgusting doctrines of apartheid. I got up and began walking out. When I reached the door I turned around. 'By the way Dr Watermeyer, you can tell the parents – and your superiors – who've complained about the black boy in the intensive care unit, that they don't have to worry any more. Johnny has left.'

Two months after I'd proposed to Barbara we became oficially engaged at a big party, planned by Ulli and held in the Zoellners' home, with about 150 invited guests. Barbara wore the dress chosen by Princess Luciana and I wore Litrico's smoking jacket again.

Don Mackenzie was there taking photographs, which were published in magazines all over the world. We'd decided to have only one photographer at the party – even though there was a large contingent of them virtually camping outside in the street. I'm sure that Don was well rewarded financially for his brilliant photographs – I had not realized that publishers paid so handsomely.

When Bill Pepper took a photograph of Barbara and me kissing just after we were married, the photograph sold for $2 500 – which was a huge amount of money in 1970.

The date of our wedding had been set for the 14th February. Barbara was superstitious about the number 13 and it was also Louwtjie's birthday on the 13th February. I thought it insensitive to get married on the birthday of my ex-wife.

The arrangements were to start the party on the evening of the 13th, but to get married after the clock had struck midnight. We were to be married by a magistrate at her parents' home.

We invited only a handful of guests which included Dr Diederichs, the minister of finance and his wife, Dr Tommy Miller, the managing director of Iscor and his wife, my daughter Deirdre, and Bill Pepper – who had returned to South Africa to put the final touches to *One Life*. He was also going to take photographs of the wedding.

I'd invited Dr Diederichs because we had become very close friends and I often turned to him for guidance and assistance.

Dr Nico Malan, the administrator of the Cape, who had just presented me with the Gold Medal of the Province, was also invited, but he couldn't make it. I had been good friends with him and his wife back in the days when I was still married to Louwtjie. He knew how to enjoy life and I was very fond of them. I knew that Louwtjie had turned to them in an effort to stop my philandering – before we were divorced. Maybe that was the real reason they'd declined? I sincerely hoped they hadn't been turned against me.

The event was receiving wide coverage by the media and the big question, of course, was what Barbara's dress would look like. The excitement leading up to the great day was marred by several threats that Barbara received from anonymous callers.

One told her that he would 'scar her pretty little face by throwing acid in it'. Another pretended to be Deirdre and asked Barbara to meet her in town. The police took this threat seriously enough to put a blonde wig on a burly policeman and, with Barbara, keep the arranged rendezvous with the caller at the City Hall. In the end it turned out to be a hoax.

I laughed about these threats, but for a 19 year old girl they were very frightening.

Fortunately, 'Three Fountains' was well secured by a high wall and armed guards at the gates day and night – a great reassurance.

I had to attend one more professional engagement before the wedding. I'd been invited to address the South African Sakekamer (Afrikaans Chamber of Business). I was quite apprehensive as I'd been receiving mostly negative publicity about my divorce from Louwtjie (herself a staunch Afrikaner) and my marriage to a 19 year old girl (who was generally perceived to be an English-speaking 'socialite').

The problems in South Africa have always been oversimplified and it was very convenient to divide the country into white oppression and black subservience – but that's not true. Among the black people there has always been traditional enmity between the tribes. The white tribes, too, had their differences – the Afrikaans-speaker often has very different values from those of the English-speaker. Tolerance between all groups is stretched.

The audience that evening would comprise mainly Afrikaners who, traditionally, have a narrow outlook on life and have their own peculiar interpretation of morality. Also, they would probably all be members of the Dutch Reformed Church, according to whom I had committed every sin in the book.

I never prepare a talk ahead of time especially when I haven't been given a specific subject. What I normally do is to look around when cocktails are being served and assess the audience – only then do I start formulating ideas on my talk and make a few notes.

When I arrived at the President Hotel in Cape Town, I couldn't have been received more warmly. Everyone appeared delighted to see me and said how proud they were of my achievements as a fellow Afrikaner.

We sat down to dinner and the *bonhomie* continued. I would be speaking after the main course, so I found it difficult to enjoy my food. I couldn't even ease my nerves with a glass or two of wine, because I've found it unwise to drink alcohol until after the speech has been completed.

After unenthusiastically pushing some food around my plate someone introduced me as 'one of the greatest Afrikaners South Africa has ever produced', which was greeted with loud applause and cheers.

At that moment I was extremely proud of my Afrikaans heritage and also to be among such sincere people. So, feeling much more comfortable and confident than when I'd first arrived, I began (in Afrikaans), 'Ladies and Gentlemen, I've been very nervous and apprehensive about this evening, as I thought all the recent stories about my escapades may have made me unwelcome to my fellow countrymen.'

'Never!' Some of them shouted.

'But, after arriving here tonight, I realize I'm among friends and honour between friends and loyalty to our country is obviously a strong Afrikaner bond, not easily broken by the media.' I smiled.

There was loud applause – and cries of 'hear hear!'.

Happily I continued, 'You are the people who will always stand by me and help me. And it's for that reason I will be so very happy if you can help me answer some questions that are frequently posed to me in my travels overseas.

'The first question I'd like you to help me with is that people say to me, "You have black and coloured women working for you at home as servants – now, when your child is ill they wash and feed him and they sit at the bedside – but if your child is admitted to hospital and that same coloured or black woman is a nurse, she's not allowed by law, to care for your child." How do I explain that to them?'

There was some uneasy chair-moving and coughing among the guests and I began to realize the cold truth – that I'd probably miscalculated their mood, and that their overtures of welcome were probably only superficial. But it was too late to stop now so I decided to press on.

'The second question that you must help me with is when I'm asked to tell them why a black or coloured medical student has to pass the same exams, pay the same fees to qualify – and yet when he gets a job in a provincial hospital after qualifying, his salary is less than that of his white counterpart. How do I answer a question like that?'

There were now loud whispers and mumbled dissent in the

audience. A man at the back shouted something I couldn't hear properly. It wasn't polite I'm sure.

'The third question you have to help me with,' I continued quickly, 'is that they say, "You tell the newspapers and magazines how the white kids play with their black and coloured friends in their little towns yet when they grow up, they aren't allowed to compete with each other on the sports field." And these people often quote the case of d'Oliveira, an ex-South African who, as you know, wasn't allowed to accompany the MCC to South Africa because he was coloured. You'll agree, I'm sure, that's also a tough one.'

I wanted to ask several more questions but, as the jeers were now louder than I was, and large groups in the audience were beginning to leave the room, I was afraid that if I continued I would eventually be talking to myself.

So, with a last request for their help in answering these questions, and thanking them for their attention, I sat down.

There was silence – except for some isolated, light, applause.

Somewhere from the back, a lone voice suggested an answer, 'Tell them we do these things because it's our business, not theirs – and you can go and join them if you want to!'

The president of the chamber decided to end the evening and I stood up, preparing to leave. The animosity was all around me. One man told me he'd never seen anyone behave as rudely as I had.

I couldn't understand the acrimony, because I had told them nothing they didn't already know, but I realized that evening how quickly 'sincere friends' can become insincere enemies.

Bob Molloy, my journalist friend, told me later that he realized I'd dropped a huge bomb-shell and he'd immediately rushed out to phone a report through to the *Cape Times*.

I certainly did drop a bomb because, for the first time, I had spoken out against apartheid in public.

The local nationalist newspaper, *Die Burger*, was howling for my blood. The English newspapers, on the other hand, applauded my stand.

The government, meanwhile, put an immediate stop to all the VIP treatment I had been receiving at the airports. When I approached the PRO at South African Airways about the change in attitude, he said that they'd had instructions 'from the top' to consider me from then on as an ordinary passenger.

It was their own little spiteful way of making their displeasure as obvious as possible.

Barbara glided down the stairs, on her father's right arm, dressed in a flowing white gown. She looked so beautiful and graceful. The guests, the magistrate and I were all waiting in the entrance hall of 'Three Fountains' standing in front of a large tapestry ominously called *Slaughter of the innocents*.

After a brief ceremony the magistrate pronounced us husband and wife and we kissed as the champagne corks popped.

The size of the crowd outside the garden gate had steadily swollen during the day with media people from all over the world. They tried every trick imaginable to get inside the grounds during the day. One photographer hid in the back of a milk truck, another pretended to be delivering flowers and yet another fell out of a tree.

After the ceremony, there were urgent and persistent pleas from the reporters for Dr Zoellner to allow them inside for just a few minutes. I discussed it with Bill and we agreed that that would be the only way to get rid of them. So the gates were opened and they stampeded up the driveway and into the house. Barbara and I were asked to pose for them, holding hands and kissing.

One photographer wanted a different angle and climbed on top of an antique French table – succeeding only in causing considerable and expensive damage to a very rare Louis XVI piece. The situation rapidly got out of hand as they began to jostle each other and crowd Barbara and me into a corner. The guards were called in and they escorted them back into the street.

All I remember of the rest of the celebration is that I made an awful speech.

The next day we went to Jan Smuts Airport and left on a daylight flight with Bill Pepper for Rome to begin our honeymoon.

I couldn't believe my eyes when the plane taxied to the terminal of Fiumicino airport. There were *thousands* of people waiting at the arrivals terminal.

Bill Pepper's son reached us before we stepped out of the Alitalia 707 and warned us that there was pandemonium inside the airport building. He didn't know how we would ever get through the crowds without being hurt.

'You can't walk under them or over them so you'll just have to walk through them,' some bright-spark suggested helpfully. Which is what we had to do. With a few burly Alitalia personnel in front of us, we bulldozed our way through the seething mass – the noise of the cheers and whistles was absolutely deafening.

Some of the people in the crowd even pulled at Barbara's long hair to see if it was real – and someone pinched my behind, an Italian custom I had thought reserved exclusively for women.

With escort cars in front and behind, and hooters blaring, we made our way to Trastevere to spend the first night of our honeymoon with Bill and his family.

During the four days we stayed in Rome we hardly ever left Bill's house because the *paparazzi* did their best to make our lives a misery. Cameras were focused on the windows and balconies 24 hours a day.

Bill gave a party at his home – to which he invited several celebrities including Robert Audrey and his wife, Sophia Loren and Carlo Ponti. The fashion editors of *Harper's Bazaar* and *Vogue* magazines were also there. They were wildly excited about using Barbara as a model – and they finally succeeded in persuading her.

The next day they arrived with an assortment of garments which Barbara modelled for them. She looked absolutely stunning and I was the proudest husband in the world to see her beautiful face on the front covers at news-stands all over the world.

When the time came for us to leave for New York, Bill backed a car close up to the front door, packed in all the suitcases, and we all made a dash.

An old man was trying to speak to us through the window. He looked so eager and harmless that I asked Bill to open the window so that we could hear what he had to say. Bill stopped the car and spoke to him for a while. As he drove away, he said, 'Typical Italian. He said he was the man who sweeps the street in front of the house and that he'd tried his best to keep it especially clean for the time you were here.'

We booked into the Waldorf Astoria in New York and that evening went to a cabaret by Liza Minelli. I enjoyed this very much. She was such a polished professional and I was delighted when invited to go backstage and meet her.

I told her how much we'd enjoyed her show and she was genuinely pleased – how her dazzling eyes lit up as she chatted animatedly with us. She'd put such a tremendous amount of energy and effort into her performance that I could see she was exhausted. I reminded her that I was a doctor and that she should get some rest immediately. Everyone laughed and we said goodnight – returning to our hotel room for our first night alone since being married.

Early the next morning we left by train for Philadelphia, where I had been cooperating with General Electric on some space programme projects for quite a while.

Barbara was invited by some women to a meeting and afterwards they took her to lunch where she had a very unusual encounter.

When they asked her what she would like to drink she ordered a gin and tonic. The waiter returned a little later to advise her that she was too young to be served alcohol – but that there was a man who wanted her phone number. When she asked why, she was told that the man worked for *Playboy* magazine and wanted to talk to her about becoming a bunny-girl and modelling for the magazine.

Barbara turned to our hosts and said dryly , 'That's very interesting. I'm too young to drink, but not too young to pose naked for a centrefold.'

We returned via Oslo to Cape Town after a six week honeymoon and moved into the two roomed flat at La Corniche. Fortunately, we were frequently invited out to dinner, because at that stage my young bride hadn't had much experience in the kitchen. It didn't worry me at all, as I remembered hearing a comedian say that a man who married a beautiful woman *and* a good cook was a bigamist.

Barbara's parents came down to Cape Town to see how we were getting on and, proudly, she invited them to our flat for dinner one evening. That afternoon she told me that she wanted to serve roast chicken, but didn't quite know how to do it.

I explained that cooking is just common sense and we scampered around the tiny kitchen, shrieking with laughter and giggling hysterically in our own, private and cosy, domestic haven.

Between the two of us we served a perfectly browned roasted chicken. Unfortunately there was no dessert on the menu as Barbara had tried to transfer the jelly from the mould onto a plate over the sink and it had wobbled off and slid like a red snake down the drain pipe.

A few days later I discovered a side of Barbara that I'd never suspected. Her parents had asked us to dinner at the Mount Nelson Hotel. We were enjoying a lovely evening in the Grill Room until I remarked that the couple on the floor were dancing extremely well. She immediately accused me of making eyes at the girl and worked herself into such a jealous and hysterical state that she stayed with her parents at the hotel that night – and, for the first time in my second marriage, I slept alone.

How wrong I'd been to think Barbara wasn't jealous or possessive.

The year 1970 was not a very productive one as we didn't perform any heart transplant operations at all – but one of our patients, Pieter Smith, died. He'd lived for 622 days after the operation. Four months before his death he was admitted to hospital with a perforated stomach ulcer. During surgery, the perforation was closed without difficulty, but unfortunately the surgeon didn't notice that it was a malignant ulcer.

A few weeks before his death the ulcer perforated again. When we explored the abdomen we found an inoperable carcinoma of the stomach.

Experience has demonstrated that malignant tumours occur more frequently in patients who have had transplants than in the population of the same age group as a whole. This is especially true for certain types of malignancy such as that of the skin, the lymph glands and the female reproductive and genital organs. We don't quite understand why, but the suppression of the patient's immune system probably plays a role.

This theory is substantiated by the findings that patients who suffer from Acquired Immune Deficiency Syndrome (AIDS) are also more likely to develop certain tumours. The post-mortem on Pieter Smith revealed that the immunosuppressive regime that we were using had been very successful in controlling the rejection. It was tragic that he should have developed this complication, as he probably would have had several more enjoyable years.

Dorothy Fisher, however, the fifth heart transplant patient, was doing well two months after surgery.

I was getting into serious trouble with the government and the Nationalist press for my anti-apartheid statements. As an employee of the Cape Provincial Administration I was supposed to shut up – but I just couldn't idly watch the destruction of my country and the lives of so many people without at least telling the world that I, like many others, was totally against segregation.

I was invited to Johannesburg to address a lunch-time meeting and decided to use the opportunity to denounce the government's policies again.

You can imagine the shocked amazement of the audience – mostly members of the Broederbond (Afrikaans: 'band of brothers', a secret society of Afrikaner Nationalists committed to securing and maintaining Afrikaner control over important areas of government) when I stood at the microphone and told them that the title of my talk would be 'Why we deserve to be called Nazis'.

I began, without pausing to allow interruption, by illustrating how closely our apartheid laws resembled some of the laws made in Nazi Germany to restrict the freedom of the Jews.

I told them that the Nationalists had passed the Group Areas Act where coloureds and blacks and Indians could only live in certain areas – the Nazis had herded the Jews into ghettos.

I reminded them we had laws which reserved certain jobs for whites only – in Nazi Germany the Jews were also prevented from taking certain positions in government and commerce.

Everywhere in public in South Africa you could see the Whites Only signs – in Nazi Germany they had *Juden Verboten*.

I quoted a few more examples and then told my audience that they shouldn't be surprised at the acrimonious opposition from the outside world, as we were giving every impression that we, the white South Africans, were the 'superior race' and that the whole world was watching the demeaning way we treated our fellow countrymen.

The chairman told me that he was sure my speech was so hot it had melted the ice-cream being served as dessert. I told him I didn't think the subject deserved to be joked about.

A few days later I had a phone call from my friend, Dr Diederichs, who told me he couldn't defend me any more at cabinet meetings. I also had a summons from Dr Nico Malan, another old friend, to come and see him in his office.

I will never forget that meeting because it almost reduced me to tears. From the moment I walked into his office he slated me for my unchristian-like behaviour and political ignorance. He said they were sick and tired of reading about me in the newspapers all the time and that he was very sorry he had been obliged to present me with the Gold Medal of the Cape Provincial Administration, because I didn't deserve it.

As I was leaving his office, I stopped at the door and said, 'Would you please convey my best wishes to Mrs Malan?'

He replied that he doubted that my best wishes would be welcomed.

My last words to Dr Malan were, 'Moet nooit sê fonteintjie, van jou water sal ek nooit weer drink nie,' which, when translated, means you should never say to the fountain that you will never drink from its water again. This was a light-hearted attempt to make a future reconciliation possible – although highly improbable.

I never spoke to him again. Shortly after that he retired as administrator of the Cape and died of a heart attack some years later.

Although I was an outspoken critic of the Nationalist government's policy, I always remained a loyal South African and, wherever possible, I defended my country when I thought it unjustly accused.

This approach made me unpopular both in South Africa because I was 'anti-government' – and outside its borders because I was 'pro-South Africa'. It was a lose/lose situation.

Barbara and I were still travelling extensively – especially as *One Life* was appearing on bookshelves throughout the world. It was eventually translated into 13 different languages and contributed over R500 000 to the Chris Barnard Fund. This was a lot of money if you consider that, in those days, the rand was worth $1,35 and that the price of an average house was R 15 000.

For the launch of the book in the United States, I was invited to appear on the programme *Meet the Press* and we were all excited that this exposure on TV would give *One Life* wide publicity.

Unfortunately the members of the press weren't interested in hearing about my biography and confined the interview to the progress of heart transplantation – so I found it hard even to mention the book at all.

I was angrily criticized by the publishers for this but I could hardly do so when asked about my results with cardiac transplants. It would be like saying, 'We have three long-term survivors,' then picking up the book and saying, 'My biography, *One Life*, has just been released – pick up a copy tomorrow.'

But, then again, I have never pretended to be a good salesman.

The whole country was looking forward to the MCC cricket tour. South Africans are sports-mad and, although rugby is really the national game, any international sport was a tonic to the ostracized society.

Because non-whites were not allowed to play either with or against whites in South Africa and because their sports facilities were much inferior to those of the whites, any non-white sportsman with promise tried to leave South Africa and settle in another country where better opportunities existed. One such South African was a coloured cricketer, Basil d'Oliveira, who had settled in England.

The MCC announced their team and, against all expectations, he was left out. I happened to be on a plane with a Nationalist cabinet minister at the time and suggested that it would be a great public relations gesture if they invited d'Oliveira to accompany the team – just as an observer.

'No,' he replied, 'we will never interfere with the decision of the MCC selectors.'

A few days later, a member of the English team announced that he wouldn't be available and Basil d'Oliveira was chosen to take his place.

Now the Nationalists had no hesitation in interfering with the MCC selections and told them that the team would not be welcome in South Africa with a coloured player.

The tour was cancelled, of course, and the new campaign for the total isolation of South Africa in the field of sport was launched, quickly gathering momentum and support. One of the leaders of this campaign was a white South African by the name of Peter Hain and another was an ex-MCC cricketer, David Sheppard.

I was, like many others, both indignant and utterly miserable about the situation. I've always been a great sports fan and, while I could see their side of the story, I thought then that the boycotters were only going to deprive the people they were trying to help. I've since changed my opinion.

Aware of my view, the BBC invited me to London to debate the issue with Peter Hain, David Sheppard and others on the Malcolm Muggeridge show, *The Question Why*.

Before leaving for this engagement, I went to Mr John Vorster, the prime minister and told him about this coming confrontation. I was adamant, and made it very clear, that there was no way that I would ever attempt to defend their apartheid policies but that I *would* try to defend South Africa.

I knew that John Harris, a close friend of Peter Hain, had been hanged because he'd planted a bomb which exploded at the Johannesburg station.

In fact, this had been the first violent demonstration – or 'act of terrorism' – against apartheid and many were to follow in subsequent years. All it had done was kill and maim innocent people. I managed to get some slides of the station explosion, which included a child who was badly burned.

Barbara wished me luck and nervously took a seat in the gallery above the studio.

Malcolm Muggeridge was the chairman of the discussion but, before the show started, I persuaded the technicians and producer to get ready to show some of the slides if I needed them.

In my opening statement I said that all of us agreed that apartheid was unacceptable and must go – and that the only differences we had were the methods to be used in achieving this.

I said that I believed in the continuation of contact, friendship and quiet coercion, knowing all too well the Afrikaner 'laager mentality'. Some others believed in breaking all contact and isolating the people, some others even believed in violent confrontation.

'I'm not a politician,' I said, 'I'm a doctor and I can only treat people if I have contact with them. A point of contact is a point of pressure and South Africa needs *pressure* to bring an end to apartheid. Nothing will be achieved by isolating the country and its peoples. And you would do well to heed the words of Abraham Lincoln when he said, "You cannot strengthen the weak by weakening the strong".'

Then I asked for the slides of the destruction caused by the explosion at the railway station. One slide was of the horribly burned child. This brought gasps of horror from the studio audience and was an extremely effective statement in support of my argument.

'These photographs,' I said, carefully choosing my words, 'show the death and mutilation of innocent people – and *this* is the type of action advocated by many as a way of overthrowing the South African government. It's inhumanity at its very lowest level.' And I stared directly at Peter Hain. The silent insinuation wasn't lost on him – nor the others.

Peter Hain was furious and, when his turn came to speak, all he could manage was to say that he could see why the South African government called me its 'best ambassador'. He certainly wasn't at his eloquent best that evening – I think the slides had had a devastating effect on his argument.

Lord Alport interjected at this stage and said that he agreed with what I was saying. He, too, was a passionate opponent of apartheid but that demonstrations like Peter Hain's *Stop the Seventy Tour* had only obscured the issues, and had caused a hardening of British public opinion *against* the anti-apartheid viewpoint. 'Still worse,' he added, 'is that pressures of a violent nature, such as the pictures we've just seen, serve only to strengthen the hand of extremists in South Africa. It is vitally important that we maintain contact with South Africa because the only solution to the country's problems will be brought about by South Africans themselves – no one else.'

Everyone, including the live audience, eventually joined in the discussion. I don't know whether we achieved very much but in the years to come it became obvious to me that isolation in the field of sport contributed significantly to stimulate the reform process.

I've never been afraid to admit my mistakes and, whenever the opportunity arose, I've said publicly in South Africa that when we are eventually accepted back into international sport, we should erect a monument to Peter Hain. I mean it.

Our inability to continue with the heart transplant programme, due to the lack of recipients, was very frustrating and in a press interview I mentioned that we were not getting the support we needed from the cardiologists.

Pamela Diamond, a local reporter who'd always resisted saying anything good about me or my work, was very quick to publish a story with as much criticism of me as she could scratch together.

She found a soul-mate in Norman Shumway who was only too pleased to rattle off a few disparaging remarks, 'Actually I didn't know Professor Barnard was still interested in heart transplant surgery. I got the impression that he had changed his interest to political and social fields.'

Diamond added that Shumway 'had laid the foundations for transplant surgery' and that one of his patients had already survived 'four months longer than Professor Barnard's only surviving heart transplant patient'. What she didn't mention was that Norman Shumway's success rate was alarmingly low.

But I'd become quite hardened to these vitriolic attacks by reporters trying to make a name for themselves. I stopped worrying about what the press said about me long ago.

Meanwhile, the newspaper report – as damaging as it tried to be – actually saved a man's life because a week or so later, Mr Dirk van Zyl phoned me and said that he'd read in the newspapers about heart transplantation and wondered if this operation would help his condition.

I asked him to come and see us and he turned out to be an excellent candidate – only 37 years old and in the terminal stages of ischaemic heart disease. I knew we could save his life – and it was, of course, an excellent opportunity to show those who'd made such nasty remarks, that I was still *very* much involved in heart transplantation.

Fortunately, a suitable donor was offered to us one week after Mr Van Zyl's admission. Damon Meyer, a 35 year old farm worker, had died after falling from a tree. His widow, Elizabeth, immediately agreed to the use of his heart as a donor.

On 10 May 1971, as with previous transplants, the donor and patient were moved into adjoining operating rooms. Ozzie was putting Van Zyl to sleep and preparing him for surgery, while Marius and I were waiting in the tearoom.

Suddenly we heard someone running urgently down the corridor (when you've worked in trauma units you soon learn to tell the difference between the sound of someone just running and the sound of someone running in an emergency).

'Prof! Ozzie wants you in A-Theatre – he's in trouble!' It was the floor nurse who spun around on her heels and rushed back into the operating room.

We both jumped up together and slipped our masks over noses and mouths as we hurried into the theatre.

We were greeted by absolute pandemonium. Ozzie was struggling to get the intratracheal tube in position and was peering through the laryngoscope, Dr Coert Venter was applying external cardiac massage by pushing hard down on the breastbone every four or five seconds, Johann and Dene were connecting the tubes of the heart-lung machine, so that we could go on by-pass if necessary, Pikkie, the operating room nurse, was hurriedly putting on her gown and gloves and a few other nurses were just running around in ever-decreasing circles.

'What's happened?' I asked – rhetorically – because I could see that, during the induction of anaesthetic, the heart had fibrillated.

'It just suddenly fibrillated!' Coert Venter replied, trying desperately to compress the patient's heart between the breastbone and spine to keep up some circulation to prevent brain damage.

Ozzie soon had the intratracheal tube in position and was able to ventilate the patient adequately.

'Oh Jesus, Ozzie! We desperately need to transplant and now the patient's going to die before we've even had a chance to open his chest!' I cried, taking over the cardiac massage from Coert.

'Does he have any blood pressure?' I demanded, increasing the rate of massage.

'Yes – a mean of about 45 – and his pupils haven't dilated at all.'

'So you think his brain's okay?'

No reply.

'If only we can get this heart beating for five minutes we can open the chest and put him on by-pass! Marius, you and Coert scrub – Johann, are you ready to go on by-pass?'

'In two minutes, Prof.'

'Ozzie, give some lignocaine and bicarbonate – Sister, let's have the defibrillator paddles. I stopped massaging and grabbed the paddles but there was no electrolyte paste on them (which is vital to conduct the electricity) and was about to shout a few choice words not suitable for the operating room, when I checked myself. Everybody was in panic. There was no use in shouting and making it worse.

'Some electrolyte paste, please,' I asked as calmly as I could and squeezed some on the front and sides of my patient's chest and positioned the paddles.

'Okay Ozzie, let's go! Defibrillator on!'

Van Zyl's body jerked as 3 500 volts passed through his chest for 10 milliseconds, producing a power of 122 500 watts.

I watched the electrocardiograph screen. There was a straight line and the flat monotone pitch of the monitor echoed around the room, except for a few seconds, when there were two or three QRS complexes and then back into fibrillation.

I started to massage again. 'Let's get an emergency Astrip done, he's probably still acidotic.'

'I've just taken some arterial blood.' Ozzie was carefully monitoring the problem. 'The blood appears well oxygenated,' he added.

'Give some more lignocaine and bicarbonate, Ozzie, and let's try and defibrillate again.' I sounded confident, but was slowly becoming resigned to the fact that we were not going to restart the heart.

He'd probably had a heart attack during the induction of anaesthetic.

I waited a few minutes for the medication to take effect and then tried defibrillating the heart again. Nothing.

If only I could connect him to the heart-lung machine! But the problem was that I couldn't apply external cardiac massage *and* open the chest at the same time.

The arteries of his legs were so severely narrowed by the same disease that had affected his coronary arteries that I couldn't even use these vessels to go on partial by-pass that way either. I just *had* to get the heart started again before we could continue.

Thirty minutes had now passed since the heart arrested and we had made at least 15 unsuccessful attempts to defibrillate it. How long should we go on before deciding the situation was hopeless and stop treatment, allowing the brain to die?

This was the decision I now had to make.

I looked up at Ozzie. 'What do you think, Oz?'

'Chris, I think it's hopeless,' he said, looking down with deep sympathy at Van Zyl's face and gently stroking our patient's head.

'Do you think his brain's still okay?'

That was a vital issue. It would be of no use to transplant a heart only to discover the patient would never wake up after the operation.

'I don't know for sure – his pupils did not dilate.'

I continued the massage. My decision now would mean life or certain death for this courageous man who came to us full of hope, as a result of an article he'd read in a newspaper.

'Let's try once more, Oz,' I said, taking the defibrillating paddles again. On the outside of his chest Dirk van Zyl already had two dark red marks from the repeated shocks.

'Okay, Oz – hit it!'

The body convulsed again. There was a flat line on the ECG. Then a beat ... a long pause ... another beat ... and then the response became more regular and more frequent. The monotone suddenly changed from its high-pitched flat drone to a merry 'ping...ping' sound.

'It's beating!' I heard somebody whisper loudly, as if afraid the heart would hear the voice and stop again.

'He's maintaining a pressure of about 50 millimetres,' Ozzie said.

I ran to the scrub room, shouting over my shoulder on the way, 'Okay, let's get him on by-pass! Marius, don't worry about bleeding – just open him, we can stop the bleeding later.' I started scrubbing my hands furiously. Please God, just give us enough time to get him connected to the oxygenator.

When I took up my position at the operating table, the heart that had so stubbornly refused to beat was already exposed. 'Give the heparin, Oz.'

We placed a single venous catheter in the right atrium and a catheter in the ascending aorta and connected these two to the heart-lung machine. 'Pump on!'

It had taken seven minutes.

We completed the transplant without any further complications and Dirk van Zyl woke up without any brain damage.

He had a completely uncomplicated post-operative course, without any evidence of rejection and was discharged four weeks after the operation.

This man had great courage and will. He went back to full-time employment two weeks after discharge from hospital.

Twenty-two years after the operation Dirk van Zyl was the longest heart transplant survivor in the world. I shudder when I think I was so close to giving up.

Barbara and I travelled a lot because it was easy. All we had to do was lock up the flat. There were no children, no garden and no pets to see to.

We had a small circle of friends in Cape Town, as most of Barbara's friends were in Johannesburg. The result was that we socialized very little. Emiliano Sandri, in the meantime, also married and had moved with his wife, Monica, into the house where we'd had the wonderful party during the first world heart transplant congress.

As this wasn't too far from La Corniche, Barbara and I often strolled along the coast to their home in the evenings.

Monica was expecting her second child and Barbara was also very keen to become pregnant.

I was worried because, from the time we got married, we had not taken any precautions as we thought that, due to my age, it would be better if we had a baby as soon as possible. It was now more than a year and still she wasn't pregnant.

I used to lie awake at night contemplating what I would do if I failed Barbara and we couldn't have children. I knew how vitally important it was to her.

There was a team of water-skiers from Europe in Cape Town and Deirdre had asked me to entertain them one evening. We took them to dinner at La Perla and afterwards we all went back to our flat in Clifton.

The party went on until way past midnight and as Barbara wasn't feeling well, she excused herself and went to lie down.

I decided that the party had gone far enough when I went into the bedroom and found that one of my young guests had passed out on the bed next to her.

After I'd herded them all out of the flat I went back to the bedroom. Barbara was sitting on the floor crying.

'I'll never have a baby!' she wailed and repeated it over and over again as she rocked back and forth on her haunches, huddled in a little bundle. Little did she know that she was already two months pregnant.

It was a monumental relief to me when Jacques, my old friend and Barbara's gynaecologist at the time, confirmed it.

Fred and Ulli were ecstatic about the news that they would soon have a grandchild and, although they never said so, I'm sure their secret wish was that it would be a boy – an heir who could continue Fred's dynasty.

The South African Chamber of Mines had made a grant of R1 000 000 available to help in the building of a research centre that could concentrate exclusively on transplantation and immunological projects. This building had now been completed and we were ready to expand our search for solutions to some of the many problems confronting the transplant surgeon.

Winston Wicomb, a young student who had just completed his B Sc and wanted to write a thesis for a Ph D degree, came to see me. I discussed the difficulties we were encountering as a result of not being able to store hearts for any reasonable length of time after removal from the donor. This problem fascinated him and he started work immediately on methods for protecting the heart muscle, during the prolonged period of ischaemia.

A few years earlier, we had been engaged in similar research on protecting kidneys after removal from the donor. Dr Ackermann, who was then working in the laboratory, came up with a novel idea. He took the kidney from donor A and then temporarily transplanted it into animal B for about 24 to 48 hours. Then removed it again and transplanted it into patient C. Animal B was then, one could say, a foster mother for the kidney for the time that it needed to be stored. As it was in B for only a short time, anti-rejection treatment was not required.

Although this worked very well in the laboratory, the idea was never used in humans.

During the few months I worked with Dr David Hume in Richmond, Virginia, we had discussed the problem of treatment of patients in coma with severe liver failure. A kidney machine had already been developed, so that the circulation of the patient in severe kidney failure could be connected to this machine, which would purify the blood until the kidney recovered spontaneously, or a transplant could be performed. This technique became known as haemodialysis.

Due to the complexities in the function of the liver, an artificial liver had not yet been developed and the only method to purify the blood of a patient in failure was to connect the patient to another liver. At that stage a pig liver was tried – with limited success.

In our discussion, I said that it would be better to connect the patient to an intact animal and that a baboon, being a primate and readily available, would be most suitable for this purpose – especially if the baboon's blood was replaced with human blood of the same group as that of the patient.

Dr Hume thought this was a great idea and I started working on it, but left Richmond before we could apply it clinically.

Just by chance, at Groote Schuur one day, I overheard Professor Saunders in a group discussing a patient who was in coma from liver failure, so I spoke to them.

'I think I have an idea which will bring your patient out of coma.'

They all looked at me. 'Do you mean by connecting a pig liver?'

'No, by connecting a live baboon,' I answered confidently.

'You must be joking!' Professor Saunders scoffed.

'No, I'm not'. And I briefly explained my idea to him.

'It won't work,' someone else said.

I looked at them thoughtfully and said, 'You know, the world of surgery is progressing so far and so fast, that the man who says it can't be done is usually interrupted by someone actually doing it.'

After some further discussion it was agreed to try out my idea, as the patient was terminally ill and there was really nothing to lose.

The lab was now alive with excitement. A big male baboon was already anaesthetized and Boets, the coloured lab assistant, was busy shaving its chest. No one had any idea of what we were about to do so I explained it to them, 'The first step is to connect the baboon to the heart-lung machine.' That was easy, as we had been using baboons instead of dogs in our transplant research for some time.

'Then, once on by-pass, we'll cool the animal down to 10 degrees Celsius.' Everyone was quiet and eagerly waiting for more information.

I turned to Hamilton, one of the Xhosa lab assistants, 'Do you have lots of ice-cold Ringer's solution?' I asked.

'Yes, Prof.' Hamilton was as good as any young doctor at surgery.

'Okay. James, at that temperature you stop the heart-lung machine and we bleed all the blood possible out of the baboon. After that you pump only Ringer's lactate through the arterial line and allow the venous blood to turn to waste.'

'We sort of wash and clean then, Prof?' Boets laughed.

'Yes, Boets, and when he's clean we don't fill his veins with wine like yours are – Boets enjoyed his *dop* (drink) – we'll use human blood through the second oxygenator. I've already asked James to prime it with the blood sent up this morning.'

There were no further questions so we went ahead step by step as I'd explained to them.

When the time came to warm the animal after his blood had been replaced with human blood, the heart slowly started beating, increased in rate and maintained a good pressure. We now had a baboon with human blood.

The animal was disconnected from the heart-lung machine and, still anaesthetized, taken up to the hospital where the patient was lying in a deep coma in a private ward. Little did the visitors in the corridor watching us pushing the trolley know that, under the white sheet, was a very unusual patient.

The venous and arterial systems of the baboon and the patient were joined through small pumps to regulate the flow.

As soon as the clamps were released, a small portion of the patient's blood was circulated continuously through the baboon – allowing its healthy liver to remove the impurities present, as a result of the patient's own liver not functioning.

We monitored both patient and baboon, and soon blood tests showed that the impurities from the patient were being eliminated. After about six hours the patient showed signs of coming out of coma. We were now faced with a dilemma that no other doctors in the world had ever had to face.

It suddenly dawned on me. 'Jesus! What's this guy going to think when he wakes up next to a baboon?'

This caused a mild sensation.

'Maybe he'll think he's been reborn as a monkey!' Someone joked.

But it *was* a serious problem. In the end we sedated him and kept him dozy and oblivious to what was going on around him. After twelve hours the tests indicated that the patient's condition had improved significantly. We waited another three hours before disconnecting the animal and taking him back to the laboratory.

The baboon showed no ill-effects from the ordeal except that he developed slight jaundice. The patient came out of coma completely.

I wasn't surprised when I read in the newspapers a few days later that the American doctors were up in arms again, claiming I'd stolen the technique from them.

'It *was* my idea,' I said to no one in particular as I read the papers, 'but who the hell cares anyway – it worked.' And I whistled happily all the way home.

'Don't you get upset about people's accusations that your ideas are theirs – when in fact, they're stealing *your* techniques? Barbara asked.

'No, not really,' I smiled. 'They'll always be able to copy what I've done – but they'll never be able to copy what I'm *going* to do.'

About a year later, we were given the opportunity to perform a major operation – the transplant of a heart and both lungs. After considerable research we decided to operate on Adrian Herbert, who had a terminal lung disease which had also affected his heart.

Although only two of these operations in the world had been performed before, and both patients survived only a few hours or days, we decided to explore and examine the problems involved.

A reported complication was bleeding – due to the fact that in the patient, both lungs with connecting arteries, veins, left upper chamber and bronchi were removed. This required a lot of dissection in the region behind the heart, often very rich in blood vessels, especially in patients who had been cyanotic for a long time.

We developed a new technique where, instead of joining the trachea, we joined the left and right bronchus separately. In this technique, the lung arteries and veins and left atrium would remain in the patient after they had been ligated and oversewed, eliminating all the previously necessary dissection that often resulted in bleeding.

It was all very exciting because we had the old team in the operating room again. Marius would remove the heart and lungs from the donor and Rodney would help me with the transplant. I was pleased to have Rodney at my side as I'd never done lung surgery and I wanted him to do the joining of the windpipes.

There was, however, a new member in the audience, my pregnant wife.

Barbara was keen to watch me operate so I took her into the operating room to see the heart and lung transplant. I was fairly sure she wouldn't last long and would leave after the skin incision. But I was wrong. She watched the whole operation with great interest. I think I was as proud of her as she was of me.

The new technique proved to be very straightforward and the operation was completed without any problems. But, a little mistake can make such a big difference to the final outcome!

Dr Hannes Meyer, a very capable surgeon training with me, was closing the chest and when he was finally checking for any bleeding points which might have been left, he noticed that near the right bronchial anastomosis there was brisk bleeding from an artery. He asked me if he could cauterize it to stop the bleeding and I agreed.

The patient had a smooth post-operative course. Both lungs and heart were working well – until the seventh day when, on routine chest X-ray, air was noticed in the left chest cavity. Although I was searching for less ominous reasons to explain this complication, the real reason was obvious. The right bronchial anastomosis had come apart and that's where the air was leaking from.

Rodney and I immediately explored the patient and found a separation of suture lines just at that point where the artery had been cauterized. What probably happened was that the cautery had not only stopped the bleeding, but had also devitalized the tissue in this area. We closed the leak and wrapped it with a muscular flap taken from the chest wall.

The patient tolerated this reparative operation well although I could see he was not doing as well, clinically, as he was before. I prayed many times a day that it would now heal, but my prayers weren't heard. On the thirteenth post-operative day there was air in the right chest cavity again.

Rodney suggested that we should put a tube in the chest and connect it to an underwater drain – there was a possibility that it would close on its own.

For the next few days I watched the bottle, hoping that the bubbling would decrease or stop – but it didn't. It got worse and worse. Eventually the leak was so severe that it interfered significantly with the patient's breathing. There was only one way to stop it and that was to remove the right lung and close the bronchus – which Rodney did.

There was no further leak, but the patient went downhill very rapidly after that operation and died on the 23rd day.

Although I blamed myself for the cautery being used at the site where the bronchi were joined, something else may have contributed towards the complication – the high dosage of steroids which the patient received. It's well known that steroids inhibit healing.

Adrian Herbert remained the longest survivor of a heart-lung transplant until the discovery of a new anti-rejection drug which made it possible to reduce the dose of cortisone. Cyclosporin was introduced in clinical practice in 1980 and, while it didn't totally prevent rejection, it reduced the severity and frequency. Heart transplant patients now have more than a 75% chance of living longer than five years – which is far better than most cancers.

Four months later our son was born. For about a week before she was to go into labour, Barbara started tidying all her cupboards. All her clothes were neatly packed away. She filed and paid all her accounts. This made me very nervous and I wondered if this was an ominous premonition.

At the first sign of labour, in the early hours of the morning, I phoned Jacques and rushed her to the Mowbray Maternity Hospital. Jacques arrived soon afterwards and after examining Barbara, said she was in weak labour.

That day, the son of Captain Friedmann, a good friend of mine, had to appear in court before a judge on a charge of Illicit Diamond Buying (IDB) which is an extremely serious offence in South Africa – much more serious than tax evasion.

I was convinced that the young man had been tricked into this crime by a police trap. What happens is that a special squad in the police force continually hunt those involved in IDB. So, in the best interests of De Beers, which monopolizes the diamond industry, they catch these crooks regularly. Unfortunately the people they catch are, more often than not, ordinary law-abiding citizens who, when short of money, are baited by undercover policemen with the opportunity of making some quick cash.

He was a big talker and may have gone around boasting that he was dealing in uncut diamonds but I'm sure he'd never done so – until then.

What happened was that he'd had a phone call from two strangers who said they knew he was in financial trouble and that they could help him. They had some beautiful, big, uncut diamonds that he could buy very cheaply and sell at a great profit.

Although he told the callers he wouldn't know how to get rid of the stones they persisted with the temptation and told him they could even help him with this.

The stupid boy fell for it and arranged to meet these two men at a parking garage in the middle of the night. They could have given him pieces of glass for all he knew about diamonds, but as soon as he took them and handed over the cash, the bastards arrested him and locked him up in a cell at the police station for the night – until his distraught father could bail him out the next day.

I felt very strongly about the injustice of this event. To me, it was like going to a man who was very hungry and telling him he could buy a loaf of stolen bread for a few cents, then arresting him for receiving stolen property.

So, despite my own concerns about Barbara, I went to court that morning to give evidence in mitigation of the sentence.

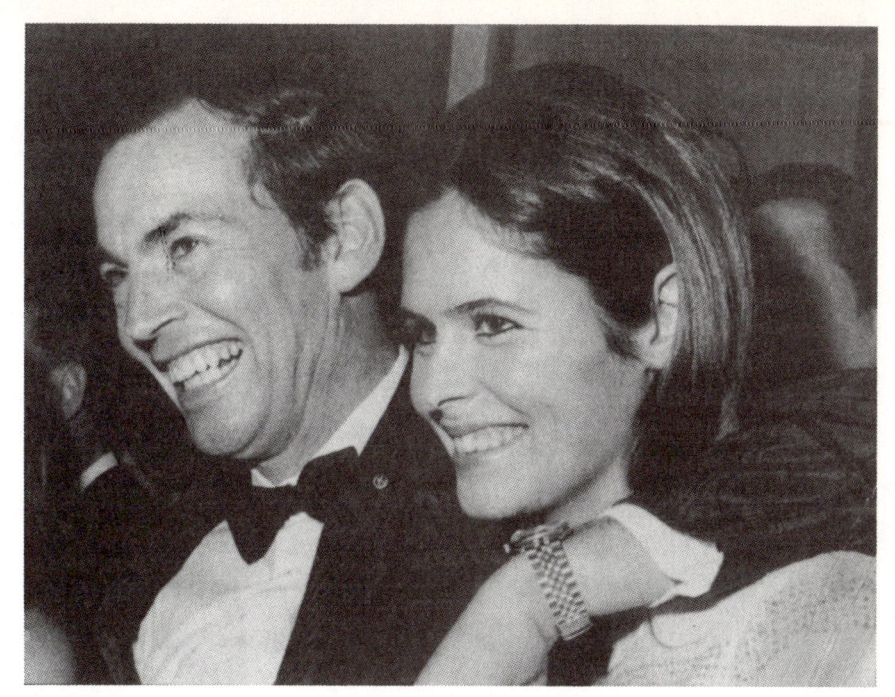

Barbara and I

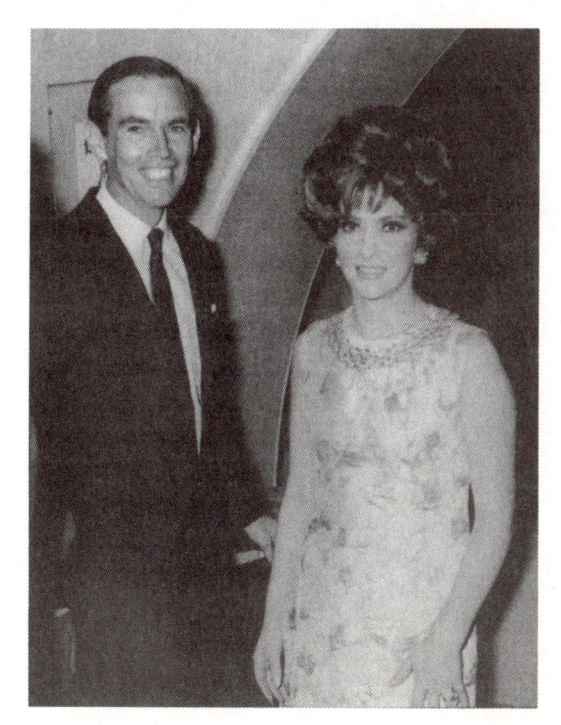

An evening with
Gina Lollobrigida

I was quite nervous in front of the judge and, having had no sleep that night, I don't think I impressed the court but I said what a good boy he was, that he came from a respectable family and that the entrapment was only a temporary lapse of his honesty.

They sentenced this unfortunate young man to one and a half years in prison – to live among hardened criminals. The judge obviously had to protect the interests of big business from such a dangerous villain.

It was a disappointing start to the beginning of what should have been a very important and happy day but I shrugged off the depression as best I could and went back to the maternity hospital quickly.

The contractions were still fairly infrequent and not too strong. I held Barbara's hand, trying to encourage her to relax with each painful contraction.

When the membranes ruptured I thought that labour would increase in intensity but it didn't. At 6 o'clock that evening Jacques examined her again and asked if he could consult another gynaecologist as he was worried about the fluid coming from the womb being stained with meconium – the baby's bowel content – and also the increased foetal heart rate.

After a while he came back saying there was foetal distress and that the baby should be delivered immediately by Caesarian section.

I went to Barbara and explained the position and said that Jacques suggested she should have the C-section. She was exhausted by that time and had been in labour for 18 hours so she readily agreed.

I grimly remembered her getting all her affairs and papers together recently, as she was wheeled into the operating room and I went to sit in the waiting room. I was anxious – almost to the point of complete hysteria.

We, as doctors, so often tell relatives of patients, 'Don't worry.'

What a stupid bloody thing to say! I promised myself I'd never say that again to anyone.

After about 15 minutes the head nurse came in to tell me that Barbara was anaesthetized and that Jacques was about to start.

'How long does it take?' I didn't know because things had changed so much since I was last at a Caesarian section nearly twenty years previously.

Will the baby be alive? Will the baby's brain be damaged by the distress? Will Barbara be all right?

All these questions flashed through my mind a hundred times as I waited. It seemed an eternity before the nurse returned with a smile.

'It's a boy, Prof!'

'Is he all right?' was all I could say before tears of gratitude filled my eyes.

'He's perfectly normal – come along,' she urged. 'They're just about to take him to the nursery – come, come and see your son.' And she pulled gently at my arm.

The operating room door opened and the nurse wheeled in the cot in which my baby was lying. He was so tiny and still smeared with caseous material.

His head was elongated from the pressures of the long labour but, to me, he was the most beautiful thing I'd ever seen – and I thought he looked like me. 'Welcome to the world, my beautiful, beautiful son.'

I wondered absently whether I'd live long enough to see him grow up.

I went back to the waiting room to wait for Jacques and to see Barbara when she was returned to the ward.

I had just seen a perfect little human being with little fingers, each with a little nail – a nose, a mouth, and eyes that could see. Billions of cells all grouped and arranged into organs, glands and tissues with such complicated functions – most of which man, with all his knowledge and wisdom, still cannot understand – and probably never will.

The wonder of conception, gestation and birth.

To think that two cells – so minute they can only be seen under the microscope – fused to initiate the process that finally produced my baby. That these two cells harboured all the instructions to control the millions of processes that would sculpt him. And that every cell in his little body *still* stored all that same information and, if called upon, could produce another human being – like him.

What a piece of work is man. There must be a God.

'Hello, Chris,' Jacques interrupted my thoughts. I looked up.

'Thank you. Thank you very much,' was all I could say, wringing his hands tightly in mine before my voice broke and the tears came.

'The little boy and Barbara are both doing fine – I think we did the right thing. We nearly lost him.' He put his arm around my shoulder and spoke gently as we walked.

After briefly visiting Barbara, who was still dopey from the anaesthetic, and phoning Fred and Ulli, I went back to the flat, doing my very best to get past the various members of the media who were only interested to know how a man of my age felt about having a baby in the house again.

'Would I feed him?'

'No, I don't have tits.' Laughter all round.

'Would I bath him and change the nappies?'

I just laughed and said I wouldn't know how.

At home I tried to sleep. The traffic noises had stopped and there was only the sound of the waves crashing on the beach below my window. I phoned the hospital in the middle of the night – suddenly very concerned – only to be reassured by a sleepy nurse that everything was fine.

My thoughts went back to that perfectly formed baby in the basket. I thought about life and death and realized I knew much more about death than about life.

Death was a clinical diagnosis made in the presence of certain symptoms and signs, just like the diagnosis of acute appendicitis or a perforated stomach ulcer.

But what is life? I once had a discussion with the late Mr Ben-Gurion who told me that even tables and chairs have life. I disagreed because, in my way of thinking, only something that can reproduce itself can claim to have life. But is that all?

The next morning, on my way to Barbara, I stopped quickly at the Red Cross Children's Hospital to see some of my patients whom I hadn't had time to visit the previous day.

I found the answer to my question there. Somebody had carelessly left a food trolley in a corner of the ward. A moment's inattention by ward staff, and it was commandeered and manned by an intrepid crew of two – one driver and one mechanic. The mechanic provided the motive power by galloping along behind pushing with his head down while the driver squatted on the lower deck of the trolley, clinging on with one arm and steering by scraping one foot on the ground. The choice of roles was easy: the mechanic was blind and the driver had only one arm.

They forgot that even the most lengthy race must end. This one did, in a crescendo of crashing and smashing plates – followed by an outraged scolding from the sister who brushed aside the protests of, 'Ag sister ons practise maar net vir die grand pree,' (Oh Sister we were only practising for the Grand Prix) and ordered the offenders back into bed.

The mechanic was all of seven years old – a shack fire had taken his sight and most of his face with it. He was part-way through a weary round of operations to release his jaw from the massive scar tissue which had gripped it so tightly to his neck, that he could only raise his head by opening his mouth. At the time of the 'grand prix', he was a walking horror with an ugly, ruined, face and a long flap of skin hanging from one side of his neck to his body. This was the skin graft which was intended to release his head from the fleshy trap and give him some neck movement.

The graft had been scalped from an unburned section of his body, rolled into a tube with one end still remaining attached – to maintain the blood supply – and the other end swung up and grafted to his neck. When it became attached firmly enough to the neck and had found an alternative blood supply, it would be cut away from the body, the tube unrolled to make a flat skin flap. Scar tissue would be cut away from under the jaw and the skin grafted on top – a very long and painful procedure involving a great number of delicate operations.

If all went well he would have good neck movement and most of these terrible scars would be covered. But it would take weeks of being wheeled in and out of operating theatres, healing scars and all the discomfort of heavy bandaging – a 7 year old's worst nightmare.

'We won!' he told me, appearing from under the bed-clothes minutes after ward discipline had been restored and Sister's awful threats of punishment were still hanging in the air. His sunken eye sockets fixed sightlessly on me in that uncanny way of the blind – and his head bobbed up and down. Incredibly, he was laughing.

The driver was 9 and had had the full book of maladies thrown at him by the time he was 7 – so he was a 'veteran' – beginning with an illness-ridden infancy and childhood, an operation for the correction of a faulty heart valve, an amazing recovery – then polio and a loss of leg action, broken bones and, recently, an operation to remove his right arm because of bone cancer. He explained that the 'grand prix' crash had been caused by the mechanical failure of a 'vrot trollie' (useless trolley).

As I left the ward he was trading insults with the mechanic. It struck me like a thunderbolt – here were two of the most terribly deprived people I'd ever met and they'd just given me a lesson in getting on with the business of living.

Life is the joy of living – the celebration of being alive.

Barbara and Frederick (we'd decided to name him after Barbara's father) came home seven days after the birth. I soon realized that there was a new boss in the house – especially after the nurse, whom we'd hired for a few weeks, had left.

Dr Rapkin, one of my teachers in paediatrics when I was still a medical student, once said that a baby cries only for three reasons – he's uncomfortable, hungry, or naughty. I could never diagnose why Frederick cried virtually every night for the first three months. They said it was colic – so it must have been discomfort, but what I couldn't understand was that he had very little colic during the day – it only started when I wanted to sleep at night!

Barbara's mother sent her maid, Lizzy, down to Cape Town to help us. She was an overweight, lovable woman with shiny black round cheeks and had an irrepressible chuckle. She was a big cosy nanny and knew exactly how to calm Frederick.

Barbara and I were frazzled and exhausted after three months. Fortunately I had an invitation to be a guest lecturer on a cruise ship, the *Chusan*. Frederick was four months old and the colic had, fortunately, disappeared. Barbara took him to Johannesburg to stay with Ulli and Fred so that we could take the cruise.

The first stop was Luanda, the capital of Angola – then under Portugese rule. Then we sailed across the Atlantic to South America.

On this trip I met a wonderful little man, Davey Kaye. Little, because he was only 5'3" tall. Wonderful, because he wanted nothing more in life than to make others happy. He was the entertainer and every night he did a cabaret which I enjoyed immensely.

When I was at primary school my mother insisted that I take piano lessons – as most mothers did in those days. My eldest brother took jazz lessons with Felix de Cola. I often watched him and listened to him playing jazz and after a while, I'd learned some of the chords and could play a few of the popular tunes. One of the tunes I played rather well was 'Red Sails in the Sunset'.

Davey Kaye insisted that I accompany him on the piano one evening and I have to admit that I was even more nervous before that performance than I ever was before an open-heart operation. I missed a few chords but I don't think anyone noticed – although I wasn't asked for an encore.

During the cruise, Barbara and I had lots of time to spend together. In the South American ports we hardly ever left the ship as we were mobbed by the crowds in the streets.

Eventually, after four weeks of bliss we returned to Cape Town and our son. He had grown a lot and it was time to have him baptized. This would definitely not take place in the Dutch Reformed Church.

I had turned my back on the church that had stood idly by while my father's coloured congregation was moved to the outskirts of Beaufort West and his church converted into a sports hall. I wanted nothing to do with the 'men of God' who turned a blind eye when the Nationalist government disobeyed the second most important of the Ten Commandments, 'Love your neighbour as yourself'.

The Dutch Reformed Church had the power to stop Dr Daniel Malan, himself a former preacher of that church, and the man responsible for the introduction of the segregationalist policies of apartheid – because he saw the Boere as the 'Elect of God'. The church could also have stopped his other wise men when they embarked on this policy created in hell. But instead, it busied itself finding passages in the Bible to allay their consciences.

There's a story about a little black boy who played in front of the door of the Dutch Reformed Church in a small country town every Sunday morning. When he saw all the people entering the church he was inquisitive and followed them. The man at the door stopped him and told him he was black and that this was a church for whites only.

This happened Sunday after Sunday until one morning the man at the door noticed that the little boy no longer showed any interest in entering the church.

He was curious to know the reason so he asked him why he'd stopped asking to come inside. The boy replied, 'Last night I had a dream that I was crying outside this church because you didn't want me to come in. I was still sitting there when God came and asked me why I was crying – so I told Him I was sad because you didn't want me to come inside the church and he told me not to worry because He hadn't been welcome inside your church for the last few years either.'

It would be scurrilous to suggest the Dutch Reformed Church had lost sight of God and humanity but they do have a great deal to answer for they *were* powerful enough to stop apartheid. Why didn't they?

Frederick Christiaan Zoellner Barnard was baptized in the Anglican church and afterwards John Schlesinger gave a party at his house, 'Summer Place'. John was the only son of a very wealthy businessman of the Schlesinger dynasty and didn't have to work much. He became a good friend of ours and was very kind to both Barbara and me.

Most of the guests thought that my speech was terrible. It was an off-the-cuff talk and I'd only decided on the main point when I saw some black children laughing as they walked past the window. I wondered what these kids had to laugh about in this country.

When the time came for me, as father of the child, to say a few words I told the people gathered in the magnificent Schlesenger mansion surrounded by every conceivable luxury – that I hoped my son would grow up to contribute to the changes in our country so that these black and brown children *would* have something to laugh about.

Barbara was very angry and Fred ignored me for the rest of the evening. But John Schlesenger thought it was very funny – maybe it was the Jack Daniels that helped him appreciate it.

I was furious!

Ugly rumours were flying around that Vel Schrire was telling physicians my results with coronary artery surgery were poor and that they shouldn't refer patients to my department at Groote Schuur Hospital any more.

Terry O'Donovan had started a small private practice in open-heart surgery at another hospital and, according to Vel, his results were much better than mine.

Matters deteriorated to a point where I had no option other than to request a meeting with Vel to confront the issue and, hopefully, put it to rest.

I gathered together all the details I could about the gossip and accusations. I was determined to go to the meeting and tell Vel what a big shit I thought he was and demand to know why he was so intent on stabbing me in the back.

On the way to the superintendent's office I met Eugene Dowdle, whose opinion I valued immensely. I told him that I was on my way to the meeting and also the gist of what I intended saying.

'No, Chris,' he advised me, 'that isn't going to achieve anything – rather try and make peace, use a more gentle approach.'

I thought about this advice very carefully and decided that Eugene was probably right. I'd be as tactful as I possibly could.

'Would you like to start?' the superintendent asked me. We were all sitting around a table in his office. A semicircle of very serious faces – all senior doctors, about to discuss childish behaviour.

'Yes, Dr Burger, I'm a very sad man today. The success we've had in the past 13 years is due to the close cooperation between the surgeons and the cardiologists – that is, between Vel and me.'

Vel's face remained impassive.

'I remember how Vel gave a party at his house with a cake and one candle to celebrate the first year of open-heart surgery here in Cape Town. There was a time when my day was not complete unless I visited the cardiac clinic and had a chat with Vel – we've always been colleagues and friends.'

Vel still didn't show any emotion, so I continued recalling events of the past years – to illustrate the strong bond that had existed between us.

'I've come here today to extend my hand in friendship to an old friend, and to ask him if we can work together again and put an end to the petty squabbling and rumour-mongering.'

There was deathly silence and everyone looked at Vel.

His reply was brief. Clearing his throat, he answered me by talking directly to Dr Burger, as if I wasn't even in the room, 'I'm prepared to cooperate with Professor Barnard again – but we will never be friends.'

At first I was bloody angry that I'd followed Eugene Dowdle's advice and been so conciliatory – I should have told him what I thought, as I'd planned to do, but I didn't know then that Vel was due to be operated on the following day for abdominal pain and jaundice.

The surgeons found an inoperable cancer of the pancreas.

I'm convinced that Vel's inexplicable behaviour was due to the terminal illness he was suffering. After everything that had happened, I was glad I hadn't lost my temper with Vel.

He fought the cancer with all the determination he was renowned for, but died two months later.

I still remember him fondly – and as one of the very best cardiologists I've ever known.

Three men then entered my life who had a profound influence on my future. They were Armin Mattli, Peter Sellers and Aris Argyriou.

Out of the blue, Armin Mattli phoned me from the President Hotel in Cape Town. He said he'd like to see me for a few minutes and we arranged to meet each other in the bar. When I arrived he was sitting outside on the stoep enjoying a beer and the sunset.

He was a Swiss-German from Zürich and told me that he admired me and my work immensely.

'I've heard you suffer from arthritis, Professor,' he said. My immediate thoughts were, Oh, not another cure!

'I'm the owner of the Clinique La Prairie in Switzerland,' he continued, obviously unaware of my initial disappointment. 'We treat various diseases by injecting the patients with live cells harvested from the foetal lamb, and my doctors tell me that we'll be able to help you too.' He took a long sip of the beer and wiped the froth from his lips with the back of his hand.

'I've vaguely heard about the clinic Mr Mattli, but the medical profession considers your treatment idiotic, and your claims unfounded.' I remember thinking that perhaps I'd been a bit tactless, but what the hell – sometimes it's best to tell it like it is.

Mattli wasn't insulted and smiled when he said, 'But the thousands of patients we have treated feel quite differently and, after all, that's what really matters.'

He had a point.

'I would like to invite you to my clinic so that you can see it firsthand. You have nothing to lose. I will pay all your travel expenses and we won't charge you for any treatment. We'd value your opinion.'

'You're right, I don't have anything to lose – except my life! If I develop a serious allergic reaction from the animal proteins you inject, then I'll die.' I said severely.

But I was becoming intrigued by the idea.

'Professor, in our 40 years of existence we have treated over 30 000 patients and we've never had a death. Each patient is carefully tested for allergies before any treatment and, if positive, we desensitize him and take special precautions.'

We studied each other silently for a while. He certainly had all the answers and spoke very confidently and persuasively. I knew then that this was a very smart businessman.

'The treatment also results in rejuvenation of various systems in the body,' he smiled impishly and finished his beer.

'Well, as you say, I have nothing to lose – so I accept your generous offer,' and we shook hands.

One Life had sold extremely well but, as I've mentioned before, I hadn't gained financially from its success so I decided to write another book and to donate only 50% of the income to research this time.

Coronary artery disease had always been labelled as the number one killer in the Western world – because it couldn't be totally prevented and the real cause was undetermined. People were scared stiff by its ominous name and, until the AIDS epidemic, the most fearsome words were 'heart attack', 'stroke' and 'cancer'.

I decided to write a book of hope to explain the disease in detail and say how modern medicine could help those unfortunate enough to be struck down by it.

With considerable help from my colleague, Eugene Dowdle, *Heart Attack – You don't have to die* was soon published.

To launch this book in England the publishers gave a cocktail party and, because he had suffered a massive heart attack a few years earlier, Peter Sellers was invited.

This man fascinated me because he was acting all the time. I'd never met anyone so hilariously funny. He could imitate anyone and was brilliant at mimicking my own accent. The only role he couldn't play was that of Peter Sellers himself, which I thought was very sad. We had dinner together after the cocktail party and promised to keep in touch, which we did, and we were to enjoy each other's company many times during the next few years.

The third man, Aris Argyriou, was a very likeable, overweight young Greek in his early thirties. The doctors told him he had an enlarged heart and he arrived at my office, one morning, unannounced.

Aris was a civil engineer and it was obvious that he came from a very good family. He was immaculately dressed – Gucci shoes, Pierre Cardin jacket and Hermes silk tie. He immediately invited Barbara, Frederick and me for a holiday on the island of Rhodos, where he was part-owner of two hotels.

I referred him to the cardiac clinic where he was examined. They confirmed that his heart was indeed enlarged – probably due to too much Chivas Regal. He was fortunately, however, not in any serious trouble then, so we advised him to ease up on the good life and to take things a little easier.

Before leaving for Athens, Aris came to see me again in my office and told me he wanted to open a health spa on the island of Kos – because that was the birthplace of Hippocrates.

He said that he'd very much like me to become involved in this project. After two hours of discussion, I persuaded him to create, instead, a centre for preventative medicine as I wasn't keen on being involved with a quasi-medical institution.

For this centre we would have to build five-star accommodation and a medical centre equipped with the most modern facilities. Our guests would have a thorough medical check-up – mainly aimed at detecting risk factors that could lead to heart attack, cancer or stress disorders.

We would also need a treatment centre where patients could be taught to change their lifestyles to reduce any risks we had detected.

Aris was very happy with this idea and after returning to Greece, he formed a company, of which I was made president, and the building of the Hippocrates Health Centre started.

Little did I know that the friendship with these three men would all eventually end in bitterness and acrimony.

'Let's go out – we've been sitting at home every night for the last month now,' I suggested to Barbara one unseasonably miserable summer's evening.

'What about the baby?' she asked, taking the bottle from his mouth.

'I'm sure Lizzy can take care of him for a few hours, we won't be long.'

I was eager to get out for a while, and was feeling restless with the routine of the hospital during the day and the flat at night.

Barbara didn't really feel like it but, if that's what I wanted, then we should go, and she handed Frederick to Lizzy to finish feeding him.

We had received two invitations for that evening so we went to a cocktail party at the President Hotel first and then set out for the opening of a new steakhouse. As we were driving along the main road in Sea Point Barbara suggested that we skip the steakhouse and rather have a quiet dinner at our favourite restaurant – Florentino's.

I stopped my car at a parking meter opposite the restaurant and we walked across the road to the warmth and oven-baked cosiness of this little family-run business. We brushed off the rain and sat at a candle-lit corner table.

Barbara ordered spaghetti and I had my favourite – a pepper steak. The owner, who was also the chef, brought us a special bottle of chianti to celebrate – as we hadn't been there since Frederick's birth.

We had a beautiful evening together. It was one of those evenings when everything was perfect: the romantic atmosphere, the food, the drink, and just being together. Life was good and I realized that Barbara meant more to me at that moment than ever before, if that was possible.

She wasn't just my wife and lover, she was also the mother of my child. We had a common bond, something more to live for. To say we were deliriously happy that evening would be a gross understatement.

I paid the bill, popped a few peppermints into my mouth and we walked out onto the busy pavement. It was still drizzling so I put my left arm around Barbara's waist and we hurried across the street to our car.

We paused in the middle of the road to allow some oncoming traffic to pass. I remember looking to my right and thinking 'those lights are very close' and the next thing I heard was Barbara shouting.

'Chris! *Chris!*' she screamed.

I was aware of other people gathered around me. 'What's going on?' I moaned.

'Lie still, you've been hit by a car,' someone told me.

Then I heard Barbara again, 'What about my baby!'

'Is Barbara all right?' I tried to say but could hardly speak due to the pain in my chest.

'Yes, she's okay, but she's hysterical.' I heard another voice say and then I sank into deep, merciful unconsciousness.

The next thing I remember is lying in the ambulance with someone placing a mask over my face. I couldn't breathe properly and had this unbearable pain on the left side of my chest. I put my hand on my chest and could feel air in the fatty tissues under the skin – it felt like eggshell crackling. Now I could begin putting together the pieces of what had happened and diagnose my condition.

I'd been hit by a car on the chest. Some ribs had fractured and one or more of them had stabbed my lung and perforated it. As a result of this, the punctured hole was allowing air to escape from the lung into the subcutaneous tissues under my skin.

According to the voices I'd heard, Barbara was okay. I only discovered later that one of those voices had been a doctor who'd been quick on the scene.

I felt my chest again. God, I thought, I'm going to get a pressure pneumothorax and die. A pressure pneumothorax is when a leak in the lung acts like a one-way valve – air can blow out, but the valve stops it from going back. Substantial pressure in the pleural space quickly builds up, which compresses the lung and pushes the heart over to the opposite side. This can lead to respiratory and circulatory embarrassment and often to death.

I told myself to take very shallow breaths, so that as little air as possible would be moved when inhaling – I was trying to reduce the pressure and the leak.

'Be careful! Hold his arm! Where's the oxygen?' Everyone was shouting and running around me, as I was being taken from the ambulance on a trolley to the multiple injury unit at Groote Schuur.

'Call Rodney!' I wheezed to the doctor when he came to look at me.

The pain was unbearable, like a red hot knife being twisted in my side every time I took a breath – as the ragged ends of eleven broken ribs grated over each other. Each nerve-ending screamed its own agony – a dentist's drill churning into a raw nerve was mild by comparison.

Fortunately, the pain caused me to black out every few minutes.

I now know why patients in these circumstances don't want to live, because there is only unspeakable pain, the escape from which, even if it meant death, would be welcomed. But the difference between my condition and that of the terminally ill cancer patient is that medical treatment *could* return my health and joy for life.

Rodney told me he'd looked at the X-rays and that it wouldn't be necessary to do a tracheostomy or put me on a respirator. Although I did have many rib fractures the chest was stable.

I could feel the pressure on my chest as he introduced the trocar and cannula. Then the tube was inserted and connected to an underwater drain. My breathing improved immediately – but not the pain.

I kept asking about Barbara, although I'd been told that she wasn't badly hurt. I had no way of knowing that she was *seriously* injured and it was only by the grace of God that she wasn't killed, or totally paralyzed from a broken neck.

She had fractured several vertebrae in the neck, but fortunately there was no spinal injury. Her left shoulder blade was also smashed, and she had multiple bruises and abrasions.

As they were taking me to a ward I said I wanted to go to C2 – my own ward – because I had more confidence in the quality of care there.

During the night I could hear the heart monitor and, each time it slowed, I thought, Oh well, this is it then – the end.

Marius came to the hospital as soon as he heard about the accident and stayed with me the whole night. I wasn't sure whether I was glad or not to be alive when the sun rose the next morning. I felt like death but wanted to know how Barbara was.

'Barbara was also admitted to C2 and is lying in a ward next to this one,' Marius said. 'She's going to be fine.'

'What happened to us?' I groaned – even the slightest movement was acutely painful.

'From what I've heard it was a hit and run,' he said. 'Some people say it may even be politically motivated, as they saw a car which had apparently been "waiting" outside the restaurant for some time. When you left the restaurant and crossed the road it suddenly screeched away from the kerb, knocked you down and disappeared.'

I remembered all the death threats I'd received and how complacent I'd become about them.

'It hit you with such force that you ricocheted into Barbara and you both flew through the air across the road into oncoming traffic. Fortunately for Barbara, she fell on to the back of a car – otherwise she would have been killed outright.

'By the way, one of the people at the scene of the accident was a doctor, and when he saw you had difficulty in breathing, he put his fingers in your mouth to see if there was any obstruction to your airway. He found three peppermints in your throat.'

I would have laughed if it hadn't been so painful when I imagined what the death certificate would have said: 'Death caused by three Mint Imperials.'

Marius looked at me for a while in silence and I could see the deep concern and brotherly love in his face.

'There's one more thing,' he added finally. 'They think you've ruptured your right kidney. There's a lot of blood in your urine.'

'Oh Jesus,' I groaned, 'what else?'

'The urologist wants you to come down for an intravenous pylogram.'

'Oh please, Marius, can't they leave it?' I begged. 'It's absolute bloody agony for me to move!'

Before Marius could answer, Sister Geyer appeared in the doorway, 'Prof, the porters are here to take you down.'

'Down where? Down to *hell*!' I cursed. And I continued hurling abuse at everyone all the way down to the urology department.

In order to see the kidneys under X-ray, an iodine preparation is injected in a vein. This radiopaque dye is concentrated by the kidneys and then excreted in the urine allowing visualization of the kidney and the urinary passages under X-ray.

'Are you allergic to iodine?' the radiologist asked.

I shook my head. The pain was so severe I couldn't speak.

He looked for a vein in my right arm and I felt the needle puncture.

'Okay, we have to wait ten minutes.'

I lay back on the X-ray table thankful for just a few minutes' respite and then the nausea started welling up from the pit of my stomach.

'I'm going to vomit! Bring me a kidney dish!' I cried. It was all I could say before I began heaving and straining, increasing the pressure inside my abdomen and chest cage to expel the contents of my stomach. The bitter taste of bile filled my mouth and a hundred daggers stabbed my lungs each time I threw up.

Beads of sweat ran down my forehead, and when I wiped it away I felt as cold and clammy as a corpse. I didn't know how long this torture continued, as I lost consciousness several times.

'Your kidney isn't severely damaged,' the radiologist announced. 'You can go back to the ward.'

'Can't you give me something for the pain?' I pleaded with a doctor.

'We don't want to give you too much Omnopon. You may become addicted,' came the unsympathetic reply. Bloody fool! I cried soundlessly.

Fortunately my brain did what the Omnopon was supposed to do – it interrupted the impulses that fired that part of my brain where awareness is registered, and I welcomed the swirling blackness each time it came.

My recovery was slow, and complicated by repeated accumulation of fluid in the right chest after the tube had been removed. Terry had to 'tap' it by putting a needle between the ribs.

I also developed one of the most degrading complications: faecal impaction. Due to the inability to strain, it was impossible to have normal bowel actions. The faeces accumulated in the large bowel and became so hard that Dr Birkenstock had to remove it by hand under anaesthetic. It was the ultimate humiliation – having one of my colleagues do this – but I was beyond caring, and thought I'd never recover to become a normally functioning human being again.

This experience taught me to appreciate the little things in life which one normally takes for granted every day. To be able to get out of bed in the morning, walk to the bathroom, use the toilet, wash, shave and have a bath without assistance.

As I regained my strength and the ability to do these things returned, each new step was like a major victory. The pleasure of being able to bathe myself again will always be a vivid memory.

I think that being a patient also makes you a more caring physician. I learned how important it is for a patient to have complete confidence in the doctor taking care of him. Also, the trust in the nurses is an incredibly important factor – a frequent change in nursing staff can be very distressing, because a bond develops between patient and nurse – in fact it's a kind of maternal love that should be interrupted as infrequently as possible.

The plastic surgeon set Barbara's nose and she had to wear a collar for the fractured vertebrae in her neck.

After a few weeks in the hospital she was discharged – only to be readmitted for the removal of a piece of shoulder blade that was almost sticking out through her skin.

Ulli came down from Johannesburg and she and Lizzy looked after Frederick.

The police arrested a black man and charged him with knocking us down and driving away from the scene of the accident. A few weeks after my discharge the case was heard in the magistrate's court in Cape Town. After I'd told the magistrate what I could remember and the police had told their story, he was found not guilty due to lack of evidence.

To this day, we still don't really know who knocked us down.

7

Deirdre, after wandering around the world skiing, had returned and was now at the University of Stellenbosch, studying to become a teacher. André, after a year wasted in the Navy doing his national service, was at the University of Cape Town Medical School – he wanted to be a doctor like his dad. Louwtjie was living alone at Zeekoevlei with two dogs, Sixpence and Ringo, and my mother was still sitting in a wheel chair at the old age home waiting for the inevitable.

One of my mother's few pleasures was the weekly visit made by Barbara. She took her cream doughnuts, which my mother loved, and stayed talking with her longer than any of her sons ever did. During my short monthly visits she would often clasp her hand over her mouth in disbelief and say, 'Chris, you are so lucky – she's such a *good* woman!'

'Hi Dad.' I immediately recognized the voice of my son.

'André! How's it going? How's the studying?' Because of my competitive nature I had always been interested in the progress of my children – especially now at University, where my son was following in my footsteps.

'It's tough, Dad – but I'm phoning you for a different reason.' I could hear the concern in his voice and he continued miserably, 'Martin is very, very sick – he's in heart failure and the doctors in Pretoria say there's nothing that can be done for him. Can you help?' His voice trailed away and I guessed he was close to tears.

'Do you know what they say is wrong with him?' I asked.

'According to the cardiologist it's not the mitral valve that you replaced seven years ago – that's working fine – the vein grafts you did afterwards are also still patent, but his heart is enlarged and they say that the left ventricle is hardly contracting at all.'

They'd told him this was due to the death of a lot of the heart muscle, which usually indicated that only a transplant could save him.

'How old is he now?' I asked. I was already thinking quickly, as we had a rule not to accept patients for transplant over the age of 50. André was aware of this rule too.

'He's only 52 – and in very good shape.' I could hear the plea in his voice.

'Then get him down to Cape Town immediately – I'll arrange a bed for him in my ward. Let's see what we can do.'

'Oh thanks Dad! Thanks a million. I *knew* you would help him!'

Martin Franzot and his wife Kitty had been pillars of strength for André during the divorce, when he lived with them in Pretoria. He'd been 'adopted' as their own son and I'm sure he loved Martin like a father.

Heart catheterization indicated that Martin's heart had been considerably damaged by the blockage of the arteries supplying it with blood. The quantity of blood pumped with each beat was only 20% of the normal quantity, and it was obvious that only a transplant could save his life.

André was so proud that his father could help this man he loved so much. 'You're the best heart surgeon in the world, Dad.' And he often visited me in my office where we discussed the operation in detail.

I had always been close to Deirdre through her water skiing but André had unfortunately taken a back seat – now we were close like fathers and sons should be. We had a common interest: medicine and surgery.

Luckily, a suitable donor was soon referred to us. I phoned André and told him that we were going to do the transplant and that, if he would like to watch the operation, he was very welcome.

'No Dad, I'm too close to Martin, I'll wait in the doctors' room. Best of luck.'

I had great difficulty in dissecting Martin's heart free, as it was severely stuck to the chest wall and surrounding structures due to the adhesions that had formed after the two previous operations but once it was free, the operation was no problem.

'Okay Johan, you can start re-warming. Ozzie, start ventilating.'

I was rather nervous about this transplant, although there should have been no further complications. Martin Franzot was not only André's adopted 'father' – he was also a very dear friend of mine.

'Sinus rhythm!' Somebody shouted happily, as the transplanted heart started beating spontaneously. The contractions were regular and strong.

'Okay Johan, reduce the flow.' This would reduce the support of the heart-lung machine. A portion of the circulation would now be pumped by the transplanted heart.

'Flow is down, Prof,' Johan confirmed. The heart filled and contracted with ease. Everything was normal.

'Okay, stop pump.'

'Pump off!'

Now the heart had to manage the full circulatory load.

'Pressure down, Chris,' Ozzie warned.

'Damn it,' I said mildly. I could see the heart swell up, but it was unable to expel all the blood it was receiving. This wasn't an unusual problem though, so I wasn't unduly alarmed.

'Okay Johan, help it again.' I wanted to ease the new heart's burden for a while.

'Pump on – quarter flow,' said Dene who'd taken control of the heart-lung machine.

Immediately, the heart picked up and was contracting fully again.

'Let's give it five minutes to recover. Oz, give some bicarb and isoprenaline,' I instructed. 'It's probably still suffering from the period it was without blood supply.'

In the meantime, I inspected the suture line for any evidence of bleeding.

'Send a message to André,' I told the floor nurse. 'Tell him the operation's finished and everything looks fine.' I was confident of the result.

'He's outside in the corridor and has been watching most of the operation' she said. 'He looks very happy and wants to congratulate you.' Her eyes were smiling.

'Okay, pump off!' I watched the heart responding and it was at that moment that I started feeling scared – the heart wasn't handling the increased work very well, which it should have been able to by now.

'Pressure's down again, Prof,' I heard as I watched the heart struggling more and more.

'Pump on again, Dene.' Fear gripped me like a cold iron vice. I struggled to breathe myself. Was I going to be unable to save my friend? Was I going to let my son down again, as I had when I left his mother and he was without a father?

It increasingly appeared I was going to lose him and I struggled for over an hour to get the heart to take over, but every time I stopped the support, it would fill up and fail.

Again and again it failed. This had never happened before. Why did it have to happen today? I kept trying but I knew – and could see in the eyes of those around me that they knew it wasn't going to work either.

The donor heart must have suffered severe damage due to periods of low blood pressure before I could do the transplant. I now had to make, probably, the most difficult decision of my life.

With a deep sigh I said, 'Dene, stop the heart-lung machine.' I had no choice.

I watched the heart swell up again. The beat became slower and slower until it fibrillated.

Martin gave a few gasps as his brain died. There was silence in the operating room as I turned around and took off my gloves, walking out to where André was waiting for me.

His wide, brown eyes were swimming in tears. 'What happened, Dad?' he sobbed.

'He died, André,' was all I could get out before my voice choked and my own tears came.

'But *why* did he die, Dad? You gave him a new heart!'

'He died because the heart couldn't carry enough of the circulation to keep him alive,' I explained miserably.

He looked into my eyes before saying, 'Then why didn't you put back his old heart? At least that kept him alive.' He turned and walked away. Away from his real father and the dead body of his adopted father.

I couldn't sleep that night. My son's words 'Why didn't you put back his old heart? At least that kept him alive,' echoed in my brain.

Why didn't you put back his old heart? At least that kept him alive.

In the early hours of the morning I made a new decision. I would devise an operation where the patient's own heart is left in place – to do whatever it still could – and connect the donor's heart in such a way that it would help the old heart instead of replacing it entirely. In this way, if anything should ever go wrong with the donor heart, the patient's heart would keep him alive.

So, that morning the idea of the heterotopic heart transplant was born (later to be dubbed the 'piggy-back').

It was still dark when I got up, shaved and dressed. I was obsessed with this idea and couldn't wait to start exploring the possibilities of the two hearts beating inside the chest of one man.

This concept wasn't new. Ten years previously I'd visited the laboratory of Professor Demikhov in Moscow. He could correctly be called 'the father' of cardiac transplantation because of the extensive research he did in this field, even before the development of the heart-lung machine.

During that visit he showed me a dog that was walking around with two heads – the second one in the heterotopic position. 'Heterotopic' means that it's not in the anatomical site of the organ – an abnormal or wrong position.

I also read in the medical journals of other researchers who'd explored this idea in the laboratory.

What I didn't like about the techniques used to that point was that they tried to place the heart in the left side of the chest and, because the patient's heart was already over to that side, there wasn't enough space. This meant they had to remove a portion of the left lung to make room. My idea was to do the operation in such a way that, if the donor heart should fail, it could be taken out and the patient would be no worse off than before the operation.

That morning I was at the anatomy museum before it opened. I took two plastic models of the human heart and positioned the one as it would normally be positioned in the chest. The second one I placed in various positions on the right side and, within ten minutes, I had the technique worked out in my mind for the operation that would make it possible to have a second heart in the right chest, without interfering with the function of the right lung.

My next stop was the animal laboratory. I didn't wait for the elevator but leapt up the steps to the fourth floor.

Without greeting Boets I asked whether Dr Losman was there. He was a doctor from Belgium who had trained with me and was now doing a year in our laboratory.

'I'll call him, Prof,' said Boets as he left an anaesthetized baboon on the table.

Jacques came in a few minutes later. 'Sorry to hear about last night,' were his first words.

'I don't know what went wrong, but I think I know the answer. I want you to stop all other projects and work full-time on the heterotopic transplant.'

Jacques looked at me mystified.

'Let me explain,' I said, bubbling over with enthusiasm. 'Call the other guys, too.'

We all gathered around the sleeping baboon.

'If you have a horse pulling a load up a hill,' I began, 'and he starts struggling, you can correct the situation in two ways: either remove the tired horse and hitch a fresh horse in front of the cart, or you can leave the old horse there to do whatever he can and hitch the fresh horse alongside him – to help.'

They all looked at me as if I'd finally gone off my rocker. But I continued anyway. 'The tired horse is the failing heart. The first approach is the orthotopic transplant where the tired horse has been outspanned and the fresh horse now has to pull the full load.

'The second operation is the idea we are now going to try, where the second heart is just an assist device – the old heart will still do some of the work.'

'D'you think there's enough room for two hearts in one chest?' asked Jacques with his French accent.

'That's what we are going to find out. Now listen carefully.' I turned to the blackboard and explained.

'First we will use baboons as our experimental animals – their chest cages are closer in shape to human chests and are much better for our purposes than dogs.

'Do you have enough baboons, Boets?'

'Ja, Prof, no problem.'

'This will be the surgical technique; the chest of the patient is opened in the mid-line, the heart sac is opened vertically. So, at this stage it's the same as any transplant. But now the difference comes. The left lung space is opened and the left side of the heart sac is detached. This should create a space between the lower part of the right lung and the patient's own heart – for the new heart to lie in. We'll have to see whether the right lung will be compressed, but I don't think so. Do you follow so far?'

My eyes swept the room – everyone seemed to understand and look interested.

'Now the connections to the donor heart – this is simple. We join the left upper chambers side to side, and the right upper chambers side to side as well. These openings will function as escape valves, for whichever heart is failing.' I turned from the blackboard where I'd drawn a schematic representation of the anastomoses.

'For the outflow to the lower chambers – on the right side we join the pulmonary arteries end to side and, on the left side, the aortas. *Voilá!* You have two hearts in parallel. Simple, don't you think?'

I didn't think I'd convinced the lab staff – they were standing awkwardly and no one spoke.

'Jesus! Are you so bloody dumb you can't see the advantages of this procedure?' They knew I was getting angry. 'Let's take the example of the problem I had last night. When I helped the transplanted heart just a little bit with the heart-lung machine it managed well, but only when it had to carry the full load did it fail. Now, if I'd left the patient's heart to give what little support it could to the new heart, Martin Franzot would be alive today. And I'm sure that whatever the problem was in the donor's heart, it was only temporary anyway and would probably have recovered, within a few hours, to take over the complete job.'

Jacques now came to life, '*Oui!* We'll start straight away, Prof.' He turned to his colleagues and clapped his hands enthusiastically, 'Okay, let's get going!'

In medicine it's often possible to assess quite quickly whether a new idea has a future or not. If you had to struggle months and months – even years – and couldn't get it to work, then the chances were that you were on the wrong track to begin with.

The piggy-back operation worked from the very first experiment.

I discussed this idea with Professor Wally Beck who had now taken the place of Vel Schrire. He pointed out that as right-heart failure in patients is usually not due to disease of the right pumping, but secondary to left-heart failure, all you have to do with this operation is to assist the left heart.

With our first two operations, we modified the technique slightly so that the patient's own right-heart would still be responsible for circulation to the lungs and the donor heart would assist only the patient's failing left ventricle.

This proved to be a mistake.

The political system in South Africa depressed me more and more as there appeared to be no one strong or powerful enough to do anything about it. I, like so many other South Africans, felt helpless and despondent.

The Nationalist party had dug themselves in by taking the coloured people off the common voters' role and rezoning constituencies, so that a few thousand votes in a place like Beaufort West – where the Nationalists were almost exclusively supported – would have the same power as over ten thousand votes in a suburb of, say, Cape Town where the Nationalists were strongly disliked.

In all the key administrative and local government positions they appointed 'Broeders' – members of the Broederbond which was, and still is, an extremely exclusive and secret Afrikaner organization. The motto of the organization was *Wees sterk* (be strong) and, in 1921, three years after its formation, it became highly secretive. It played a significant role in determining the National party's apartheid policies, especially as most of the key politicians and high-ranking officials were sworn members.

How such an organization could ever have existed is baffling, and even more inexplicable is how such a bunch of God-fearing moralists could ever have supported apartheid, given their piety. (One of the more serious 'crimes' a broeder could commit was to attend church only infrequently.)

Their policy of 'Separate but equal' was so obscene that I just *had* to do something more than just talking at dinners and banquets.

I decided to write a novel.

In many respects it would be based on my own experiences and those of my colleagues. I am primarily a storyteller and find it easy to formulate ideas, but I'm not a novelist. So I searched for someone to help me write *The Unwanted* and I met Siegfried Stander.

I decided there would be two characters in the book – a black boy and a white boy. They would both become doctors and the book would deal with all the injustices that the black boy was subjected to: inferior education and also the fact that, once at medical school, he was not allowed to examine white patients – he wasn't even allowed to watch a post-mortem done on a white corpse.

The story would follow these two characters during their careers and the plot would have some bizarre twists to it and a very surprising conclusion – but I suppose you'll have to read the book.

I was very pleased when it was finished, as I thought it was quite a good book, but the Afrikaans press slated it. It was never a bestseller in the United States or Europe but it was very popular in countries behind the Iron Curtain, strangely enough.

Although the royalties from *The Unwanted* helped augment my meagre salary of R1 200 per month, it wasn't enough to take care of my wife and my son. Fortunately Barbara received a substantial monthly allowance from her father so we were able to move into a bigger flat in La Corniche and her mother helped us furnish it. For the first time in my life I lived with wall-to-wall carpeting and antique pieces around the sitting room.

Barbara was used to a good life where she was short of nothing and she enjoyed dressing in designer garments. I felt guilty that I couldn't give her all these things – although she never complained. She had a husband and a son and would have lived in the greatest poverty to keep her little nest secure and undisturbed, I'm sure.

Emiliano Sandri, who'd come to South Africa after the war and worked as a steward on the trains had eventually, through shrewd investments in restaurants, become a wealthy man – and he gave me an idea.

I pestered him until he sold me one of his restaurants in Newlands close to the famous cricket and rugby grounds. Now I was going to become rich! At least that's what I thought.

My friends agreed. 'With your name the restaurant will be full every night,' they enthused. I soon found out, however, that a name is of little value if it's not backed by quality and professionalism – even a packed restaurant doesn't necessarily mean it's profitable.

Monica, Emiliano's wife, told me when I took over the restaurant from her husband that I was 'mounting a wild horse'. In the next few months I found out what she meant. The restaurant business was more than just preparing and serving food and banking the money.

Every month my books stayed firmly in the red. Instead of augmenting my income, it was draining it. I had sleepless nights trying to work out what I was doing wrong.

I thought I had the best staff available – two highly experienced Italian restaurateurs and a qualified Belgian chef with assistants and waiters.

In my spare time I went out of my way to buy the best quality fresh vegetables, fruit and fish.

The restaurant appeared to be well patronized but I was still losing money. I knew there had to be something seriously wrong – but what?

Every Saturday night I went there in person and mingled with the customers to find out what they thought about the food and the service – I also listened to their complaints. Later in the evening Barbara would join me and we'd have dinner together.

One such evening, everything appeared to going smoothly and I was very happy when Barbara arrived. We sat at a table in the corner where I could still watch the customers and the general activity of the restaurant. Then it happened.

The waiter had just served the man sitting at a table opposite me with an order of linefish (this is supposed to be fresh fish, caught by line – unlike fish caught by net and frozen).

I watched him look at the fish for a while, then he raised his plate to his nose and smelled it. Then he passed it to his lady friend who also sniffed at it. She pulled up her nose and then pinched her nostrils closed between her thumb and forefinger.

I leaped from my chair like a racehorse out of the starting gate. Passing the table, I scooped up the plate of fish without pausing or even breaking my stride and, like John Cleese in *Fawlty Towers*, rushed straight to the kitchen. Only when I was out of sight of the customers, did I stop to smell.

There was absolutely no doubt. I grabbed some of the other fish about to be prepared; they were the same. I turned to the chef who was watching my feverish antics in the kitchen with great curiosity.

'Is your fucking nose blocked, you stupid fat slob! Can't you smell the fish is off!' I shrieked.

I turned to the waiters, 'Has anyone else ordered the linefish?'

'No Sir, that was the first order,' one of them said, backing away from me in case I hit him over the head with one of the fish.

'Take the linefish off the menu and tell anyone who wants it that we don't have our usual fresh fish available.'

I left the kitchen and walked back to the customer who had been sitting without food for a minute or so. I apologized profusely and said he could order anything he liked – except linefish – as well as any wine he wanted and it would all be on the house.

I returned to Barbara and sitting down, was just in time to see my Belgian chef putting on his jacket and disappearing from the restaurant, issuing a torrent of Flemish insults on his way out.

So there I was, a famous heart surgeon, in the kitchen helping to prepare a wide variety of food. I don't know quite how we got through the evening, but the customers appeared satisfied and the experience confirmed that I had to make some changes in the staff. A few days later – fortunately for me as it turned out – both the Italian restaurateurs resigned as well.

So now I was without *any* staff. How could I run the restaurant? But my luck was in, Tony Ingala came to see me and suggested that I should let him and a friend, Aldo Novati, run the restaurant on the basis that they'd pay me a monthly salary and what was left over they would take.

Since that day I've had no problems with the restaurant and it immediately started making money. I still couldn't prove what I suspected were the reasons for the previous losses – but the profits and instant success under the new management seemed to confirm I was probably right.

The news that Barbara was pregnant again was unexpected but ecstatically received. Christiaan Alexander Zoellner Barnard was born by elective Caesarian section in the same hospital where Frederick had been delivered just two years previously.

Fortunately Barbara encountered no complications and was back in the flat with our baby within a week.

Although we were very happy living at Clifton, another baby meant the flat was just too cramped – so Barbara started house-hunting.

After months of searching and viewing she eventually decided on 'Waiohai' – a beautiful three-bedroomed house with two acres of ground in the rural suburb of Constantia. This was an area for the well-to-do and way beyond my reach. Fortunately, Fred and Ulli also liked the place and they gave it to Barbara as a gift.

A week before we moved in, a woman was bludgeoned to death in a house not far away from our new home. I've never been the bravest of men when it gets dark, and I dreaded leaving the security of the little flat – with so many people around me – and moving into this large, secluded house surrounded by so many trees. But eventually we moved in.

This was *real* luxury, which I could afford only because we had considerable financial support from Barbara and her parents – but, at night, I was as scared as hell. Every little noise woke me up.

A phone call in the middle of the night is always bad news for a heart surgeon. Now these calls were even more unwelcome, as it meant I had to face the dark walk to the garage alone.

Because of my friendship with Peter Sellers, some businessmen asked me to invite him to South Africa for the opening of a Backgammon Club in Johannesburg, which he readily accepted.

Peter arrived and a few of us went to meet him at the airport in Johannesburg. There was great excitement among some Indians when they spotted him, and he posed for a few pictures and imitated their accents to perfection, which reduced them, and us, to hysterics.

The opening of the club was a bit of a flop and again it was obvious that when Peter wasn't working from a script or acting the role of somebody else he was very dull.

Our party then set off for the Chobe Game Lodge in Botswana.

Peter was smoking a lot of pot and one night, I also tried a few puffs. I think I did feel more relaxed afterwards, but it was unnecessary for me to rely on any foreign substance to escape from the realities of life, so I never smoked it again.

We had a very embarrassing experience one night when the manager decided to screen *The Party* – one of Peter's movies. But halfway through, most of the guests decided that there were better things for them to do and began leaving the room. Peter was very upset and sulked for the rest of the evening.

From Chobe we went to Cape Town via the Victoria Falls. I had to get back to work and it just so happened that the first operation was a vein by-pass for a patient with severe coronary artery disease, which seemed to interest Peter so much that he asked if he could watch the surgery. He also took several pictures during the operation.

Arriving at the hospital with someone as famous as Peter Sellers caused quite a commotion, of course – and he signed autographs for the staff as I showed him around. Some of my colleagues were so envious that they decided to avoid us.

One of the sisters told me later of a conversation she'd overheard between two specialists:

'Isn't that Peter Sellers with Chris Barnard over there?'

'Yes, I wonder which one of them is the bigger actor?'

My son, André, was a Goon fan and was very keen to meet Peter, so Barbara gave a little party at our new home for my son and a few friends to meet Peter Sellers. At that stage we didn't have all our furniture, and we sat on the floor for dinner.

André and his friends were mesmerized by Peter and his Goon

stories. He obviously enjoyed himself too and kept us in stitches of laughter.

When he went back to London, I felt sad for two reasons. We had all grown very fond of this talented yet complicated man. But I also felt sorry for the man himself – he appeared to be a very lonely person, made even more lonely by the fact that he didn't enjoy his own company.

Armin Mattli had organised my visit to La Prairie as promised. I I would stay there for a week, and then meet Barbara and the children in Athens for a holiday in Rhodos – which had been arranged by Aris Argyriou.

A limousine and driver met me at the airport in Geneva and after a very scenic drive, I was admitted as a patient to the clinic.

The luxury of the accommodation impressed me much more than the knowledge of the medical staff. After some tests, it was decided that I should receive cells from eleven different organs, including placenta, thymus, gonads, liver and heart. Why I had to get these organs I wasn't quite sure.

From what they had told me on the morning of the injections, a pregnant ewe from their famous 'black flock' was slaughtered at the abattoir. The lamb was removed with every precaution taken to prevent the foetus from being contaminated. It was then taken to the clinic's laboratory. There, the various organs were removed and the cells separated. These cells were then suspended in normal saline.

The doctor arrived with three assistants and a tray with eleven syringes. I learned that the cells from each organ had to be injected separately – I could never understand the reason for this because, if they were going to be absorbed and transported by the circulation, they would mix anyhow. I think it was done more to impress the patient with the extent of the treatment when he got his bill.

Anyway, I didn't argue and received five injections in my left buttock and six in my right. They weren't done very well and, as a result, I couldn't sit down comfortably for days.

I don't know if the treatment was of any benefit but, except for a little fever, it didn't do me any harm – at least, not that I was aware of.

Before leaving the clinic, I had several discussions with the doctors and with Armin Mattli. They had already treated thousands of patients – many of whom claimed to have experienced benefits from these injections. But my concern was that they had never performed any controlled studies and that they were open to wide criticism by sceptics.

In order to make any acceptable deductions from clinical studies, they should have taken two comparable groups of patients – each receiving exactly the same number of injections. One group would receive the actual treatment and the other group would receive no cells at all.

In experiments such as this it's vital that the patients are not aware of whether they are receiving the treatment or the placebos. If, statistically, one can then show that the group receiving treatment with cells did better than the others, the medical profession would accept that the treatment was of value.

It wasn't enough just to say it's of benefit 'because the patient feels better'. He may have felt better just because he'd spent a few thousand dollars for the treatment!

I wasn't interested in getting involved in the clinical programme, but I agreed to embark on a research project which could clear up the situation. Maybe we would find experimental evidence for the claims made clinically?

Armin Mattli appointed me as the scientific adviser, at a substantial salary, and the two of us became very close friends.

The theory formulated by Dr Niehans, who started the clinic many years ago, was that the foetal cells, because of their immaturity, would not evoke an immune response from the patient.

The cells would stay alive and after absorption, repopulate the diseased or depleted organs and in that way, cause rejuvenation and benefit certain diseases.

It was therefore also recommended that, after the injections, the patient should not be exposed to sunlight or take alcohol or do anything which might damage these little cells.

I knew this was a lot of bullshit.

These foetal cells, being from a lamb, would soon be recognized by the immune system of the patient as 'non-self' and be destroyed.

I suggested that if the treatment was of benefit then it wasn't due to the cells remaining alive, but due to them releasing substances that had healing and rejuvenating properties when they died.

I was soon able to prove that I was correct, by showing that the blood of patients who had received treatment had a much higher concentration of antibodies against sheep cells than the average population. This indicated that the patient's immune system *did* react to the presence of the sheep cells.

There was, however, enough clinical evidence to make me curious and, with the help of Armin Mattli, I joined forces with the Schafer Institute in Basel to continue the research.

I met Barbara and the children in Athens and she was very suspicious of my blue and tender bottom. We stayed for a few days in the Astor Palace Hotel and then left for Rhodos.

Aris and I spent a lot of time together discussing the project on Kos.

Soon after arriving home in Cape Town, we were ready to perform the first heterotopic heart transplant on Ivan Taylor, a man of 59 who was in the terminal stages of heart failure, due to extensive destruction of his heart muscle.

'Prof! They want you in the operating room.' It was Dene who came to call me from the rest room, where I was having a cup of tea with Marius.

I slipped my mask over my face and went into A-Theatre. I'd decided on Jacques Losman as my first assistant, as he had done a lot of the research. 'What's the matter?' I stopped at the head of the operating table and peered over the linen screen that separated the anaesthetist from the operating field.

'No, nothing, Prof,' he replied without looking up 'I just thought you should have a look.' He'd opened the right lung space horizontally and the heart sac vertically.

'Do you want me to go on?'

'Yes, I'll start scrubbing. In the meantime, detach the right side of the heart sac below from the diaphragm and above where it reflects onto the roots of the vessels – and be careful of the phrenic nerve.' I turned and walked to the scrub room.

The phrenic nerve runs along the side of the heart sac. If damaged, it would cause paralysis of the right side of the diaphragm and this would interfere with breathing during the post-operative period and delay his recovery. The diaphragm would also rise up into the thoracic cage and reduce the space for the second heart.

When I finished scrubbing and drying my hands and arms, I put on a gown and gloves and walked into A-Theatre to perform an operation that had never been done before on a human being. If it was a success Mr Taylor would have two hearts – I would have inspanned the 'fresh horse' next to the old tired one.

We performed the operation just as I had planned it more than a year previously in the anatomy museum, after the death of Martin Franzot.

The only modification in the technique was that instead of joining the donor's lung artery to the patient's lung artery, I joined it back into the right upper chamber of the patient's heart. The donor's heart could now assist the patient's left side, but his own right side would still carry the circulation to the lung.

When we had completed the full anastomoses, each heart was simply started with an electric shock and everyone in the operating room came round to peer over the anaesthetic screen, to see the strange sight of two hearts beating each at their own rate in the one chest.

We closed the sternum without any evidence that there was interference with the ability of the hearts to function adequately due to lack of space. The anaesthetist also reported that the right lung expanded freely.

By recording the pulsation in one of the arteries of the patient, we were able to get a rough idea of how much blood each heart was pumping. It was obvious that the new heart had already taken over most of the load.

What impressed us was the excellent circulation of the patient and also the low venous pressure. This was probably due to the fact that the patient's own right pumping chamber, used to the high pressure in the lung, was still carrying that part of the circulation.

Unfortunately, when Mr Taylor had recovered from the affects of the anaesthetic it was obvious that he had severe brain damage. I couldn't understand how this could have happened, as I was sure I'd expelled all the air from both hearts before starting them, and at no stage did the patient experience a severe drop in blood pressure which could have damaged his brain.

Because the main artery from his heart was badly affected by arteriosclerosis it was suggested that, when we cross-clamped this vessel during the operation, pieces of the diseased lining must have broken off and lodged in his brain. This complication didn't improve and it was tragic to see my patient with his heart repaired but his brain unable to celebrate and enjoy the improvement in the quality of his life.

The news of a 'successful heterotopic transplant' hit the headlines around the world and most science writers hailed it as another medical breakthrough. The local South African press were much less enthusiastic about the medical side, however, and concentrated their reporting on the fact that the hospital wouldn't pay for the burial costs of the donor.

By the time I'd become aware of this nonsense, it was too late. I was furious with the irresponsible reporting and only slightly less angry with the bureaucrats in the hospital, who stubbornly refused to pay.

If I'd been asked, I'd have readily covered the funeral expenses – even out of my meagre doctor's salary. How expensive could it be anyway?

One month later we also gave Mr Goss, a 47 year old male, a second heart. His heart muscle was seriously affected by rheumatic heart disease. A few years earlier, we had replaced the aortic valve to correct its severe dysfunction due to the same rheumatic fever.

It was absolutely imperative that a patient's own aortic valve should close without leaking; otherwise the blood pumped by the other heart would flow back into the patient's left pumping chamber, placing it under an intolerable burden.

Again, we were very impressed with the excellent circulation the patient had as soon as the two hearts started to beat. And the patient went home a month after surgery.

Some weeks later I had an anxious phone call from him, 'Prof, I feel dizzy and I'm sweating – it just started suddenly.'

I couldn't think what had gone wrong. 'It's probably something you ate that's upset your stomach,' I said, trying to reassure my patient and calm him down.

'No Prof, I think there's something wrong with my heart. It's not the same as before.' (Strange how these patients never referred to their two hearts – just about their 'heart'.)

'Can you drive to the hospital or should I send an ambulance?' I wanted him to be under our care as soon as possible.

'No, I can come in by car.' And he drove himself to hospital where we admitted him to the intensive care unit immediately.

On examination, it was obvious that his circulation was poor and what was unusual was that he had a very high venous pressure (the pressure in the vessels bringing the blood from the body to the right heart). I still couldn't make out what had happened until I saw the electrocardiograph tracing – his own heart had gone into ventricular fibrillation. He now had no right-sided pumping chamber because the right side of the donor heart hadn't been connected. The flow of blood into the lungs was inadequately managed by contractions of the two right upper chambers.

We immediately defribrillated his heart and, like magic, the circulation immediately returned to normal.

This complication convinced me that it was essential to support both left and right sides with the donor heart, so that if the patient's own heart stopped beating then the donor heart could take over the full circulation.

Mr Goss, however, had the dubious honour to be the first man to drive his car without his own heart beating inside his chest. He lived for more than 10 years with the two hearts – but not without further problems.

I received an invitation from Imelda Marcos, the wife of the president of the Philippines, to be her guest at the inauguration of the All Asia Heart Institute in Manila.

It was an unusual invitation, because President Marcos was one of the strongest critics of apartheid and the lack of political freedom in South Africa. I had been told that at Manila airport there was a big sign that said 'Dogs and South Africans not allowed'.

I didn't see this notice when we arrived two weeks later. Someone said they'd removed it temporarily, out of respect for me.

We were taken to the guest house of the palace and quickly dressed for the dinner that night, where we met the other invited guests. From America, there were Dr Denton Cooley and his wife, Dr Don Effler and his wife, and Christina Ford – the very attractive Italian wife of Henry Ford. She wasn't accompanied by her husband and, to Barbara's chagrin, I sat next to her during dinner.

My old friend from Madrid, the Marquis de Villaverde, was there in all his splendour and several members of a very well-known and extremely wealthy Spanish family by the name of March. Also included on the guest list was the Italian film producer, Franco Rossellini.

Apart from the dinners and sight-seeing trips, I had two major engagements. One was the inauguration of the centre and the other was to lecture at a medical conference.

On the day of the inauguration, Barbara and I sat on the raised platform with President Marcos, his wife and other VIPs.

There were parades of military bands, schoolchildren, nurses and other social groups. Then the four surgeons present each had to say a few words.

When my turn came I was quite nervous. and everyone was wondering what the doctor from the land of apartheid was going to say. I opted for extreme diplomacy. I knew, for example, that the beautiful Imelda Marcos had previously been a 'Miss Philippines'; Ferdinand Marcos was also regarded locally as a big war hero.

And so I began, 'Mr President, Madame Marcos, Honoured Guests, Ladies and Gentlemen, as South Africans we know very little about the Philippines; we only know it as a country of beautiful women and brave men. Now that I've spent a few days here I know this is true. My own country also has beautiful women and brave men and I hope you will, one day, come and visit us so that you can be given the opportunity to see for yourself.'

I had the loudest applause of all, which just goes to prove that to deliver a successful speech in circumstances like that, all you have to do is keep it short and flatter the hell out of your hosts.

At the medical conference things didn't go so well for me. The lecture hall was packed and even Mrs Marcos attended.

As we had just done the first two heterotopic transplants, I decided to talk about this operation. I discussed the advantages and disadvantages of the procedure, surgical technique and the limited clinical experience.

When I'd finished, the chairman of the session asked if there were any questions. Dr Effler stood up and could not have been less medical, or more personal, in his vitriolic attack.

He first blamed me for all the publicity received in the press and accused me of reporting my medical experience with the lay press instead of the medical journals. He then predicted that no other surgeon would ever attempt this operation and that even in my own clinic, it would be gone and forgotten within a year – if success was to be the goal.

I have been blessed with a fairly quick and agile mind – as well as a sharp tongue – and was careful, in this case, to make his insults work against him. When I responded, I politely reminded him that he seemed to know a lot about heart transplants for a surgeon who had no surviving transplant patients after two attempts.

I also said, 'I can't control what the newspapers write – they report on whatever they consider to be newsworthy and I'm often the last one to know about it. They obviously had their own sources who'd told them what we had done – and that was their main news of the day.

'I can, however, assure you that when we feel we have sufficient experience, we will write a full report for the medical journals. But, Dr Effler, I do not intend making the same mistake as we did after the first orthotopic transplant – when people like you accused us of writing a "premature" report!

'It also occurs to me,' I added, 'that it's very difficult to satisfy the demands you make. We're either reporting "too early" or "too late" – perhaps you can give me the benefit of your advice in future? Then maybe everyone will be happy.'

As to his predictions that nobody else would ever attempt the heterotopic transplant, I said, 'My instinct tells me, that as medical science continues to move forward, the heterotopic operation will be used – rather than allowing progress to stop as you seem to suggest. However, I'm not a fortune teller and cannot predict the future. Finally Dr Effler I would remind you that "success" is not "a goal"; it's a result.'

Time proved Dr Effler to be a very inaccurate fortune teller, as the operation was subsequently performed by many surgeons all over the world and I recently spoke to a leading surgeon in the field of heart transplantation, Sir Magdi Yacoub of London. He told me that he still frequently performed the 'piggy-back' operation when he thought that the donor heart was too small and needed support from the patient's heart until it had developed sufficiently.

In my own hands the operation also had good results. Out of the first five operations that we performed, three lived ten years after the operation and one of these, a fisherman, is still doing well 17 years after receiving the second heart.

The conference ended and Effler hurried away. Imelda Marcos apologized on behalf of the centre for the rudeness and we all got on with the serious business of having a holiday.

We spent a lot of time with the president and his wife, and we became friends – playing tennis and racquet-ball together. I even accompanied the president to a military passing-out parade.

The whole party spent the night on the president's yacht and paid a visit to Corregidor Island, where so many young men died in the Second World War. The Bataan Peninsula in Manila Bay left a lasting impression on me; I could almost hear the echoes of gunfire and the cries of the soldiers as I stood alone on the deck gazing across the water.

It was to this peninsula that General Douglas MacArthur finally retreated. Two thousand troops escaped to the island fortress of Corregidor – the formidable 'Gibraltar of the East' – but 78 000 surrendered and were forced to make the 65 mile 'death march' from Mariveles to San Fernando.

Suddenly cold, I joined my hosts inside the yacht and shrugged away the ghosts.

On what was to be our last night in Manila, Barbara and I went to the palace to say farewell to the president and his wife, and to thank them for their wonderful hospitality. 'No, you are not leaving tomorrow,' Imelda Marcos announced, to our surprise. 'You will be part of my party to Kathmandu for the coronation of the king of Nepal.'

Barbara started to refuse because of the children, but out of the corner of my mouth I told her to be quiet. 'We'll never get another opportunity like this!' I whispered urgently. But I did point out to Mrs Marcos that we had a few problems: first we wouldn't be allowed into Nepal with South African passports and, secondly, we didn't have the necessary clothes with us for all the functions that would be part of such an event.

Imelda Marcos dismissed these comments as of no consequence. Early the next morning, we were taken to the president's office and after swearing allegiance to the Philippines, we were made honorary Filipinos and presented with Filipino passports. So one problem was solved.

The question of clothes presented no difficulty either as we were about to discover. From the palace, Barbara and I were taken to the airport by limousine where we were joined by Franco Rossellini and a few officials. We were taken by plane to Hong Kong, and then to a suite in the Peninsula Hotel. There, a Chinese tailor was waiting to take my measurements for a morning suit, evening suit and tails. There were also several ladies with a range of garments to see that Barbara's needs were taken care of.

Halfway through the dress rehearsal for the coronation ceremony, I managed to get Barbara alone and asked her, 'How the hell are we going to pay for all these clothes and shoes?'

One of the officials overheard my conversation and immediately put me at my ease, telling me Mrs Marcos would take care of everything.

Franco Rossellini spent the day having his chest decorated with a big colourful dragon by a Chinese tattooist. The next morning all the garments and accessories were ready and we flew back to Manila.

The following day the Marcos' private jet took us to Kathmandu, Nepal. The party consisted of Mrs Marcos and her entourage, Franco, the Marquis de Villaverde, Christina Ford, Barbara and I.

The flight was very pleasant. Although Franco was still in pain from his new tattoo he entertained us with stories – especially his experiences with Maria Callas when making a movie with her.

We booked into the same hotel as Mrs Marcos and she went out of her way to get us invited to all the functions and to take care of us.

Before every function we would gather in the foyer of the hotel. On one of these occasions she noticed that Barbara had very little jewellery. This was immediately corrected when she instructed one of her ladies-in-waiting to take Barbara up to her own suite. Fifteen minutes later my wife appeared wearing a diamond tiara and the most beautiful diamond earrings I'd ever seen. This actually put a damper on the rest of my evening as I was worried about what would happen if one of these incredibly expensive items was lost.

One evening Imelda gave a dinner party to which she invited Prince Charles and Lord Mountbatten who were also in Kathmandu for the coronation. During the evening, I chatted to Prince Charles who explained to me that both his mother and father had told him a great deal about South Africa but that he could never, of course, visit the country because of the political problems.

Lord Louis Mountbatten thoroughly enjoyed himself and danced with Barbara a few times. She was very popular and, at one stage, there was a good-humoured argument between Mountbatten and Prince Charles as to who would have the next dance. I noticed that Prince Charles had a keen eye for a beautiful woman and he paid close attention to Barbara, whispering in her ear as they danced.

I very much enjoyed the company of Lord Mountbatten. He was extremely interesting company and we talked about his experiences during the war as admiral of the fleet. He was able to tell me a great number of interesting facts about Nepal, Burma, India and the Philippines as he had, of course, been supreme allied commander in Southeast Asia and was appointed viceroy of India.

I, along with most of the free world, was horrified when four years later he was blown to pieces with eight pounds of gelignite by a gang of Irish terrorists.

He and Prince Charles were obviously very close. Charles called Mountbatten 'Dicky' and I learned later that they referred to each other as 'HG'. Mountbatten was known as 'Honorary Grandfather' and Prince Charles as 'Honorary Grandson.'

The next morning we went shopping with Imelda Marcos and all the rumours about her extravagant shopping habits are absolutely true. In a carpet shop, she bought virtually every carpet.

Finally it was time to leave the company of princes and kings and presidents so we returned via Calcutta and Bombay to South Africa. We had no problems in India as we were, at that time, citizens of the Philippines.

I had made some professional visits in Bombay and a private audience was arranged with Mrs Indira Ghandi.

I was flown to Delhi – and stayed in one of the most beautiful hotels in the world, the Oberoi Hotel.

We had a very friendly chat, discussing medicine – especially birth control – which Mrs Ghandi was enthusiastically endorsing at that time to combat poverty. We also spoke about South African politics.

She said that the big problem was the apartheid in South Africa and I agreed, but that it wasn't unique to South Africa – there was discrimination everywhere in the world.

'Mrs Ghandi, I know there's a lot of wrong in South Africa but people don't realize there's a lot of good in South Africa too.

'I promise you that I will persuade our government to cover all the costs for you to send a delegation to my country to look at things for themselves. They will be allowed to go anywhere – especially to meet the people of India who came to settle in South Africa, and see what they're doing and what's happened to them. The only condition would be that before they leave South Africa they make a press declaration on what they found.'

I wanted it to be completely objective.

She looked at me and said, 'I'm sorry, I can't do that.'

On reflection, I think my timing was bad. Only a few months previously she'd been found guilty of electoral corruption by the high court and had been disbarred from holding any public office for six years. What she'd done immediately afterwards, just before my arrival, was to authorize the arrest of 676 political opponents

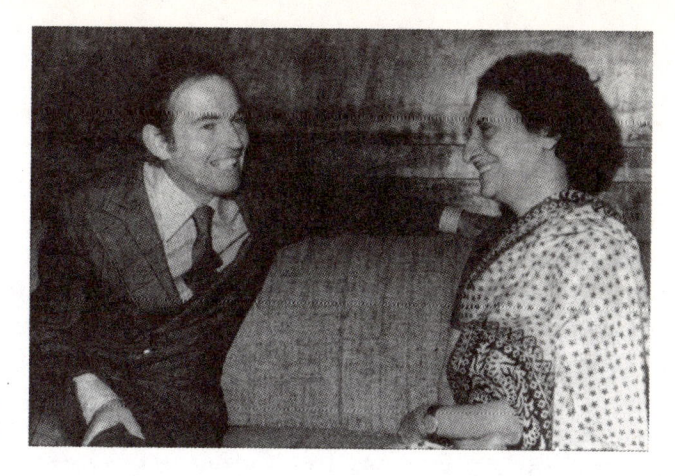

A visit to Mrs Ghandi

in pre-dawn raids, she banned most of the political organizations and rushed an Act through parliament virtually giving her dictatorial powers.

I couldn't help but wonder at the gall – the infernal hypocrisy – of political leaders like she was, who were so quick to criticize my country while their own was a complete disgrace. In fact, while I was there she was still busy censoring news of crime and economic problems. She harassed editors, jailed journalists and closed down newspapers.

What she'd done in India could *never* have been done in South Africa.

Anyway, I didn't fancy the idea of languishing in an Indian jail very much, so I kept my thoughts to myself and said a polite goodbye to Mrs Ghandi.

Bad news awaited me when I arrived home. Mr Goss was running a high temperature and the indications were that he had an infection in the artificial aortic valve of his own heart which we'd left behind.

I couldn't think of a worse complication to deal with. We had had experience with infection in artificial valves and we knew that it was extremely difficult to treat, as the valve wasn't supplied by blood vessels and high concentrations of antibiotics could not reach the bacteria or fungi responsible for the infection. But now things were even worse, because the patient was immunosuppressed and we could get very little help from his own immune system.

After discussing the problem at length with my colleagues, we decided that the only way to save his life was to remove the valve and close the root of the aorta – but then there would be no outflow to the left pumping chamber.

I had a plan, so we went ahead with surgery.

When my patient was connected to the heart-lung machine and this had taken over the circulation, I made a large incision in the left pumping chamber to expose the valve from the bottom. It was covered with infected clots and the sewing ring had already partly detached from the aorta.

We removed the valve, sutures and as much of the infected tissue as possible – leaving a large hole between the aorta and the left ventricle. I closed this opening by using one of the leaflets of the mitral valve (the valve between the left lower and upper chamber).

The opening of this valve was then stitched closed so that blood couldn't flow into the left lower chamber. As this chamber would be excluded from the circulation, I resected most of its muscle and carefully stitched the large wound in the heart.

After re-warming and removing the aortic clamp, the heart took over without hesitation.

Mr Goss now had a unique circulation in that the blood returning from the body was pumped to the lungs by his own heart, but the oxygenated blood returning from the lungs was pumped to his body by the donor heart.

My patient now had, anatomically, one and a half hearts, with which he lived a very full and active life for 3 906 days.

'Guess who's just been admitted to our ward?' Marius greeted me one morning just before starting our ward rounds. 'Mr Robert Sobukwe, the leader of the banned Pan Africanist Congress (PAC)!'

The Nationalist party had carte blanche in those days and, since the early sixties, had been banning organizations and either putting their leaders in jail, or restricting their freedom.

Most whites stood idly by. Why should they get involved? Life was good to them, it was easy, so why complicate the matter? We all had a comfortable existence.

So many of us accepted this – except for a few lost voices – and turned a blind eye to the daily injustice committed around us. I admit, in all honesty, that I should have done more. So, when

Robert Sobukwe became my patient, I had the opportunity to learn, first hand, from a leader of one of the black African resistance movements, what their fears and aspirations were.

Robert was suffering from an inoperable carcinoma of the lung. He was a dying man, but he still believed that he would see the day when our country would be freed from the unholy influences of apartheid.

I spent many hours with him and tried, wherever I could, to lessen his suffering. Because he received no treatment during the weekends, we allowed him to leave the hospital, but even this small gesture of compassion was restricted by a totally unsympathetic security machine. When I explained to the officers on guard that he was a dying man and was unable to harm anyone any more, I was told to stick to medicine and leave the security of the country to them.

The officer in charge said, 'Sobukwe is a dangerous man and the restriction order must be strictly adhered to.'

Robert took all the humiliation and suffering without complaint, and I only once saw him rise to anger – when I compared him with Nelson Mandela. 'Don't ever compare me with Nelson! He's a criminal and I'm not!' he shouted emphatically.

I gathered from this that there was a big gulf between the PAC and the African National Congress (ANC) and didn't discuss the subject with him again.

Eventually I flew up to Pretoria to see Mr Vorster, then prime minister, in an attempt to do something for Mr Sobukwe. After telling him of my talks with Robert and explaining what an intelligent and understanding human being I found him to be, John Vorster agreed to meet him and asked me to make the necessary arrangements.

I was besides myself with joy about what would be a historic meeting and couldn't wait to bring my patient the good news.

'Robert, I have wonderful news for you,' I said breathlessly, after running up the stairs to Ward C1. 'I've just seen the prime minister and he's agreed to meet you!'

His expression darkened and the ominous fire came back into his eyes. 'I have nothing to talk to Vorster about. I will only see him when he's ready to hand over the country to me!'

He lay back on his pillows and closed his eyes. Subject closed.

He died a few weeks later and I heard his two children were staying in the United States with Andrew Young – the United

States ambassador to the United Nations at that time. I phoned him and asked if they could send the children over for the funeral.

He said there was no money available to pay for their air tickets so I told him I would organize the money for their fares myself.

'Eschel, it's Chris Barnard.' I'd met Eschel Rhoodie on one of my overseas trips and knew that he was fighting a losing battle trying to improve the image of South Africa overseas.

'I don't know whether you can help me – but I'm trying to find two air tickets from New York to Johannesburg.' I said hesitantly.

'What for, Chris?'

I continued, 'Promise me that no one will ever know if I tell you.' I knew that such a gift would cause a major political storm – both from the right-wing Nationalists as well as the black movements. 'I think you'll agree with me when I say we whites have exploited the blacks unashamedly. Let's show some remorse by flying out the two Sobukwe children to their father's funeral.'

Robert's two children flew to South Africa to be at their father's funeral. I never heard from them again but Mrs Sobukwe thanked me later for making these arrangements. Nobody knew where the money came from.

The time I spent with Robert Sobukwe made a lasting impression on me. I was so sad that this wonderful human being should die so consumed by hate.

I lay awake at night haunted by the knowledge that I should be acting more positively. That I should play a much bigger part to overthrow this wicked regime – and be unafraid of the consequences.

I should really become a terrorist.

But I didn't. I sat on the fence, afraid to fall into either of the two camps. Like Gary Player, Anton Rupert, Jan S. Marais, the Oppenheimers, and many other Afrikaners like myself, I only did enough to assuage my conscience but not enough to rock the boat. Very few of us were prepared to stand up and be counted. We were all cowards, taking care of our own safety and comfort before anything or anyone else.

Of course, we had excuses. I had a family and children to look after. I wasn't a politician. Whenever I could, I spoke out against apartheid. But what the hell did we *really* do to bring about the fall of the South African government? Nothing, except not to vote for the Nationalist party. Big deal.

But certain events caused me to change my strategy to more positive action. Unfortunately, many people assumed that I worked *for* the government – when, in fact, I was using the system itself to work *against* it.

The suffering of South African blacks, coloureds and Indians was exploited internationally by politicians, prime ministers, presidents, pop singers, actors and many others – mainly for their own selfish reasons: to get good press exposure, and fill their own coffers. It was a sure way of getting your picture in the newspaper.

I really began to despair for the entire human race when that pompous Teddy Kennedy visited South Africa. Full of political rhetoric he arrived with his equally ignorant flunkies and proceeded to lecture *us* on morality!

He was desperately searching for some virtuous publicity – and he found it among the deprived citizens of South Africa. He got plenty of coverage as he cluck-clucked about discrimination and strutted around the townships – careful not to get his shoes muddy but equally careful to be in full-frame of the TV cameras.

And what did he do for the black people of South Africa? One big, fat zero. Zilch. Zip. Nothing.

Hypocrisy was the order of the day and the leader of the orchestra of hypocrites was the United Nations. While condemning South Africa as a threat to world peace, they welcomed Idi Amin with open arms.

Amin, a former sergeant in the King's African Rifles, seized control of Uganda and promptly began his rule of murder and mayhem. As Alan Palmer, the historian, said, 'No other political figure in modern Africa so blatantly championed the interests of a small section of his people against the rest.' Yet, at that time, he was chairman of the Organization of African Unity!

And, while the Kennedys and Amins of the world were doing their worst, South Africa – the original bad dog with the bad name – was vilified everywhere.

Donald Woods, a South African newspaper editor, after fleeing to 'freedom' was allowed to address the United Nations on his arrival in New York on 'The South African Situation'. Even Stevie Wonder, the black pop singer, was given this opportunity, but when it was proposed that I be given the same hearing – and having provided them with my credentials and qualifications, I was told I would be 'put on the waiting list'.

I'm still waiting – twenty years later.

I decided to write a book, with only five chapters, dealing with the complexity and ethnic diversity of South African society, the international hypocrisy, the misuse of freedom, a political solution and the future.

The book was not well received in South Africa because it asked for the abolition of all discriminatory laws and a one-man, one-vote system for the selection of government.

The book was not popular outside South Africa either – because it insisted that the world should also look at, and condemn, other countries where there was discrimination and lack or absence of freedom.

The chapter on the misuse of freedom was especially unpopular among the members of the so-called free Western press.

My views are that freedom is a privilege and not a statutory right and, like any other privilege, there is always a responsibility associated with it. Freedom can't just be dished out ad hoc without those receiving it being prepared or capable of accepting the responsibility attached to that freedom.

One of the biggest myths is 'freedom of the press'. The only 'freedom' should be that reporters' access to news and events isn't restricted. This is where the freedom ends because the interpretation of the news is determined by the editor, sub-editors and owners of the newspapers. What you and I read every day is not the news, but the views of these newspapermen who often live without conscience, honour or any sense of moral responsibility.

Freedom of the press? By all means. But freedom with a responsibility that news should be accurately reported with the emphasis on *communication of information* – not creating sensation.

When *South Africa – Sharp Dissection* appeared in South Africa, many news editors were furious. I'd hit a very sensitive nerve and they couldn't leave it undefended. Several newspapers published scathing reports on both me and my book – the *Natal Mercury* published a particularly blistering attack, misquoting me and taking sections totally out of context.

I lodged a complaint with the Newspaper Press Union and the editor and I were summonsed to appear before an enquiry.

The editor arrived with his legal advisers and I came alone. I explained why I objected to the article and the newspaper attorneys presented their own case. The outcome was that they had to publish an apology and a retraction. But it was a Pyrrhic victory, as the damage had already been done.

Publishers in other countries didn't want to touch the book – except Pierre Belfond in France.

I was invited to France and Belgium for the launch of the book, and several reporters refused to attend my press conference or to interview me because I was labelled as a 'racist'.

What confused them was that being pro-South Africa didn't mean being pro-apartheid.

During this visit, one of the major French television networks invited me to discuss the book on a live programme – which I was very happy to do. When I arrived for the interview, the director of the station expressed his pleasure of having me as a guest and said it was so fortunate I was there that particular evening because it 'just so happened' they were going to screen a programme made about South Africa, by an Austrian documentary producer.

He said that he'd appreciate it very much if I would watch the documentary and make a few comments afterwards. I agreed to do this, but asked for a preview first so that I could organize my comments.

'That's not necessary,' the director told me. 'We've seen the programme and it's a very good film – just an honest reflection of South Africa.'

I should have smelt a rat, I suppose, but taking the man at his word and having high regard for the credentials of the French TV station, I sat there as the programme began.

When the film was screened, my jaw dropped in utter amazement. I'd heard about this type of reporting but never really believed it existed. It was, from beginning to end, a total fabrication. One blatant lie after another. I just couldn't believe what I was seeing. When it was over, the director turned to me and asked if I had enjoyed the programme.

'I want to sob,' I said, 'when a man like you, who has so much power and influence to mould opinions throughout your country, believes that what we've just seen is an honest reflection of South Africa.'

He looked surprised and asked, 'Why do you say that, Professor?'

I looked at the studio audience and then back to the director, as I shook my head in disbelief and disgust.

'I'm the first to admit that there are a lot of terribly wrong things in South Africa, and that black people are often treated worse than animals. But why does a film like this have to rely on such ridiculous distortion and blatant lies to illustrate the point? By using this technique the film loses all its credibility because anyone with any intelligence can see that it's one lie after another. It would have been so much better to report *truthfully* on my country, so that the French people can base their opinions on truth rather than this dreadful deception.'

'Those are very strong accusations, Professor. Can you prove that it was full of lies?' He was obviously upset.

'Of course I can prove it!' I was so wound up that the words tumbled out.

'You remember the scene where the commentator talked about the growing hate among blacks for the whites, and how they prepared themselves to overthrow the regime by force?'

'Yes,' he nodded.

'You'll also remember, that it showed a mass of black men standing waving their fists and shouting?'

'Yes, I remember that.'

I paused, so that the studio audience and viewers at home would remember my reply. Then, slowly and deliberately, I said, '*That* scene was filmed at a Johannesburg football stadium during a match – it had *nothing* to do with political violence!'

I heard some murmurs from the audience.

'You remember the scene where young white men were practising target shooting with pistols, and then the sound of gunfire continued while the picture changed to a black woman's face in great agony?

'That woman was giving birth to a child – it had nothing to do with shooting at all!'

Now the studio audience was obviously on my side and I verbally took the film apart scene by scene.

The head of the French TV station was highly embarrassed because he'd been fooled by the Austrian, so they invited me to make a programme, with a French crew and at their expense, on South Africa – the way I saw it.

I later did it and it was called *The Open Heart of South Africa*.

The same Austrian programme was also bought by the BBC for screening and, when the South African embassy in London heard about it, they strongly suggested that my comments also be shown. The BBC refused this request outright.[*]

During the filming of my views on South Africa, I had the privilege and honour to interview Mr Breyten Breytenbach in Pollsmoor Prison.

He was one of South Africa's most respected Afrikaans poets and had lived for many years in Paris – where he married a Vietnamese woman. Since 1949 interracial marriages had been illegal in South Africa, but parliament, quick to spot an inconvenient loophole and piqued about Breyten's wedding, passed an amendment to the original Act. This made a marriage between a male South African and a woman of a different race, outside the country, invalid.

He had been arrested, in 1975, for marrying an Asian woman and for illegally entering South Africa on a French passport. He was also charged with eleven other illegal acts under the Terrorism and Suppression of Communism Acts, which included smuggling weapons, plotting violent acts of sabotage, spying in the ports and conspiracy. ('Conspiracy', at that time, was less concerned with what *had* been done but more with what the accused *intended* doing. A successful conviction needed only to show that the accused had associated with known subversives.)

Breyten Breytenbach, quite unexpectedly, pleaded guilty (maybe as an act of petulant defiance) and was sentenced to nine years in prison. Most of this was spent in solitary confinement.

The civil service was staffed mainly by Afrikaans-speaking South Africans so he could expect to be treated worse than most in prison. Many Afrikaners, at that level, would have labelled him a traitor.

My heart went out to this deeply sensitive, fine man who was the victim of circumstances. It was so sad to see how his spirit had been broken by the crude and ill-mannered wardens to whom he had to 'yes sir, no sir'. These jailers reprimanded me for addressing him as 'Mr' – to them he was just 'Breytenbach'.

I went to see John Vorster and begged him to release Breyten as he was no danger to South Africa or South African society.

He refused.

Taking the TV crew with me, I also interviewed the minister of police at that time, Mr Jimmy Kruger. I had only one question for him, 'We read a great deal about prisoners being ill-treated by the police. I don't want to be like the Germans one day, who said they knew nothing about the concentration camps. Are prisoners being tortured and beaten by the police?'

The minister answered, 'The police aren't children and sometimes they may manhandle a prisoner, but I can assure you that prisoners are never beaten or tortured.'

Only a few weeks later Steve Biko's name hit the international headlines.

Biko was a major exponent of the Black Consciousness Movement (BCM) and became president of the South African Students' Organization (SASO), which was later banned.

He had been arrested on suspicion of distributing 'inflammatory pamphlets' and was held in a Port Elizabeth police cell for 18 days.

Some reports said he was kept naked to 'prevent him from hanging himself with his clothes'.

Police swore that Biko had 'hit the back of his head against a wall' in a scuffle during interrogation. The district surgeon examined him and found 'no evidence of abnormal pathology', but admitted later that, in fact, he'd found extensive injuries.

Four weeks after his arrest Steve Biko was driven 1 200 kilometres to Pretoria, still naked and chained, lying in the back of a police van. He died 'a miserable and lonely death on a mat on a stone floor in a prison in Pretoria'.

Kruger's first public response to Biko's death was a shrugged, 'Dit laat my koud' (it leaves me cold). Then he said Biko had died 'following a hunger strike'. He later denied saying that Biko had died *of* a hunger strike.

The subsequent investigations and trial were closely followed by the international media and to my country's shame, it was obvious what had happened.

And this was after Jimmy Kruger had looked straight into my eyes, filmed by a TV camera, and said, 'I can assure you that prisoners are never beaten or tortured.'

By the time we'd celebrated the tenth anniversary of the first heart transplant, the team had only performed 31 transplants in all. Of these, 20 were piggy-back operations and of those, two were extreme emergencies where we couldn't find human donors and had used animal hearts as a temporary assist device – in the hope that the patient's own heart would recover before the animal heart was rejected. Both failed.

In the first case, using a baboon heart, it failed within hours. In the second patient, where a chimpanzee was used as the donor, the patient lived for four days before the heart was rejected.

I decided not to use apes again as donors, especially not a chimpanzee – as sacrificing this animal was an extremely emotional and traumatic experience both for its mate – and me.

In fact, it was the weeping chimpanzee which gave me my greatest insight into animal intelligence. The chimp was crying because I had just taken away his mate and cut her heart out.

Before that, if anyone had told me that chimps could weep for love of one another, I would have smiled and asked if they'd read any good books lately. I no longer hold that view.

I suppose I could defend myself on the grounds of legitimate scientific research and the health needs of my patients. Other surgeons do so – but I now know there is a line which, once crossed, makes us lesser human beings.

That chimp not only wept. He cried loudly and pitifully. He pined, lost weight and sat for days staring into space during his mourning.

Fortunately, we abandoned the use of chimpanzee hearts and so his life was spared. We even managed to find another mate for him in spacious quarters on a beautiful game farm near Cape Town.

I was thrilled when I heard, much later, that the pair had been blessed with a new baby.

Of the other 18 piggy-back operations, where human hearts were used, 13 patients were still alive – of whom 12 had been discharged from hospital and were doing well.

It was a normal day, until the telephone rang. 'Prof, Jack Smith's doctor just phoned from Johannesburg; he's not well at all.'

This was bad news, as he was only 27 years old and had done exceptionally well after receiving the second heart to help his own, which was badly damaged from a muscle disease of unknown origin.

'Jannie, get him down to Cape Town as soon as possible.' I told Dr Jannie Hassoulas, who had taken over from Bossie Bosman in the transplant unit.

The next morning, Jack Smith arrived in a serious condition. Studies showed that the transplanted heart was hardly pumping at all, due to acute rejection.

What had happened was that the young man hadn't liked the round ('moon') face that inevitably resulted from the high doses of cortisone and he'd simply stopped taking his anti-rejection drugs.

He was now being kept alive only by the output of his own heart which we had left in place. We immediately re-started the immunosuppressive drugs and the next morning, when I visited him, he told me he was feeling a little better. But to my horror, the electrocardiograph tracing showed that the donor heart had stopped beating. His old heart was now on its own.

'What are we going to do now?' I asked Jannie, hoping for some helpful advice.

'I don't know, Prof. I suppose we'll have to take the rejected heart out.' Jannie had his usual worried expression on his face.

'Then we may just as well slit his throat – he'll never survive the operation unless we give him a second transplant.'

'I'll notify the multiple injury unit immediately, as well as the neurosurgeons, that we urgently need a heart donor.' Five days later we were still waiting for a new heart.

Jannie looked as if the whole world had turned against him. 'Cheer up Jannie! We're going to defibrillate the heart,' I said encouragingly, having just made up my mind.

The five days of anti-rejection treatment had, in all probability, reversed the situation and a shock should start the donor heart beating again.

'Jesus, Prof! What happens if the shock fibrillates his own heart as well!'

This was a possibility. An electric current passing through the chest could fibrillate the heart, especially if it was diseased, in which event he would probably die.

'Then we just shock them both again – have you got any better suggestions?' I replied.

Jannie was deep in thought. 'What about a clot?'

This was another danger. The donor heart had not been contracting for five days and the blood in it may have clotted. If it started beating again it would expel the clot, with the disastrous results of a cerebral embolus. I should have thought about it more carefully and put him onto anti-coagulants but it was too late now.

'Let's get the defibrillator and call Ozzie, in case we have to incubate and ventilate,' I said, although this procedure wasn't a surgical one and no anaesthetic would be necessary – only sedation. We'd use the defibrillator in the ward of the intensive care unit.

We were ready. I had the defribrillator paddles positioned in front and at the back of the right chest so that the current would mainly pass through the donor heart.

'Okay, Oz – hit it!'

Jack's body jerked violently as the power surged through his body and he moaned. All eyes were on the electrocardiograph screen. There was just a straight line, the most depressing sight for a heart surgeon.

Then, both hearts started to beat.

'Christ, Prof! I thought you thumped me on the chest with a sledgehammer!' Jack complained, painfully rubbing his chest. The mere fact that he was conscious was proof that no clot had gone into his brain. I felt the pulses in his legs and they were all present.

'Jannie, we were lucky.' I said simply, smiling at my colleague. Jack Smith would certainly have died during this episode of rejection, but the old horse was still there to continue pulling the cart up the hill – further proof that the heterotopic transplant is a good surgical option.

He lived for nearly ten years with his two hearts but unfortunately he stopped taking the anti-rejection drugs again and the next time we weren't so lucky. He died.

8

Barbara and I received an invitation from Peter Sellers to join him on a yacht for a few days' cruise along the west coast of Italy. He would send a car to collect us from Rome airport. The invitation couldn't have arrived at a better time. I had been working and travelling a lot, so a few days on the Mediterranean with Peter Sellers and Barbara would be heaven. I accepted immediately and a few weeks later we left for Rome. The driver was at the airport to meet us as promised, and we all met at the harbour.

The yacht was very luxurious and chartered by Peter, who was with his daughter and his new girlfriend, Lynne Fredericks.

We had a wonderful time. The weather was perfect and every evening we berthed in a different little harbour, and went to one of the local restaurants for dinner.

During one of these stops, we visited Roger Moore's house and spent several very interesting hours with him and his gorgeous wife.

A day before the cruise was to end, Peter took to me to one side and showed me an electrocardiograph tracing. 'What do you think of this, Chris?' he quietly enquired and I could feel his gaze on my face as I examined the graph.

I silently prayed that it wasn't his. There were a lot of extra beats evident, initiated from different areas in the left lower chamber. These ventricular extrasystoles were often a warning sign that the heart could, without warning, go into ventricular fibrillation with sudden death, if the patient was not at that very time in an intensive care unit.

I looked at the tracings again and again, putting off asking him the obvious question. He was not, in my opinion, in the best mental condition to cope with such a severe problem. As a probable hypochondriac it would be his worst nightmare.

'Is this yours, Peter?' I asked gently.

He nodded with a tight-lipped smile.

'I'm afraid this isn't very good; you should let somebody have a look at you.' He knew this already, of course, because whoever did the tracing must have told him.

'Where do you think I should go, Chris?' I knew he trusted me and that I would give him an honest opinion.

'Well, there are many good places all over the world, but why don't you come to Cape Town? We have excellent cardiologists there and you'll be among friends.'

He agreed.

As soon as I was back in Cape Town, I discussed it with Professor Beck and we made arrangements for Peter Sellers to be admitted to Groote Schuur Hospital.

Unfortunately, I received an invitation to New York which I couldn't refuse and it meant I would be away when Peter arrived in Johannesburg so I changed his admission date for one week later and Barbara would meet him and Lynne Fredericks at the airport and take them to the Mala Mala game reserve for a few days until I returned.

When I told Peter about this slight change to the schedule he was quite happy about it and said he was looking forward to a few days in the bush anyway.

After I'd completed my engagement in New York and returned to Johannesburg, neither Peter nor Lynne were at the airport. There was just a message from Barbara to meet her at her parents' home.

When I arrived at 'Three Fountains' Barbara told me the whole story. She'd met Peter and Lynne and they'd gone to Mala Mala as planned and enjoyed a few days there until, one morning, my future patient told her he wasn't going to Groote Schuur any more. He had decided to go and see the faith healers in Manila instead.

I could understand his concerns about open-heart surgery – but I didn't think he'd be foolish enough to even begin to think that faith healers could cure his dangerously sick heart.

I didn't hear from him again – at least not for a while.

Some months later, during a visit to London, I had a phone call from one of the staff members at the Saudi Arabian embassy. We met at my hotel and she told me that she'd been asked by a princess to invite me to Saudi Arabia – all expenses paid.

As Barbara and I had already been invited to Jordan, we decided to combine the two trips – I would first go to Riyadh and then meet Barbara in Amman.

When I left South Africa for London to collect my tickets and visa, I was troubled by a persistent cough. My chest X-ray was clear, so I took some cough mixture – which didn't help.

The trip to Riyadh was a nightmare. I think I'd taken too much of the cough mixture and felt like death.

As the plane began its descent, a young Arab sat down in the seat next to mine and said he'd recognized me and asked if I was to visit his country. I told him I'd been invited by a princess and I was also going to give a few lectures at the medical school in Jedda. He wanted to know who was meeting me at the airport and I told him that as far as I knew it would be the princess.

'Professor Barnard, you do not know my country. It's highly unlikely that a princess will meet you, but my staff will be available and, if there's no one to assist you, we will take care of things.' I'd forgotten that this country had only formally allowed women to be educated since 1960 and only finally abolished slavery in 1962.

There was no one to meet me.

The young man I'd been talking to on the plane, however, was the son of Crown Prince Fahd, and his staff took me to his guest house, where I stayed for the time I was in Riyadh. I dread to think what would have happened had I not met the prince.

He and his staff took great care of me. He even arranged for me to have a meeting with King Khalid, who was very interested in my work as he suffered from a heart ailment himself.

Before I left the palace, the interpreter told me that the king would have preferred to have come to Cape Town for a medical check-up but due to our political situation, this was not possible. He went to the Cleveland Clinic instead – where he died.

After giving five lectures in Jedda – with great difficulty, due to shortness of breath – I left for Amman, where Barbara was at the airport to meet me.

I was seen by a chest physician there and he told me I was suffering from asthma. He prescribed bronchial dilators, which immediately improved the cough.

One morning, on my way to a lecture, I was informed that Barbara and I had been invited to the king's birthday party that evening.

When we arrived at the palace, we were introduced to King Hussein and his beautiful queen. I immediately took a liking to the ruler of Jordan – he was friendly, humble and, apparently, a very brave man.

We were all standing around having cocktails before dinner, when who should arrive? Peter Sellers and Lynne Fredericks. He spotted me immediately but we didn't talk until after dinner.

'Hello, Chris – I'm completely cured!' He smiled broadly and told me the story about how he had gone to Manila, where the healer performed eleven operations on him – in his hotel room – and without anaesthetic.

At first I thought it was just another of his jokes and was desperately trying to stop bursting into laughter – until I realized he was absolutely serious.

He told me that the faith healer had entered his chest by cutting him open with his fingers. During the first operation he took out the blood clot in his heart. He said the faith healer didn't operate as deep as I did – only when he took out the oedema from his lungs did he go deep into his chest.

I asked him about the blockage in the artery supplying the heart muscle. That appeared to be no problem to the healer of Manila. 'He just cut it out!'

'How did he stitch the remaining ends together, Peter?' I asked gently.

'Oh, he just stuck it together,' and emphasized the point by placing the tips of his index fingers together.

'Yes, and at the end I asked him to take out my appendix as well, seeing as I was there. I don't have any scar but the appendix is out.'

Lynne Fredericks confirmed all that he related. She was present during the 'surgery', saw everything, and even took some photographs.

She seemed very keen to substantiate this preposterous idea and said, 'They laid a white towel on Peter, some sort of X-ray, since shadowy areas seemed to appear on it, allowing them to carry out a diagnosis. Then they massaged his skin; suddenly blood appeared and their hands seemed to slip into his body.'

'Those people are performing miracles, Chris. One day you and the rest of the medical profession will praise their work,' Peter added. He never admitted how much he'd paid them – all he said, rather shyly, was they hadn't asked for a fee.

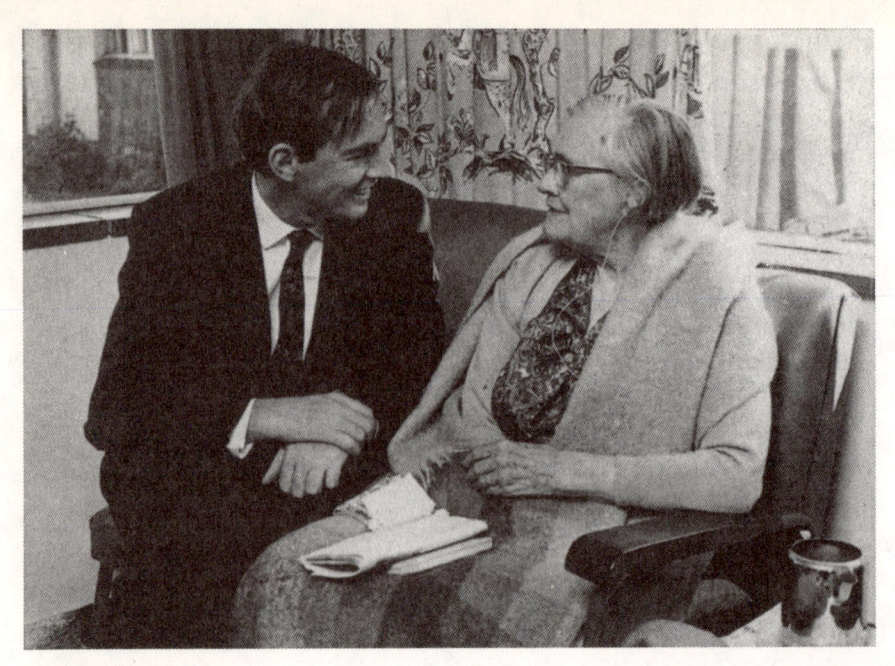

A visit to my mother

'Peter,' I asked, after listening to these ridiculous stories for long enough, 'I'm the last one to say that what you've just told me isn't possible but I really would like you to go to a cardiologist in England or America and let me see a copy of his report.'

'Yes, and I'll send you the pictures I took too,' Lynne interjected.

I never received the report, or the pictures – only a telegram a year later.

Although I was on the crest of a wave in my professional life, the happiness in my personal life was slowly being eroded.

My mother's health had deteriorated further and we had to admit her to a hospital where she could receive more professional care. Ironically, this was the same hospital where my first two children were born – then known as the Booth Maternity Hospital. In those days it was an institution for the beginning of life, but now it supervised the ending of it.

She was still asking when God was coming to take her away but God hadn't done so yet because medical technology had stepped in. Modern medicine, obsessed by specialization and preoccupied with technology continues to be driven inexorably towards heroic intervention striving, misguidedly, to keep patients 'alive'.

My mother, through medical intervention, had survived her first massive cerebral bleeding. She now had no hope of anything beyond a meaningless existence, chained to her physically and mentally deficient body.

A generation earlier, she would have died of 'the old people's friend' – pneumonia. Today, doctors, blinded from reality by technological gimmicks, sew, stitch, incubate, pump, drip, feed and intensively nurse – all aimed more at massaging professional pride, than for human consideration.

We forget that those machines cannot give love.

Life is more than just air – which is all a respirator can give. No sentient being can relate to intravenous feeding. Such heart-lung reparations are subject to hell-on-earth in the strict theological sense. Hell is a place without love and there can be no real love in a machine-supported life.

Every morning my mother was woken up, cleaned, fed, dressed, put in a chair and then back to bed – to awaken again to begin another day of frustration, boredom and humiliation.

'When is God going to take me away?'

'Soon, mother, soon – I promise you.'

Barbara was beginning to realize that the security she sought in our marriage was extremely elusive. It wasn't her fault. She even agreed to live on a lonely farm in the Karoo – out of the goldfish-bowl of our public lives and away from the threats to her vitally important family unit. We looked at farms for sale in the Beaufort West district but, unfortunately, couldn't find a suitable place to hide.

A unique set of circumstances made our lives too hectic. We were public figures and always under surveillance by the media and hounded by photographers. This was the age of the telephoto lens and no matter where we went, we were never alone. It reached a stage where, even in the most private places, we could sense the long-distance cameras. We had to be constantly aware of not giving the photographers any opportunity of a 'unique' shot.

Even everyday events gave these guys an opportunity. I'd be in a restaurant with a forkful of spaghetti and POP! would go the flash-bulb and there I'd be with a noodle hanging out of my mouth. If Barbara was looking away from me, we 'weren't talking'; if I danced with another woman, our 'marriage was in trouble'; if we went anywhere alone, then we 'had separated'.

We tried so hard to live a normal, relaxed life, but it's impossible to float gently on a river when it's in flood and you're heading for a waterfall.

I thought that, as time passed, I would be able to live my life like any other ordinary human being, but no: any girl I was seen with was a photograph and a story. This, to the newspapers, appeared to be vitally important news that the public just *had* to know about.

One evening in New York, I went to dinner with the South African consul. Afterwards one of the guests asked me if I'd ever been to Studio 54.

'I've never heard of the place – is it an art gallery?'

Everyone laughed and insisted I go with them, 'You'll enjoy it – it'll be a real experience – everybody who's anybody goes there.' So a few of us went to the night club.

When we arrived there was a long queue waiting to get in. One of the men in our group went to the ticket office and told them that I was outside and wanted to see inside the club – just for a few minutes. We were immediately shown in ahead of the waiting crowd. This was a mistake, as I found out later.

Inside, there were thousands of people enjoying the spectacular lighting effects and the loud music. I asked one of the women in our party if she'd like to dance – it seemed a fairly normal thing to do. There was a dance floor, there was music and there was someone to dance with.

Within five seconds of being on the dance floor, several dozen flash-bulbs exploded around me and all the cameras were being pointed at the girl and me. In a moment of *déjà vu* I thought, Oh God, I've been in this situation before as my mind flashed back to the evening in Baden-Baden with Uta Levka. We hurriedly left the dance floor, but the damage had already been done and the 'incriminating' photographs had been taken.

I was only told afterwards that the newsmen had been tipped off by the man in the ticket office. We should never have used my name to get ahead of the queue.

That very night, the photographs were sent by wire all over the world. The South African newspapers bought them immediately, of course, because it was such an 'important' story!

Barbara was, understandably, furious – even though I asked the consul to phone her and explain the whole story. I decided there and then that I'd beat these bastards at their own game and vowed never to give them another opportunity of photographing me with a woman – unless it was my wife. But the *Sunday Times* in South

Africa was too cunning and devious for me as I would discover a few weeks later.

The next day Mr Pik Botha, the South African representative at the United Nations, arranged a press conference for me.

At this meeting I mentioned that, in a peculiar way, it was a good thing to have the apartheid laws in South Africa – because these laws made discrimination a diagnosed disease.

'As a doctor, I know that you can only treat a disease once it's been diagnosed – so now we can treat this sickness, and continue the treatment until South Africa is totally cured.

'In many other countries the same disease exists – but it hasn't yet been diagnosed and so it remains untreated – because the governments pretend they are unaware of it and consequently do nothing.'

When we left what I thought had been a very successful encounter with the press, Pik Botha summoned all his diplomatic reserve and whispered acidly, 'I don't think it was such a good idea to call it a disease!'

My next encounter with a photographer happened when I was invited to a dinner-dance at Richards Bay, a town at the mouth of the Mhlathuze River on the Indian Ocean in Natal. It was named after Sir Frederick Richards, an admiral in the British Royal Navy in charge of attacking the Zulus when Britain was colonizing the country.

Unfortunately, for some reason Barbara couldn't come with me. Near the end of the evening, the manager of the hotel where the function was held, asked me if I would pose for a photograph with his staff. There were about six people in all and after the photograph had been taken, I asked several ladies to dance – including the waitress who'd stood next to me.

Ten days later the headline in the South African *Sunday Times* was: 'Barnard Whoops It Up With Waitress!'

To prove what a swinging time I'd had with the waitress, they published a photograph of the two of us standing together. When Barbara saw the picture she burst into hysterical tears and screamed that she'd had enough, that she was leaving and wanted a divorce.

I couldn't understand where they'd found the picture of me and the girl alone. The more I tried explaining what had happened that evening, the more suspicious Barbara became.

Finally a friend of mine, Vito, went up to Richards Bay to get a statement from the waiters as to what had happened and to prove to Barbara that it was a totally innocent evening.

He came back with both the statement and the picture. The bastards at the newspaper had simply etched out all the other people in the group photograph I'd posed for – leaving only the waitress and me apparently 'alone'.

I phoned Tertius Myburgh, the editor of the *Sunday Times*, whom I knew well and who was also a highly respected journalist. I asked him how he could condone such second-rate, sleazy reporting and allow a total lie to be published together with a concocted photograph.

I couldn't believe his reply.

'I thought it was funny.'

I knew perfectly well that that wasn't the reason he allowed the story to appear. Tertius Myburgh saw a chance to increase his circulation – and to hell with the distressing affects it would have on my wife, my children and my marriage.

It's just so damned infuriating when lies and falsehoods are published. There's no recourse whatsoever – all you have is this feeling of total helplessness and frustration.

Anyway, with the help of Vito, who produced the truth about the event, my marriage survived – but not without permanent scars.

Despite these ups and downs our marriage was still, basically, a very happy one. Frederick and Christiaan were growing up to become two handsome, healthy boys, happy to be living in Cape Town and attending the South African College School – SACS junior – the oldest school in South Africa.

Being a farmer at heart, I really enjoyed the large garden we had at 'Waiohai' and I installed an automatic sprinkling system so that the entire garden could be watered during the night and the lawns kept green and lush. At the back of the house, I cultivated my own vegetable garden where I spent many happy hours digging, nurturing and harvesting my own 'crop'.

A magnificent aviary was built and eventually I had a large collection of South African and exotic birds. I spent many happy hours watching them.

As the kids were at school for most of the day at this stage, and Barbara had two servants to run the home, she had a lot of free time. Together with Tony Ingala's girlfriend, Bertha, she opened a boutique in the centre of Cape Town, called B&B which, in the beginning anyway, was a great success.

André, my son from my first marriage, gave me a lot of pleasure. He was a quiet, good-looking young man who buckled down to the serious job of becoming a doctor and was a hard-working student. He had much better results in exams than his father ever did. I had always been very competitive – both at school and at university – so I was enormously proud of his achievements and followed them closely and enthusiastically.

Deirdre, my daughter from my first marriage, was restless. I believe that, in many ways, because of our close relationship – especially during the time she was water skiing – I was her anchor. With her parents' divorce, this steadying influence was broken and she was then like a ship floating around aimlessly in any direction the current took her. She eventually qualified as a teacher at Stellenbosch University and married a solid, down-to-earth Afrikaner, Kobus Visser.

Their wedding reception was held at my restaurant, La Vita, and Barbara used all her social and planning skills to make this a glittering occasion. We used the entire Dean Street Arcade – the restaurant is in the centre of this up-market shopping mall in Newlands.

My colleague and friend, Syd Cywes, who had a large collection of orchids, lent me about 30 pots of these beautiful plants in flower which were positioned between the tables.

It was a very splendid event and my daughter radiated happiness. I have to admit that I was so very happy for her, that I got slightly drunk that evening.

Sue Edwards, who was my new secretary, handed me a letter one morning from Amnesty International in Vienna. They pleaded with me to do something about a political prisoner, Strini Moodley. They claimed he was in solitary confinement, had tuberculosis of the lungs and was unable to see a doctor.

I wrote to the commissioner of prisons who promptly acknowledged receipt of my letter and promised he would investigate the matter.

Two weeks later I received his comprehensive reply, in which he told me that Strini Moodley had been found guilty on a charge of terrorism and was not a political prisoner. He was not in solitary confinement and he did not suffer from tuberculosis of the lungs – he also saw a doctor regularly.

I wrote back to Amnesty International and relayed the information. They replied immediately, repudiating the information – would I please investigate further? This I did – with the same result. After several exchanges of letters, I eventually told them they were wasting my time and theirs because I could do nothing more than give them the facts as they were given to me. Strini Moodley was, in fact, an active member of the black consciousness movement and he had been convicted of terrorism.

A month later, I received a letter from Mr Moodley's attorney suing me for R10 000 because I'd called his client a 'terrorist'. I was deeply hurt because I'd really done my very best to help this man and all that had happened as a result of my efforts was that I'd landed myself in a libel action.

I wasn't just going to give in and be a meal-ticket for any prisoner who wanted to make some easy money. So I consulted my friend Noel Tunbridge again – the lawyer who'd managed to keep me out of trouble for so long.

He told me this would be a supreme court case and that we would have to appoint an advocate. He suggested Mr Harry Snitcher, whom I knew well and who was a highly respected jurist. We had a meeting in his chambers and, after I'd related the whole story, he told me that my case was so strong, there was little doubt we'd win. We entered a plea to defend the charges – and claim costs.

Three weeks later, Noel phoned me with some devastating news. He said that both he and Harry Snitcher were of the opinion that I should settle out of court. Their reasoning was sound, because Strini Moodley had no funds, so even if I won the case with costs, he wouldn't be able to pay them and I'd be left with large legal fees to pay myself. I settled, for R3 000 I think, but it left a very bitter taste in my mouth. Still, it was another lesson learned.

Not long afterwards, I received another letter from Amnesty International asking me whether I would be so kind as to help them with another prisoner. I'll leave it to the reader's imagination as to what I did with *that* letter.

'Professor Barnard? Your mother's had another stroke, I'm afraid, and her condition has deteriorated greatly.' It was the sister from the hospital where my mother was being nursed.

I told her I would be there immediately and, on the way, I

thought that maybe God would now remove those barriers erected by the medical profession and grant her her wish.

My mother didn't recognize either Marius or me, but kept on repeating, 'Thank you very much, thank you very much.'

My guess is that she knew her suffering was nearly at an end and she was grateful for the release. Her lungs were very, very wet and she could no longer swallow.

'The doctor's suggested we start her on antibiotics and put a nasal-gastric tube down her throat to feed her,' the sister said.

'Why would you want to do that?' Marius demanded.

'We can't just leave her like that, Doctor!' came the reprimand and the sister looked at the two of us.

I asked her, 'Do you think that *any* medical intervention will bring her back to a condition where she'll thank us for being alive?'

The sister didn't answer.

I turned to Marius. 'Do you agree that we withdraw all treatment and just keep her comfortable?' He nodded his head and at that moment, as if she understood, my mother spoke weakly again, 'Thank you very much.' And closed her eyes.

Later that night God came and took her away.

When the sister phoned me during the night to tell me that my mother had passed away, I received the news with mixed feelings. I was sad that the wonderful woman, who had had so few comforts in her life and who'd lived only for her four boys, was dead.

I could see her in front of the Singer sewing machine which she turned by hand, as she worked deep into the night to make clothes for her sons.

I could see her in front of the Dover stove, opening the lid of the iron pot to turn over the leg of lamb for our Sunday lunch.

I also saw her in great pain and humiliation in that hospital bed.

Now Maria Elizabeth was at peace and I was pleased she had finally reached the place she'd always wanted to be – a place where she wouldn't suffer from cystitis and constipation and constant pain.

My mother had always expressed a wish to be buried alongside her fifth son, who'd died from a congenital heart disease long before I was born. When little Abraham was terminal and had difficulty in breathing my parents brought him down to Fish Hoek, a small fishing village on the Cape Peninsula, to be near the sea.

He'd died during this visit and was laid to rest in a cemetery near Muizenberg. I'd never visited his grave, but the funeral undertakers found it and my mother's wish was fulfilled.

We were all waiting for the funeral service to begin. My mother's coffin was placed in front of the pulpit. Marius and his wife Inez, Barbara and I and Joyce, my eldest brother's wife – who'd left him many years previously with a lot of bitterness and hatred – were sitting together in the front row.

My brother Barney and the woman he'd been living with walked into the church. He stopped dead in his tracks when he saw Joyce. The anger and disgust on his face was obvious. He seemed about to turn on his heels and leave, but he changed his mind and strode purposefully up to where we were all sitting, pointed his finger at Joyce and shouted so loudly that his voice echoed round the church, 'What the *fucking* hell are you doing here!'

I was so glad that my poor mother couldn't see or hear any of this and I shrank down into the pew. Marius took him aside and told him he should have more respect for his mother. He calmed down and, with his girlfriend, went to sit in the furthest corner of the church.

We buried my mother next to Abraham and this also made headlines, as we were accused of desecrating an existing grave.

My mother's suffering, and also that of one of the patients in my ward at that time, Mr Van Rooyen – who was slowly being strangled to death by a carcinoma of the lung – convinced me that there must be a place for euthanasia in the treatment of the terminally ill.

With the help of two friends, Bob Molloy in Cape Town and Steve Donaghue in New York, I discussed and examined the religious, social, medical and legal aspects of both active and passive euthanasia in a book called *Good Life, Good Death*.

After that I wrote another novel, *In The Night Season*, with Siegfried Stander. My main characters were two doctors who had totally different approaches when they were confronted with a woman who had incurable breast cancer. The one believed in heroic intervention to the bitter end and the other in humane non-intervention.

I travelled through Europe and the United States to promote these two books and this gave me the opportunity to bring the problems of the terminally ill patient to the attention of the public – and the medical profession, who often turned a blind eye.

Doctors, as a rule, are afraid to state publicly what they truly believe should be done when it comes to euthanasia – although most of them practise it anyhow. Many of them won't admit that, with a terminally ill patient, the time comes when treatment should be withdrawn and no additional treatment instigated.

The patient should be allowed to die a death with dignity.

But I've always been of the opinion that we should be allowed to go further. Society has to accept that once the legal boundaries are drawn, it should allow the doctor actively to end the life of a terminally ill patient in great suffering – after all medical means to restore his health have been exhausted.

These books brought me face to face again with David Frost, but this time I came off second-best.

This was our third encounter. At the second interview, a few years earlier, he was assisted by Thomas Thomson, the author of *Hearts* – a book that dealt with the rivalry between Doctors Denton Cooley and Michael de Bakey.

I prefer to go to an interview without any preparation and without being told the questions in advance, so that I can be spontaneous in my answers. This works best for me. Unfortunately, I didn't follow the rule this time with David Frost.

Eschel Rhoodie told me that Frost had invited an ex-South African to help him and wondered if I could use some help from his department myself?

The man was a lawyer who defended the downtrodden in South Africa and who portrayed the part of a poor but magnanimous philantropist very well.

Rhoodie's department of information told me that this lawyer had left South Africa in such a hurry he'd left behind a beautiful house with two BMWs and a Mercedes parked in the garage and that he had probably made a lot of money defending these 'poor repressed people'. When he left the country he still enjoyed an extravagant lifestyle.

So I went on the programme with preconceived ideas because I had all this advance information – a big mistake.

David Frost began, 'Professor Barnard, you've said your country's been unfairly treated. Can you give us an example?'

I said, 'There are many reasons, but let me give you one example. Recently South Africa's been singled out as the only country that is a threat to world peace and that the United Nations has declared a total arms embargo on us.

'Now, there are a lot of things wrong with South Africa but firstly, I don't think South Africa is a threat to world peace and, secondly, if we *are* a threat, we're not the only country with discrimination, suppression of people and political prisoners. What about the rest of Africa? What about India and many parts of Asia? There are so many countries where there is far worse death and destruction, so why single out South Africa as a scapegoat?'

David then turned to the other man and asked him what he thought. This ex-South African, of course, started quoting all the South African laws that made it an 'enemy of the world'.

I pretended not to know who this man was and when he was halfway through this diatribe, I stopped him and asked him if he was a South African – which he confirmed, of course.

Then, foolishly, I said, 'Oh yes, weren't you the guy who ran away from South Africa?' And I mentioned all the cars he'd left behind, the hypocrisy and that sort of thing. I thought I would easily expose him for what he was.

David Frost is not a fool – he clicked immediately that I was well prepared for this. He said, 'Professor Barnard, your memory comes back very quickly – you must surely know my other guest, although you pretend you don't?'

David Frost also has the killer instinct. He knew he had me and he slowly began twisting the knife with cutting sarcasm and ridicule.

Then I did the worst thing possible – I lost my temper.

'Mr Frost, you invited me onto this show to talk about euthanasia – now you and your friend want to use this opportunity to run down my country. I'm not prepared to take part in this exercise.' I stood up, unclipped my microphone and walked off the set.

As I was leaving, Frost made his last stinging remark, 'You know, Professor Barnard, you had a good opportunity tonight, to state South Africa's case and you goofed it.'

I couldn't sleep that night because I'd made such a fool of myself and because Frost was right – I'd goofed an excellent opportunity.

A week later I had a cable from Peter Sellers. It read, 'Dear Chris, I saw you on the Frost show and you made a real ass of yourself. It was not the way for a man of your intelligence to behave. Peter.'

The truth always hurts but, what was even more painful was that this was the last communication between us before he died a few months later.

I like to think that he didn't carry any ill-feelings about me to his grave. Anyway I was pleased to hear his son say that the last few words his father said, the night before he died were, 'I should have gone through with the operation when I had the chance – with Chris.'

Ironically, six months after Peter's death his wife, Lynne Fredericks, married David Frost, so maybe he'd got the better of both Peter and me.

'Chris, do you think you could come and see me in the Hendrik Verwoerd Building – I have an extremely important mission for you.' It was Eschel Rhoodie.

During the previous year, the Department of Information had asked me to appear on television shows and make contact with politicians and ambassadors in various parts of the world.

I never asked to be paid for this work – but they covered my expenses. These payments were also made in a very unusual way. I was never asked to submit an expense account or give statements and receipts. Eschel would just give me, every now and again, an envelope with cash – which I signed for.

I asked him several times whether I had to declare the income, but he was non-committal. This worried me to such an extent that I even went to see Owen Horwood, who was minister of finance at the time. He was also not sure how I should handle the matter and told me they hadn't decided about it yet.

I'm eternally grateful to my accountant, Mr Lotter, as he insisted I declare the money on my income tax return.

When the 'Information Scandal' rocked the South African government later, I had nothing to hide – I'd made it known to the receiver of revenue that I'd received expenses from the government and, while I thought the method of payment odd, it had all been above board as far as I was concerned.

When I saw Eschel in his office that day he told me that South Africa would lose millions if the trade unions of the US went ahead with their intended boycott of South Africa. He wanted me to go and see George Meany, the head of the union, to try to dissuade him from this line of industrial action.

When I arrived in Washington I was met by some of Rhoodie's men, who gave me all the background on the disaster that South Africa faced.

The next morning, when they collected me from the hotel and drove me to the union's office, they handed me a clipping from the *Washington Post*, in which the death of a Mexican prisoner in an

American jail was extensively reported. He'd died of injuries inflicted by the police. They'd even found faeces and urine in his hair. It sounded very similar to the Steve Biko case.

George Meany was an elderly man and greeted me in a civil but less than cordial manner. I could see he was wary.

I began telling him about my work and explained, as vividly as I could, the interesting experiences we'd had with piggy-back heart operations. I'd learnt that this was always the best approach – it usually broke the ice and stimulated conversation.

He was fascinated by these stories and I could see he was becoming more friendly.

I told him how much we needed money to continue with our work and how I'd heard he was going to cripple our economy with an extensive union boycott.

'Why do you want to do this, Mr Meany?'

His face darkened immediately and frowning, he raised his voice slightly, 'Look how you treated Steve Biko!' The previous warmth in his manner disappeared completely.

'Mr Meany, I'm very ashamed and deeply sorry to admit that this happened in my country – but do you think such behaviour is unique only to South African police? Couldn't it also happen elsewhere – even in the United States?'

He replied very quickly and laughed gruffly. 'Oh, it would never happen here – this is America.'

He obviously hadn't read the papers – so I reached into my pocket and handed him the newspaper clipping.

He read it and leaned back in his chair. There was silence.

After a suitably polite interlude, I continued evenly, 'Mr Meany, if you think the boycott will help, then go ahead. But I beg of you, before you do that, send a delegation to South Africa to get first-hand information on the situation there. You'll find that the whites are not all racists and that, generally speaking, all races work together and are changing things.

'There is a lot of bad in the country, but there's even more good and it's getting better all the time.'

The boycott never happened.

Barbara had always said, 'Chris, if you have to go out with other women please tell me. I won't be as upset as I will be if I learn about it elsewhere.' I took her request seriously and genuinely – with disastrous results.

While Barbara was overseas on a buying trip for her boutique, I had a phone call from Dr Nico Diederichs, who was then state president, inviting me to come to Pretoria to be one of his guests at a dinner he was giving for the sister of the shah of Iran.

The shah's family had emotional ties with South Africa, as their father had died in Johannesburg when he was exiled during the Second World War. There was a move afoot to change the house where he'd died into a museum.

I went up for the dinner and during the course of the evening, told the visiting party that if they came to Cape Town I would be honoured to show them around one evening. I didn't think for a moment that they'd take up my offer.

A few days later I had a call to say that some members of the party would like me to show them the night life of Cape Town that evening. I was certainly not an authority on the local nightspots, but couldn't refuse the request. So a few of the younger members of the group – with their bodyguards – joined me and we visited two night clubs.

When Barbara arrived home I told her about the evening. Although I've always loved women, I've never understood them – and this was no exception. She was furious!

'How the hell could you do that! What d'you think you're playing at? Running around with young girls the minute my back's turned!' She really laid it on thick.

I tried reasoning with her, which, as any man knows, is a thankless task. 'It was a group of visiting dignitaries, darling. The girls in the party had bodyguards next to them all the time. Even if I had had other plans, which I promise I didn't, I would have had their bodyguards as an audience, because they never left their sides. I swear it was an innocent evening.'

Barbara refused to listen and was not interested in these 'feeble' excuses. In fact, she was deeply hurt and the old fears of insecurity now became much stronger.

She was so disturbed by this that her health began deteriorating seriously. She ate less and less, and lost a great deal of weight – which, I believe, was a subconscious cry for help and a way of demanding attention and sympathy.

My world was starting to crumble around me, but worst of all, I began to lose interest in surgery. On many mornings I'd look for excuses not to go to the hospital and I allowed my assistants to take over an increasing amount of the clinical burden.

Never, in my wildest dreams, would I ever have thought the day would arrive when I'd *hate* putting on a pair of surgical gloves.

I was dealt another crushing blow when Marius resigned and left Cape Town to settle in Johannesburg. A few months earlier he'd suggested that I let him handle the clinical side, so that I could concentrate on research and administration. At that time I'd taken it as an insult – and told him so. Now, too late, I realized he was right. He'd had ample experience of running the department when I was away on my frequent trips overseas.

Now my department was to lose all that experience and our results, especially in transplantation, reflected this.

The arthritis, which for years during my marriage to Barbara had been in remission, was flaring up again. Rheumatoid arthritis is not just pain and swelling of the joints. The continued local inflammatory process is also associated with other general symptoms such as severe tiredness, mental depression and irritability – which didn't help my marriage either.

To make things even worse, the 'Information Scandal' broke and, although I wasn't really involved, some reporters tried to drag me into it by implication – without success.

The parliamentary auditor claimed that unnamed information department officials had been making unauthorized expenditures for the previous three years. The report alleged that up to $460 000 had been spent on attracting favourable publicity for South Africa, without the treasury or parliament's knowledge.

It was only the tip of the iceberg, as the amounts involved grew into millions and more and more people were named.

The scandal resulted in the resignation of John Vorster, the prime minister, the resignation of Connie Mulder – favoured to be the next prime minister and the disgrace of Eschel Rhoodie, information secretary and the man who'd come up with the idea of improving South Africa's image abroad.

His plan had been to set up a secret fund to finance the waging of 'psychological and propaganda warfare' to influence foreign 'opinion formers and decision makers.' It began with the approval of Connie Mulder (minister of information), Dr Nico Diederichs (minister of finance) and John Vorster (prime minister).

One amazing story followed another in a frenzy of media voracity. The scandals stretched from failed attempts to take over the *Washington Star* to 'hit-contracts' on people who 'knew too much'.

Through Eschel Rhoodie, I had several opportunities to meet

Connie Mulder – whom I found to be a very practical politician, and I was convinced that if *he* became prime minister he would get rid of apartheid very quickly.

I used all my contacts and influence to get votes for him but he not only lost the bid for leadership, he also had to resign from the cabinet as a result of the 'Information Scandal'.

What I never could understand was why he later became so conservative. I'm sure that he never believed, in his heart, that that was the right road for South Africa to take. I think it was bitterness that drove him away from the Nationalist party into the conservative flock.

At one stage in my life I thought it was possible to change the government's approach by gentle persuasion – which I continued doing for a long time. I was wrong.

They'd been in power for so long and had become so arrogant and dictatorial, that such an approach would never work and I turned my back on the Nationalists forever.

I tried to expand my investments in the restaurant business. Tony Ingala left La Vita in Newlands and the two of us opened a steakhouse close by. This again was well patronised but not financially successful. After a few months I sold it – and, not much later, it burned down.

Tony persuaded me that we should become partners in a pizzeria in Tokai, a suburb close to Constantia. Unfortunately we had a serious argument and parted company before this could be opened.

I was approached by the chairman of the Welgemoed Golf Club. They were building a new club house and planned to have a restaurant there. Would I be interested?

I approached Chris Lesley, who was the chef at the steakhouse and asked him if he would like to be the manager of this new La Vita for me. He agreed and we had a grand opening, to which we invited some of the prominent citizens of the area.

Chris had also asked some local schoolgirls to be waitresses that evening – I remember one of them being an outstandingly beautiful creature.

I now had three restaurants: Newlands, the one at Maureen's hotel in Tableview and the new one at Welgemoed.

An alarming number of young South Africans, and even older

professional men and women, were selling up and leaving the country to live in places such as the United States, Canada, Australia and New Zealand.

In fact, the joke at the time was the definition of a loyal South African: someone who couldn't sell his house or get a foreign passport.

Their decisions to emigrate were based on two reasons: the poor salaries paid in academic positions and the political uncertainty. Some were of the opinion that there was no future for their children in a country so full of hate and repression.

I'd had several very lucrative offers myself but always declined as I felt that I owed South Africa so much. This wasn't only the country to which my forefathers had emigrated in 1708 from Cologne, and had settled as free burghers; it was also the country that had given me my education and the opportunity to perform the first transplant.

I loved my country and was sure that the government would eventually come to their senses and abandon their racial policy that had destroyed the country with more devastation than an atomic bomb.

We had become increasingly isolated and despised by the rest of the world. On several occasions, I was offered honorary doctorates by foreign universities, but because the students objected and said they wouldn't allow me onto the campus, the invitations were withdrawn.

There were several countries which refused permission for South African doctors to attend medical conferences and funds for clinical research had dried up.

One day I received a letter from a colleague who'd emigrated. He told me that in New Zealand the media had given extensive coverage to an accusation on me in a book titled *Slaughter of the Innocents*, which had just been published.

It claimed that I had 'ripped out' the heart of a baboon 'without anaesthetic'. The author also described, in lurid detail, how the staff and patients in the hospital had been shocked and disturbed by the screams of the baboon.

I was urged to take legal action as these reports were causing considerable damage to their own research efforts.

I'd been told about the accusations in this book – but they were so ridiculous that I didn't take them seriously – and assumed no other remotely intelligent person would either.

It was obvious that the writer had never seen a live baboon – these animals are extremely powerful and vicious, with upper eye-teeth longer than those of a lion. There's no way, even in the wildest of imaginations, that a baboon could be held down while his heart was being ripped out. They are colossally strong and extremely savage.

In any case, why on earth would I want to do such a thing? In the first place, all life is precious to me. In the second place, at a major research centre like ours, there were always highly trained anaesthetists available.

So off I went to see Noel Tunbridge again and we instituted legal proceedings against the media in New Zealand as well as in England and the United States where these accusations were also publicized.

In New Zealand and England I was awarded compensation by the courts, but the lawyers in the United States advised me not to go ahead as I was a public figure and, consequently, 'fair game'. It was very unlikely that my claim would succeed in the land of the brave and the free.

It's a fact that people get some kind of morbid delight out of maliciously spreading bad news. Barbara's so-called friends relished telling her about my 'affairs' at any and every opportunity.

I don't deny that at that stage I found other women attractive and paid more attention to them than ever before, but I loved my wife and family too much even to consider having a serious affair.

Barbara had also warned me that if she ever found out I was running around with women again, she would divorce me immediately. But, somehow, I never thought she'd ever go that far. I felt supremely overconfident and didn't think she had the guts to sacrifice what security she had. A very rude awakening was heading my way.

It was one of those evenings when everything turned out just right. Both Barbara and I had a wonderful time. After dinner we had a few dances at a night club called Charlie Parkers and then, the best part of the evening, back home in bed on my 59th birthday.

I had to leave the next morning for the United States on a long tour to promote a book, *The Body Machine*, of which I was co-author.

Barbara took me to the airport as usual. Being very superstitious, she always went through a little ritual of making a cross on my forehead with her finger. She was always very tearful at these partings too. But on this occasion, it was different – just a quick peck on the cheek and a casual farewell. No cross on the forehead.

I didn't notice it at the time, but on reflection, I should have realized that something wasn't right.

I phoned her from New York and she was happy and excited to hear from me. I kept in contact by phone over the next few weeks – as I always did when I travelled alone – and I only had to visit San Francisco, Los Angeles and Seattle for some final interviews, before I returned home.

In San Francisco I checked into the Stanford Court Hotel. The following morning I was just about to leave my room for a television interview, when the phone rang.

'Hello, Chris,' said Noel Tunbridge, 'I'm afraid I have some bad news for you.'

My immediate thoughts were that Barbara or one of my children had been in an accident and my voice trembled as I asked what was wrong.

'Barbara's lawyer has just phoned me. She's suing you for divorce.'

There was silence. I couldn't believe what I'd just heard.

'Why?' was all I could say as my mind spun dizzily and I tried to think what I could have done that would precipitate such drastic action. My legs were also trembling now, so I sat down heavily on the edge of the bed.

Noel answered my question with a sad voice, 'According to Barbara, the maids in your house told her that when she was away a few months ago, they found you in bed with a girl.'

This was good news. I was relieved to hear that what prompted Barbara to take this rash course was a blatant lie. I knew I could prove it was untrue – so everything would be okay.

My pulse began slowing down and, more calmly, I asked Noel to persuade Barbara to wait until I was home and that I could explain everything.

'I'll try, but she seems very determined,' he replied uncertainly and added, 'even her father's been down to Cape Town to consult with the lawyers. But I'll try and I'll phone you tomorrow.'

The fact that Fred was already involved definitely wasn't good news, so after gazing at the silent telephone for what seemed an eternity, I struggled through the day's interviews and decided to cancel the rest of my tour and go home to rescue my marriage.

The next morning Noel phoned again with even worse news. Not only was Barbara unwilling to wait – she'd instructed him to tell me that if I attempted to go home to 'Waiohai' she would get an interdict to have me legally evicted. The harsh reality and severity of the situation suddenly hit me.

I was in a strange country with unfamiliar faces around me. I'd never felt more lonely and deserted. So absolutely devastated and alone – with no one to talk to and, now, no home to go to.

I remembered that a friend in Cape Town, Gloria Craig, had given me the telephone number of her daughter Jenny, who was living in Los Angeles. She was very beautiful and, at one stage, had been the girlfriend of Don Mackenzie.

I decided that I'd cancel Seattle and phone her. I told her my bad news and said I'd be flying to LA that day and asked if I could meet her.

So I booked into the Beverly Hills Hotel and Jenny's company did a lot to lift me out of the deep depression – I was even able to keep my appointments in Los Angeles, which included being a guest on the *Dinah Shaw Show*.

I was feeling much perkier now and even sang a little song on the show – which was a huge faux pas. I jokingly said, 'Of course, you were the Dinah we used to sing about when I was a kid: "Dinah, is there anyone finah, in the state of Carolinah..."'

I thought it was very funny but she just looked coldly at me and said, 'I'm not that old.'

The rest of the show went very well and I even told her, in front of millions of Americans, that my wife had just dropped me. She turned to the camera and made a live 'appeal' for Barbara to take me back.

On my way home I made a guest appearance on the *Michael Parkinson Show* in London and gave a lecture in Madrid. Although I received some tempting invitations, I avoided any sexual encounters – but it did make me realize I was single again.

Single again? Was that what I wanted? The thought hadn't crossed my mind before – all I'd wanted to do was avoid a divorce, but now I was uncertain about what I really wanted.

Now that I'd recovered from Noel's phone calls, I realized I might have some options.

Should I go all-out to save my marriage or should I allow events to take their course? On the one hand, I'd be free from the restrictions that marriage imposed, but on the other hand, I felt very sad for Frederick and Christiaan, both still so very young. Deirdre and André, who'd been much older when I was divorced from Louwtjie, had been left with permanent psychological scars, I reminded myself.

A divorce is often just a selfish escape from the responsibility of married life. Fighting parents, in my view, are still better for the children than a broken home.

Suddenly, in the midst of my thoughts, I sat bolt upright in my seat on the plane. I hadn't thought about my love for Barbara once.

Fritz Brink collected me from the airport and helped me avoid the press. He and his wife, Maureen, two wonderful friends, gave me board and lodging in the Tableview Hotel which belonged to them. Tableview is a coastal resort-suburb with a magnificent view of Table Bay and Table mountain.

They were also business partners because, a year previously, I'd opened a third La Vita restaurant in their hotel.

I phoned Barbara and we arranged to meet for dinner at the Hohenhort Hotel in Constantia. She was very emotional that evening and several times her blue eyes spilled over with tears.

I tried to explain the truth about the story her maids had told her. I'd had a cold at the time, and was in bed trying to shake it off. A young girl and a friend came to visit me and after a while, the friend left and the girl stayed chatting with me for an hour.

'There's no truth whatsoever in the story that she came to bed with me – after all, I wasn't feeling well, it was broad daylight, the windows and doors were open and I *knew* the maids were there. Surely you don't think a sly old fox like me would be so stupid to take a girl to bed in those circumstances?' I tried to make her see the funny side of it.

But she wouldn't believe me. 'Both maids told me, Chris – *both* of them!'

Maybe I could have saved my marriage that night – if only temporarily – because when I drove her back to 'Waiohai', she cried bitterly and asked me into the house. I refused – I don't know why – but I think that was the final straw as far as Barbara was concerned.

How often, in the following months, I regretted that decision.

The two boys were now on their Christmas holidays and I took them with me to Swartvlei (Afrikaans: 'black lake'), which is 20 kilometres from the Knysna lagoon and where Fritz had a house. My sons were to spend a part of their vacation with me.

Barbara phoned me to say that she wanted the divorce over as quickly as possible and could I come to Cape Town to meet her lawyers and decide on the terms?

Barbara, her father, the two lawyers and I gathered in Noel Tunbridge's office. It was an acrimonious meeting and I nearly stormed out when they accused me of infidelity.

Finally we agreed on the terms and once more, I was thrown out of my home – just as it had been with Louwtjie. This time I had only my clothes and three pieces of furniture: a stinkwood chair – the only thing I inherited from my parents, a chair that Barbara's mother gave us and a writing desk her father had given me. Oh yes – and the bed and mattress on which I was supposed to have screwed this girl and screwed up my marriage.

A month before what would have been our 12th anniversary, Barbara and the lawyers went to the supreme court in Cape Town and the judge finalized the divorce.

I was still at Swartvlei with the boys. Early that morning I drove up to the Knysna Heads – two large rocky sentinels at the mouth of the Knysna lagoon – where 23 years previously I had come to mourn the death of my father.

A divorce is, in some ways, worse than death. Death is final and there's nothing you can do about it. Divorce is a living nightmare – you are haunted by the lingering hope that you will get together again.

At that time I didn't understand why Barbara was in such a hurry to get the divorce over with. I'd asked her to put it on pause for a while as perhaps we'd be able to sort out our differences. But there was no stopping her.

I must admit that I was, in a way, glad to be free again and I took a vow never to marry again. The experiment had failed twice and there was no sense in repeating it.

For some peculiar reason, I'd envisioned Barbara sitting alone at home fretting over the loss of her wonderful husband. This dream was, in small measure, a cushion against the separation from her, my home and children. It wasn't so bad when I thought of it in that light.

Then it happened.

I took the children back to 'Waiohai' on a Sunday afternoon.

Barbara was lying at the pool and there was this young, bronzed, hunk of a guy, in a pair of scant red swimming briefs, strolling around as if he owned the place. Then the penny dropped.

During the next six months I became absolutely grief stricken and embittered. I was totally and utterly consumed with jealousy.

My medical activities ground to a halt. Other doctors took over my responsibilities as I became less and less active. I still went to my office at the medical school every day – just to stare into space and plot how to get Barbara back. When there had been the chance of a reconciliation, I hadn't wanted her. But now that there was another man involved – and a young, handsome, virile man at that – it became my main, if not my only goal in life. It was to become an obsession.

Fortunately, my secretary, Celeste McCann, had been through a divorce and break-up with a boyfriend herself, and she kept me from totally falling to pieces.

When I think back now on those months after my divorce, I'm ashamed of my despicable behaviour. Deep in my heart I knew that I didn't want my married life back, but on the other hand, I didn't want anybody else to have Barbara either. The male ego is very complex.

At that time it was quite all right for me to go to bed with another woman, but when I thought of Barbara in the arms of another man I wanted to die. I wanted to scream obscenities and bang my head against a wall – such was the intensity of my jealousy. On more than one occasion, I became seriously worried about my mental health.

I kept thinking that perhaps I was getting too old?

After many days of devious and demented thought and planning I had my insane strategy worked out.

First, the servants who'd spread these unholy rumours had to be punished. Next, I had to get as much background information as possible about her new lover, so that I could discredit him. Lastly, I wanted to keep as close as possible to Barbara and always present the best side of Chris Barnard to her.

I could have killed those two lying bitches, but even in that disturbed pathological emotional state, I wasn't violent. A witchdoctor would be the answer. I'd heard so much about the supernatural powers of the black sangoma. He could cast a spell over a person which would lead to a lot of suffering or even death.

I'd heard he didn't necessarily have to know his target or have contact with them; all that was necessary was to procure any article belonging to the person one wanted to have punished.

My hunt for a sangoma was on. Where could I find such a man or woman who would do this dirty work for me?

When filming the French television documentary, I'd interviewed a witchdoctor in Johannesburg – but he was more like a medicine man who tried to cure people – I needed one to do exactly the opposite.

Eventually, the black driver who worked for Fritz and Maureen Brink told me that he knew of one and a meeting was arranged in the dense bushes near Cape Town's airport. All the witchdoctor needed to work his black-magic was a bottle of gin. I thought he might need this as an ingredient to make a potion.

I was disappointed when I finally met him. He wasn't dressed in wild animal skins and had no bones to throw – let alone one through his nose. But he assured me that he *was* a sangoma and that he could call upon the evil spirts whenever he needed them. I explained my problems and asked him to deal out the worst punishment he could to these two bitches. I gave him the gin – and R500 to speed up the process.

My first task had been completed. The maids would slowly fade away. A few weeks later I quietly told them of their fate. They just laughed at me. A month later they were still in good health – I think that all my visit to the witchdoctor succeeded in doing was getting him drunk and giving him an unexpected cash bonus.

Both maids left Barbara a few months later and I believe they lived happily ever after. In the meantime, I lived from one phone call to the next – just hoping to hear Barbara's voice again.

I would have done *anything* to win her back.

But instead, when I did get the chance of taking her out to dinner, with red roses and French champagne, she told me how 'wonderful' her new boyfriend was. How handsome and well-built he was – and how exciting her 'new life' was. She was out, I'm sure, to punish me for all the tears she'd shed for me, because each comment about Joe was like a dagger piercing my heart.

One Sunday evening, when I took the children back to 'Waiohai' after they'd spent the week-end with me, he was also at the house.

He asked me if I'd like to have a drink and the three of us sat in the lounge. This 'trespasser' was now the host and I was the guest.

After a while, Barbara excused herself saying she had to get ready for dinner. Joe and I continued with our very amiable conversation.

About half an hour later, Barbara returned and asked whether I had already eaten.

'No, I haven't actually.'

'Well, you'll have to excuse us because we're going to have dinner now.' She and Joe left me sitting in the lounge.

I stood up and walked out of the front door of 'Waiohai' for the last time.

Frans Prazzl, a senior reporter on one of the newspapers in Vienna, phoned me to say I'd been invited to attend the Opera Ball and they'd asked a young Austrian actress, Evelyn Engleder, to be my partner.

Frans and his wife, Elizabeth, met me at the airport in Vienna and took me to the very grand Schwartzenberg Palace – chandeliered ceilings, marble floors and rococo furniture. This hotel had everything you'd expect from the best in Vienna, which is probably why the queen of England and various heads of state stayed there.

That evening, we had dinner together and Evelyn joined us later when she'd finished at a play in one of the local theatres. She was a stunning woman in her mid-twenties and although she denied it, I was told she had once been voted 'Miss Austria'.

The following morning was free, so I wandered around the garden of the hotel and noticed they were making a movie next door. I thought it would be fun to watch and see how it was done.

I was told that they were busy filming the life of Wagner and asked whether I would like to meet Richard Burton.

I said I'd like nothing better than to meet such a great actor and they took me into the building. Richard Burton sat in a chair dressed in the clothing of Wagner's era, waiting to be called on set.

He said he would like me to have dinner with him that evening at his hotel and would send a car to collect me at 8 o'clock. I was very excited at the prospect of spending a few hours with this brilliant man, whom I'd read so much about.

When I arrived at his hotel that evening, he was sitting in the lounge drinking huge martinis out of a water glass. It was obvious that he'd had quite a few of them, and when the subject came around to medicine, he was, understandably, only interested in liver transplants.

After a while, when we were better acquainted, I tentatively suggested that it seemed such a pity that a man with his exceptional skills was undermining his health by drinking so much.

His answer was quite blunt and straight to the point, 'Piss off.'

In my senior school days, we'd had *King Lear* as a prescribed book. There were still a few lines I could recall from this play, so I quoted what I remembered to him.

He told me I was 'murdering the Bard' and proceeded to recite from this play for at least five minutes – in his deep, resonant, Welsh baritone. He didn't stumble over the words once and was absolutely word-perfect.

I was spellbound.

In the meantime, he was supplied with fresh water glasses filled with martinis – I told the waiter to stop bringing them, but he said he couldn't refuse if that was what his guests ordered.

My dinner companion then fell asleep for a while, so I started eating the crisps and the olives. I realized that that was probably all we would be served for dinner.

When he woke up again, he was eager to carry on talking so I told him about my divorce and how I was trying to get back at my ex-wife.

'Never marry your ex-wife, I tried it and it was a disaster,' he slurred as he told me that his marriage was also over.

'But Elizabeth Taylor is one of the most fascinating women in the world, surely?' I asked.

'Elizabeth Taylor? Ha! Elizabeth Taylor *invented* vulgarity!'

It was disappointing that we couldn't enjoy a sober discussion as he seemed to be a very sensitive man.

He ordered another martini and I ordered a taxi.

The Ball at the Vienna Opera House was more glamorous than I could ever have imagined. The men were dressed in tails and the ladies in beautiful ballgowns and hundreds of couples swirled gracefully around the dance floor to the Strauss waltzes.

Seven hundred guests were invited and Richard Burton was also there, but he left early. I was told he had some problems with his equilibrium and they kept him away from the cameras and the VIPs.

I danced deep into the night with Evelyn. I couldn't have had a better female companion. She was loving and full of understanding. There was only one drawback – a boyfriend.

This visit helped restore some of my confidence, although I was still hurting badly. I was reluctant to leave Vienna as I'd met some wonderful people, but I had to keep an appointment with Armin Mattli and Dr Schafer.

Armin met me at Geneva airport and we drove straight to Basel, where the Schafer Institute was. I was interested to see the results of the experiments I'd planned with Rolf Schafer during my previous visit. If these results were positive, we would have some experimental evidence that the clinical claims of the La Prairie Clinic had a scientific basis.

Some years previously, a group of American researchers showed that ageing of cells could be observed and studied in tissue cultures – where the cells are grown in a culture medium outside the body.

They reported that certain cells called fibroblasts (which are from the connective tissues of the body) taken from the human foetus and cultured in perfect environmental conditions, would not live forever. Whatever was done, they would stop multiplying, change in shape and die. In other words, we each carry our own death warrant within our own cell structures.

Schafer's experiment was designed to prove, or disprove, that foetal cells contain one or more biological factors that would retard the onset of the ageing of the cells in tissue culture, and probably reverse it.

He took hamster foetal fibroblasts and cultured them in the same way the American researchers reported. As soon as he observed evidence of ageing in these cells, he added foetal lamb cells to the culture.

I was fascinated by the microscopic pictures he showed me – which indicated that both the changes in shape and the inability to multiply further *could* be reversed by the presence of foetal tissue.

I had one major objection to the claims this experiment suggested – that treatment at the clinic had *rejuvenating* results. That could not be proved.

In the Schafer experiment, the foetal cells continued to live *with* the ageing cells in the culture. In the patients treated at the clinic this would not happen because we had shown, in our earlier work, that the cells are destroyed by the patient's own immune system very soon after injection.

Although these initial results were encouraging, we had to run experiments in which the foetal lamb cells were destroyed soon after introduction to the tissue culture. This could be done by making antibodies to sheep cells in the hamster. If we then added these antibodies to the tissue culture at the same time as the foetal cells they would be destroyed (as in the human patient). If we could also demonstrate an anti-ageing effect then we'd know that after death the foetal cells liberated anti-ageing factors of some kind.

In other words the treatments at La Prairie Clinic *could* be clinically proved to have anti-ageing effects.

Dr Schafer also suggested that we study the ability of certain molecules in cell membranes, called glycosphingolipids, to promote genetic repair. I asked him to explain further.

He went to the blackboard and drew six small yellow circles. In the centre of each, he placed a dark red dot. 'These are cells – the building blocks of any living tissue,' he began. 'Each cell, however, is a little factory that manufactures a variety of proteins that are essential for healthy life.'

He peered over the top of his glasses at the two of us.

'Proteins, again, are made up of thousands of smaller molecules called amino acids – arranged in a variety of sequences depending on the type of protein to be manufactured. The sequences are determined by the commands from this centre.' He pointed to the red dots in the middle of the circles. 'The nucleus – a concentration of nucleic acid. Do you follow me?'

Armin nodded his head; the question had woken him up.

'Let me explain with a more simple example: A woman bakes a cake from instructions received from a tape recorder. It tells her to mix flour, sugar, butter, baking powder and an egg. The tape can be compared with the genetic material relaying instructions for the ingredients – which, in the case of the cell are amino acids – to the woman, who represents the cell. She's told how to mix the ingredients and then how to bake it.

Armin had his eyes closed again. Although I had read this explanation many times, I still marvelled at the simplicity of such a complex process. One must remember that there are only 20 amino acids, but due to the multitude of sequences in which they can be arranged, they are responsible for thousands of proteins.

Dr Schafer continued, 'Just imagine what would happen if the tape was damaged and, say, the flour is left out of the list of ingredients. The woman won't have much of a cake.

'Unfortunately, this vital command centre of the cell is the target of continual assaults from factors within and without the body. This results in damage to the genetic molecules and, if not repaired, distortion of the instructions to the cells. Luckily, various repair mechanisms have evolved over millions of years since life started on this planet.

'During youth there is a delicate balance between damage and repair. It's only when damage outstrips repair, that ageing takes place.'

Schafer stopped and took a sip from a glass of water.

'So, Dr Schafer, if we can find a substance which will enhance the genetic repair, then we have an anti-ageing factor?' I asked.

'Exactly,' he said, wiping his mouth with the back of his hand, 'and, I believe, the glycosphingolipids are such substances.'

We discussed experimental models to be used in these studies and afterwards Armin suggested we should go for a beer.

The contact I'd had in Basel with research and medicine had given me new hope again – maybe things were not so bad, maybe there were still exciting days ahead for me.

Lennie Kristal, one of the directors of Multimedia, the company I'd worked with on *The Body Machine*, had organized a conference in Haifa. The topic to be discussed was 'Mankind 2000'.

On the road from Tel Aviv airport to Haifa he told me they'd invited 12 speakers whom they considered authorities in their own field to predict and comment on how they envisaged the year 2000 in respect of their individual specialities. I, of course, was expected to talk about medicine.

Lennie had met Barbara, but he tactfully avoided talking about my personal problems.

I told him I still wanted to work on my talk and, as I'd eaten on the plane, would prefer to stay in the hotel that evening.

When he left me, the bareness of my room brought back the emptiness in my life. There was nothing in the room to comfort me. No female clothes in the wardrobe, no hint of perfume in the air or cosmetics in the bathroom. I stood there, still holding my suitcase and felt as if I was being suffocated. I had to get my head out of this cloud of doom. I had to do *something*.

I decided to phone Maureen Brink in Cape Town – maybe she had some news that would cheer me up.

The Brinks always took a long time to answer their phone but now it was ringing far too long – maybe they'd gone down to Swartvlei? I was just about to replace the receiver, when the happy voice of Maureen answered.

'Maureen, it's Chris.' As I said it tears trickled down my cheeks and I could hardly speak. 'I'm in Haifa – any news from Barbara?'

'Yes! In fact she's right here – she came to visit us.' Maureen's excitement and love for life, which was so evident in her voice, depressed me even further.

'I don't want to live any more, Maureen. There's nothing to live for!' I blurted out. I have absolutely no idea why I said that, because suicide had never entered my mind. Maybe I thought this sob story would soften Barbara's feelings.

'Don't talk like that, Chris! You have your children to think about and you've got so many friends who love you.'

'No, Maureen, all these things mean nothing to me without Barbara,' and I started to cry.

'Hold on Chris, Fritz wants to speak to you.'

'Hullo, Chris – having a good time?' my old friend said, trying to lighten the conversation and change the subject.

'Fritz, I just phoned to say goodbye. I've got a bottle of sleeping tablets and I'm going to take the whole lot,' I persisted.

'Wait! Barbara wants to talk to you.'

The voice that I knew and loved so much was suddenly talking to me. But it was cold and without emotion.

'Pull yourself together! What's wrong with you?'

I couldn't speak to her, so I quietly replaced the receiver and went to sit on my bed.

'Suicide,' I mumbled to myself 'What a lot of bullshit. What I need is a good fuck.'

The search was on for a woman – but why stop at one? Why not a dozen?

Yoram, another director of Multimedia, had his girlfriend with him. She was a beautiful Australian, Victoria Storay. She told me that her sister Karen would probably join us in Israel if I phoned her because she was about to leave her husband. As she didn't have any children or other commitments I thought that if she was like her sister she would be just the girl to drive the blues away.

I couldn't wait a moment longer to have a woman around, so I phoned the number Victoria had given me. It was probably in the middle of the night in Sydney – but what the hell. The phone rang and rang until a sleepy male voice answered, so I quietly replaced the receiver.

When I returned to Cape Town, there was an invitation for me to join the cruise ship *Rotterdam* at Singapore, for the leg of its cruise to Durban via Bombay and Mombasa.

I thought this would be the right medicine to get me back on my social feet. The romance of a cruise on the Indian Ocean, starry moonlit evenings and lots of women – could a man ask for anything more? This was the way I would finally get Barbara out of my system.

I boarded the ship in Singapore and couldn't have had a more miserable time. All I really wanted was for Barbara to join me and I kept recalling the happy days we'd spent on the *Chusan*.

I even discussed my desperation with the captain and he suggested I cable Barbara to join the ship at Mombasa. How could she refuse?

I sent a romantic cable about the cabin waiting for her – with red roses and champagne on ice – all the details of the itinerary and told her what a great time we'd have. When the ship berthed in Mombasa, I was on deck and my eyes swept over the crowd on the quay, expecting Barbara to be waiting for me.

She wasn't, of course. There's no fool like an old fool.

The next day, when there was still no sign of Barbara, I decided to visit Mr Wandera – a patient from Kenya on whom I had done a piggy-back operation a year earlier. He'd told me he lived in Mombasa and that if I ever visited the city, he would love to entertain me and show me around.

But I couldn't. The Kenyan authorities refused to allow me off the ship with a South African passport. They didn't mind Mr Wandera, a black African, living in Kenya with a white girl's heart in his chest, but the surgeon who performed the operation wasn't welcome.

It was disappointing and I was glad to leave Mombasa.

I still hated having a room without a woman in it so I asked one of the croupiers – an attractive brunette – to hang a few of her dresses in my cabin, just to have something of a woman around and I found the faint, lingering scent of perfume very comforting. On a few evenings after the casino closed, she came to my cabin, so her perfume wasn't only in the air – it was on the sheets and pillows as well.

Back in Cape Town, I decided to continue my mission of getting back at Barbara. The first stage in my plan – to punish the maids – had been a total failure. Now I was going to find out all I could about the man she was living with, and discredit him as much as possible.

I investigated his previous private life, I tried to find out whether he had a police record and also tried to get him conscripted into the army. Anything to hurt him or his reputation. All I discovered was that he'd been very popular with women, who all thought he was a thorough gentleman – very gentle and very kind. Most of the women I talked to said he was so handsome they wouldn't mind leaving their shoes under his bed any time.

All this information made matters worse. I'd failed again. But during all this, I gained one unexpected but very important ally – Barbara's father.

He'd been very disappointed when he learned that his possible future son-in-law was a Portuguese discotheque owner. In his heart, Fred had always wanted his daughter to marry into an important family, preferably someone with a title. This is very common with men who have made sizeable fortunes – they want the dignity and importance of a royal connection. Her marriage to me wasn't really what he'd wanted either – but he accepted it with good grace as, although I came from very obscure Afrikaans stock, I was at least a professor with degrees from five universities and a well-known public figure.

In his mind, Joe really wasn't good enough for his daughter.

Of course, I was delighted with this turn of events. Little did we both know that our opposition just made Barbara even more determined to fight for her man. Just as she had been prepared, once, to go and live on a lonely Karoo farm – so too she was prepared to share the good and the bad with Joe Silva.

Nothing else had worked, so in my half-crazed state, I decided to make Barbara jealous.

I spread rumours about the fabulously rich women and beauty queens who had now entered my life. I conveniently allowed the newspapers to photograph me with gorgeous girls (they were all girlfriends of my friends) and it was one of the few times I was grateful for the publicity.

I was still hurting very badly and the thought of a wet, cold Cape winter in a lonely room, facing the grey Atlantic Ocean and Robben Island, was too much to endure. I decided to take Frederick and Christiaan on a vacation to Rhodos with my friend Aris Argyriou.

I phoned him and he was very happy about our planned visit as it would also give me time to look at the progress of the health centre on the island of Kos. He booked the Adam Suite in the Paradise Hotel for me and the two children.

A few days later, I was chatting to Dene and said that I wished I could find a nice girl to come with me on this trip – both as company for me and also to look after Frederick and Christiaan when I went out at night. She suggested that I ask a young girl who had lived quite near us in Zeekoevlei. She was now living in Swellendam, a small town about three hours drive from Cape Town. I asked Dene if she'd phone her for me and sound her out.

I remembered Cathy from when she was still at school – she was a petite little blonde who, even as a young teenager, oozed sex appeal. I was sure she wouldn't be interested in this idea.

'Prof, Dene's on the phone.'

I picked up the phone, 'Hi Dene, I suppose she said "no".'

'Not at all, Prof. She said you should come and see her.'

I left for Swellendam that afternoon and booked into a local hotel.

When I saw Cathy later, working in the garden of her little cottage, I just had a feeling she would be the right choice.

She was. And the four of us left for Athens a few days later. I made sure that this news reached the press – although Cathy thought that it would be unwise for her to pose for photographs with me.

The Adam Suite turned out to be the same accommodation that Barbara and I had shared with the boys a year earlier. Memories flooded back and, for the first few days, I was in a black mood.

But Cathy was a wonderful companion and the kids enjoyed their holiday in the sun. As time went by, I grew very fond of this blonde Dutch girl but Cathy insisted that, at least while the boys were around, we should keep our distance.

Barbara, in the meantime, had joined her parents at the Villa d'Este on Lake Como, where we had also been guests of friends when we were still married. She phoned to ask if Frederick and Christiaan could join them for a week and I willingly agreed.

Aris accompanied the children on their journey to Como and I was left alone with Cathy in the Adam Suite.

A few days later, just as the memories of Barbara were slowly, if painfully, fading I unexpectedly had a phone call from her. She asked if I could come to the Villa d'Este immediately. She was in a terrible state because her father insisted that she end her relationship with Joe.

I told Cathy I'd be away for a few days and would join her in Athens to continue our holiday. I really was very attached to this unassuming, down-to-earth little girl by then.

A car met me at Milan airport and took me to the Villa d'Este. When I met Barbara, I could see she'd been crying and she told me she'd phoned Joe that morning and that it was all over between them.

I thought this was really good news, but what I didn't realize then was that both Fred and I were fooling ourselves: Barbara wasn't ready to break up with Joe.

That evening after dinner, Barbara and I went to a disco but we just couldn't recapture the joy of simply being together that we'd had previously. She was still hurt inside.

I also made a very big mistake in telling her about Cathy. She became very upset and insisted that I phone her immediately and break off the association. She said that if she had to make a sacrifice, then so did I.

After trying to get through to Rhodos for hours, I finally managed to reach Aris and asked him to explain to Cathy that I wouldn't be coming back to Greece, and also asked him to put Cathy safely on a plane to South Africa.

When we returned to Cape Town, Barbara and I saw each other fairly regularly. She wanted to make a clean break from the past and the memories that 'Waiohai' held, so she decided to sell it and buy a house in Newlands. I helped her to move in, but didn't move in myself because I knew she was seeing Joe again.

This hurt me very much. It was difficult for me to see her, knowing that she was involved with someone else.

One evening, the nanny called me to say that Barbara was out and that Christiaan was in great pain with earache. I went straight to the house and the poor kid was obviously in agony, so I phoned Professor Sellars, the head of the ear, nose and throat department at Groote Schuur, and he came to see my son. He confirmed that it was acute middle-ear infection and prescribed the appropriate treatment.

Barbara phoned a little later and said she'd heard there was trouble at home and I told her what had happened.

'Well, if the child's okay now you can go home,' she said with a steely edge to her voice.

'No, it's okay, I'll stick around for a while in case he starts crying again.'

She slammed the phone down and half an hour later, she burst in through the front door.

'What are you still doing here!' she demanded angrily. 'All you've done is to mess up a good date for me.'

'So you're still seeing Joe, then?'

'Yes. And what's more, he's going to come and live with me,' she said defiantly. 'To hell with what you or my father think!'

I had known long before that this would happen. Why I ever bothered to try with her again, God only knows.

For the next few months, I tried very hard to renew my interest in surgery – which wasn't successful. I also dated as many girls as I could – which *was* successful.

After doing an advertisement for an insurance company, in which I said the heart was really only a pump, I received an anonymous letter telling me that all I knew about 'pumping' was how to pump women.

The writer was correct – I was trying to prove to myself that I hadn't lost Barbara because of any inability to satisfy the needs of a woman, and that I was still a sexually active, virile man.

Darcey Farrell phoned and invited me to come to Perth to take part in a show that raised money for disabled children – a 'telethon'. I'd been there the previous year with Barbara and had been a big hit with my ukulele. I'd also mimed *Oh Doctor, I'm in Trouble* with Lana Cantrell. The whole thing had been tremendous fun.

I accepted and asked Darcey if he'd mind phoning Karen Storay-Dowdle in Sydney, to ask if she would join me for a few days. I hadn't forgotten Victoria and her suggestion that her sister would be just the right girl for me. Full of expectations, I went with Darcey to meet Karen at Perth airport. She wasn't as pretty as her sister but her Slavic looks, curvaceous, statuesque body and strong Australian accent were very appealing.

Sammy Davis Junior was the main performer on the telethon and I'll never forget his superb rendition of *Mr Bojangles*. Lana Cantrell accompanied me again and this time we mimed *Cinderella, Rockafella*.

Karen turned out to be a great companion, but, to my surprise, she told me that all her possessions in the world were in her suitcase and she'd come to Perth so that she could travel with me to Cape Town.

I wasn't ready for this. It would be like taking coals to Newcastle. So I told her a story that I had to go on several overseas trips and it wasn't a good time for her to come and visit me.

Back in Cape Town, my lack of interest in my work persisted – but I'd written two more books at the request of Multimedia.

One was on how you have to change your lifestyle when you suffer from arthritis, *Living With Arthritis*. The second was called *Your Healthy Heart* and dealt mainly with how to avoid heart attacks.

I also made a half-hearted attempt at another novel with Siegfried Stander. This was later published, mainly through the efforts of Siegfried, under the title, *The Faith*.

I had several midnight collect-calls from Sydney. Karen Storay-Dowdle wanted to know when she'd be coming to Cape Town. She certainly was determined.

I remained reluctant, but eventually relented and sent her a return ticket – Economy Class.

I spent my 60th birthday alone with my friends Norma and Mike Rattray at Mala Mala where a few months before Barbara and I had gone to see if we could fall in love with each other enough to get together again.

In Cape Town, Barbara invited me to her house – also to celebrate my birthday. She had, as always, gone out of her way to make this an unforgettable evening. It was a very kind gesture.

We'd just sat down at her magnificently laid table, when the phone rang. It was for me.

'Chris? It's Maureen,' she whispered, 'can I speak?'

'Yes of course, what's the matter?'

'Someone has just arrived at DF Malan airport.' She was still whispering theatrically.

I still didn't grasp what it was all about. Maureen loved to pull my leg and I thought this might be another of her jokes. Then she said, a little more softly, 'Karen Storay-Dowdle has arrived and wants to know where you are.'

Damn. This girl couldn't have arrived at a more inappropriate time. What was I going to do now?

'Maureen, please do me a favour – send someone to fetch her and put her up in your hotel for the night?' I was also whispering now. I can't imagine why.

'Trouble?' Barbara asked with an amused look on her face when I returned to the dinner table.

'No, you know what Maureen's like – she's always playing the fool with me.' And we started to eat, although I'd lost my appetite.

We were just about to start dessert, when there was another phone call. It was Maureen again, who told me I'd have to come immediately as this girl was hysterical and accusing me of treating her like a tramp off the street – and that she was going to go back on the next plane to Australia if I didn't see her straight away.

I went back into the dining room and asked Barbara if she'd excuse me, as something urgent had come up.

I could see she was hurt. She'd tried very hard to make it a pleasant evening and now I was hurrying off.

Karen refused to stay in the hotel, and insisted on moving in with me, into the room I then had at the Brinks' house. I'd moved out of their hotel to their home in Bloubergstrand ('Blue Mountain Beach'), which was the next suburb along the coast from Tableview.

We didn't have much sleep that night, so the following day I suggested we have a nap in the afternoon and I was just drifting off to sleep when some voices in the passage woke me.

'Uncle Chris and big Karen are having a rest.' I heard Maureen's granddaughter explaining innocently.

'I'm sure they need a rest,' came Barbara's sarcastic reply.

My God! It's Barbara! She's in the house!

'Get out!' I hissed at Karen and started shoving the clothes she'd just unpacked back into her suitcase. She looked at me in a state of sleepy bewilderment – probably thinking I'd gone mad and that it would be a good idea to get away from me as quickly as she could.

I opened the window above the lawn, below street level, and bundled Karen – with her suitcase – through it.

Something made me look up, and when I did, my worst horror was confirmed. Barbara was standing quite still and looking at the performance below her. The three of us were frozen in an embarrassing tableau. Barbara looking down, Karen half-in/half-out of the window and me about to throw her suitcase out after her. It was a nightmare.

Time stood still for what seemed like an eternity. Then Barbara, almost in slow motion, turned round and walked away. The last thing I noticed was her look of extreme distaste – as if she'd bitten into a lemon.

I helped Karen back into the room, where she continued to live with me for three months.

Although she was not well liked by my daughter, the Brinks, or any of my other friends, Karen gradually healed my wounds and I recovered both my physical and mental health. She even helped me stop smoking.

I have a lot to thank Karen Storay-Dowdle for.

Before she went back to Australia I invited Karen and her sister Victoria, to join me on the *QE2* from Sydney to New York – which included several stops in the East. As a guest lecturer on the Cunard liner, I was permitted to invite a companion. They'd also given me another ticket as part of my remuneration.

From the time Karen left Cape Town, until I boarded the plane for Sydney, I dated several different girls and the memories of Barbara slowly faded.

I had given Barbara and Joe my blessing and wished them well – unlike her father, who still considered their association unthinkable.

Eileen le Roux, Maureen's sister, invited me to her son's birthday party. I'd been dating an anaesthetist, Dr Sheila Etoe, to whom I'd taken a definite attraction. Here was a girl I could marry – if I ever decided to take that risk again.

She was beautiful, intelligent, medically trained, mature and single. I'd noticed her on many occasions in the operating rooms over the years, and had always taken care to look my best whenever she was the anaesthetist. So I invited Sheila to come with me to this party.

We were dancing a waltz when I noticed a young girl sitting on her own on the steps leading down to the dance floor. She was wearing a yellow dress and, curiously, I noticed she had a plaster on her big toe. I can't imagine why I should remember something like that. Then my heart skipped a beat. It was the same gorgeous creature who had waited on us at the opening of La Vita in Welgemoed.

I finished the dance and asked Lauhan, Fritz's son, to get me the phone number of the girl in the yellow dress.

Several drinks later, I summoned enough courage to ask her to dance. Her name was Karin – 'just like your girlfriend from Australia'. She laughed as her blue eyes stared straight into mine. She had a full, sensuous mouth and the magnificent body of a girl born to model bikinis. I suddenly ached to spend more time with this girl. No, she's far too young, I sighed to myself as I crossed to the other side of the room.

When I danced with Sheila again she said casually, 'You seem very taken with that girl in the yellow dress. Are you?' I shrugged nonchalantly and grinned.

Lauhan brought me her phone number, written on the back of a matchbox with a lipstick pencil. It must be her lipstick, I thought, so she obviously didn't mind giving me her number. I couldn't wait until the following afternoon when I planned to phone her.

'May I speak to Karin, please?' My mouth was dry with excitement.

'I'll see if she's here,' the young boy's voice said. Probably her brother, I thought.

'Hello, Karin speaking.'

It was probably the most beautiful sound I'd heard for years. I tried to speak but my voice had gone. I covered the mouthpiece and cleared my throat. 'Karin? This is Chris – do you remember meeting me last night?'

'Oh yes, can I help you?' I'm sure she was a little disappointed. She'd told me that she'd just broken up with her boyfriend – maybe she would have preferred a call from him?

'How about dinner with me tonight?' I nearly didn't say anything after the cool reception and was about to forget the whole idea.

'Well, I'm not so sure – I hardly know you.'

'Karin, it's the 14th of February today – my wedding anniversary to Barbara. I don't want to be alone tonight.'

She was silent, probably thinking what a lame sob story this all was but after a few moments, she said, 'Okay, where shall I meet you?'

I was so thrilled, I could hardly keep the excitement out of my voice. 'Meet me at La Vita in Welgemoed – you know where that is. I'll see you at 7 o'clock and we'll go through to Newlands.' I put the phone down quickly before she could change her mind and phoned Aldo to book a table. I also asked him to put a vase of red roses on the table.

She was even more beautiful than I remembered and, although

she was only 18 years old, she had her feet firmly on the ground – she was very mature for her age and every minute in her company was a moment to treasure.

I didn't want the evening to end, so after dinner, I suggested going to the HardRock Café for a nightcap.

As we sat down at a table, a young university student came around selling flowers for Valentine's Day. As a rule these girls irritate me intensely – the flowers are overpriced and they're experts at making one feel uncomfortable. It's difficult to refuse them when they say, 'I'm sure your beautiful companion would like a rose?'

But at the HardRock that evening I didn't even ask the price, and bought the whole basket.

I told Karin that I was going on a cruise and asked her to join me later in Italy – I would make all the arrangements and all she had to do was phone my secretary, Celeste, a week later.

I didn't attempt to kiss her when I dropped her off at her car in Welgemoed. A small voice warned me to tread carefully.

The next day, I left for Australia and the *QE2* cruise – with the other Karen.

One would think it would be boring to be at sea for days on end, but there are always so many things to do on board. During the day, one could choose between aerobics, dancing classes, card games, lectures and dozens of other things. In the evenings, after dinner, there was a movie, cabaret and Joe Loss and his band for dancing until past midnight. The disco went on until the early hours of the morning.

Being at sea gives one a very secure feeling. The ship is like a small city that cares for all one's needs. But there was still a lot of loneliness around – especially among the elderly women who'd lost their husbands and joined the cruise to see if there was still some excitement left for them in life.

I remember a particularly sad event one evening. The woman was certainly in her sixties, but the man she was with didn't look old enough to have a driver's licence. As the music ended she was involved in a scuffle with another woman of about the same age. They were fighting over the teenage twit who stood simpering on one side of the room while the women assaulted each other.

The stewards separated them before either had time to do any serious damage.

Both were very rich. They wore exclusive haute couture outfits in the small-car price range and their jewellery alone must have given the purser a security headache at every port.

The one was the widow of a wealthy professional man and the other had been a social somebody in the American Mid-West. Both were clearly from educated backgrounds; yet they were competing for the attentions of a mindless gigolo.

The winner went off happily with her adolescent prize, while the loser drank alone at a corner table. I remember the look of utter loneliness on her face as she soaked herself in the high-priced booze. She was staring into the bottom of each glass as if the answer was visible in the liquor.

She'd arrived face-to-face with the ultimate problem – that we're all finally alone, even in a crowd.

Man (or woman) is a herd animal – needing others. The original reason for staying in a crowd was simple: being alone literally meant death. Our civilization has provided for us materially, but it ignores the herd instinct, the need for others, the contact which means one is still alive.

Loneliness and the despair of age are two faces of the same coin – spiritual death. It's an instinctive reaction to flee from death, to be where the noise and the people are.

From that arises the unspoken belief that if there are enough people to reassure one of existence one can stave off loneliness. If one can surround oneself with youth, one can stave off death.

If the lonely are desperate enough, and if they have the resources, they'll try to buy what they cannot have – which is what the ladies in the lounge of the QE2 were doing that evening.

Feeling very sorry for them both, I tucked my arm around my 25 year old girlfriend and went to bed.

Karen had had a university education but had spent the previous two years working at a stable with race horses. When she'd been in Cape Town, I'd proudly walked her around the Members' Enclosure at the Metropolitan Handicap (South Africa's equivalent of Royal Ascot). The 'Met' is an important date on the social calendar and I was delighted to be there with Karen – she wasn't as stunning as Barbara – but she was still young and beautiful.

She also had a very keen sense of humour, but despite all her qualities and the wonderful way she'd helped me, I was still sorry that it wasn't Victoria who'd be sharing my cabin.

And, of course, I couldn't forget the Karin in South Africa. In order to keep in contact I sent her postcards from every port of call

– Bali, Singapore, Bangkok, Hong Kong and Hawaii – telling her how much I missed her and how I was looking forward to seeing her again.

One evening we were invited to have drinks with Madame Joska Bourgeois. She was a very wealthy woman who was on a round trip with a male companion, a handsome young Algerian by the name of Sahad.

Her suite was one of the few on the upper deck and must have cost a fortune. She laid on the best Dom Perignon and afterwards invited Karen and me to have dinner with her in the King's Lounge.

Joska and I became very close friends. She was a delightful and wise elderly lady – who hadn't inherited her money, but had made it herself. I respected and admired this woman and we've remained good friends ever since.

As the *QE2* turned back from the East towards the United States, I started scheming about how to leave the ship – and Karen. I tried very hard to get her interested in one of the sons of a wealthy family, but she insisted on staying with me – she thought I would be her future husband. The young multi-millionaire didn't seem to interest her at all.

In the evenings, I would leave her with a group of young people – hoping that something would happen. But, inevitably, ten minutes later she'd be knocking at our cabin door.

Eventually I told her that she had no future with me and that I was going to get off the ship at Honolulu as I had work to do in England. She could go on to New York if she wanted to, and I gave her an air ticket to use to fly back to Sydney.

In the meantime, I'd cabled Celeste not to make arrangements for Karin Setzkorn to join me in Italy, as I was coming home.

Karen Storay-Dowdle and I parted company in Honolulu. She was sad but accepted the situation philosophically.

A few weeks later, when I was back in South Africa, I had a letter from Victoria telling me that as soon as I left the boat Karen became involved with another man. A year or so later I saw her in New York – she was happily married and told me she was expecting a baby.

I don't know what happened to the lovely Victoria.

As soon as I arrived back in Cape Town I phoned her.

'Hello, Karin – I'm back,' I said eagerly.

She paused for a moment before saying, 'Oh, hello.'

Maybe she'd met someone while I was away? 'Have you found a boyfriend?'

'Well, not really a boyfriend – an acquaintance,' she replied.

I was so relieved to learn that the door hadn't been closed completely. 'Well, will you have dinner with me tonight?' I had already planned, in my mind, what I hoped for during the next few weeks and wanted to discuss it with her as soon as possible.

'No, I'm sorry – I'm writing exams and you know what it's like, I've left everything until the last minute. I *must* study tonight.'

When I'd dated Karin the first time she didn't seem to be one of those girls who made excuses easily. But I wondered if this was a polite way of telling me to push off so I persisted, 'You have to eat sometime. Why not spend that half-hour with me? I'll meet you at La Vita, Welgemoed – we can eat there, and as soon as we've finished you can go straight back to your books.'

She agreed and Chris Lesley, who knew Karin, of course, gave us a secluded corner table.

Karin joined me at the bar promptly at 7.30. God, I'd forgotten how beautiful she was. Be careful, Chris – don't make an ass of yourself. Handle this one with great care – she has to last – I warned myself.

Not wanting to waste any time we went straight to the table where Karin ordered Lobster and I had Langoustine.

Chris Lesley was an excellent chef and the food was prepared to perfection. I was very fond of him and his wife Anne, and had recognized his talent as a chef several months previously when he worked at the steakhouse.

I'd lent them some money to buy furniture and they'd now settled in a house at Welgemoed near the restaurant. They'd done very well for themselves, even making enough money to buy a helicopter.

Karin didn't want dessert – only a cappuccino. Time was flying by and I had to make my move.

'Karin,' I began – and the bloody waiter interrupted, saying there was a man at the bar who wanted to speak to me. I thought it might be a customer with a complaint, so I excused myself and followed the waiter to the bar.

'Hello, Chris – my old mate!' This total stranger greeted me and he had difficulty in climbing off the stool. I could see he'd given the bar a lot of business already that night.

'You 'member me shurely?' he slurred.

'I'm afraid I don't,' I replied politely – although the man irritated the hell out of me.

'You 'member old Shusie?' Was he playing the fool or did he have something important to say?

He slapped me on the back before continuing, 'No, I can shee that now you're an important man you don't remember your ol' friendsh any more,' and he fumbled with a pack of cigarettes.

Karin was watching, so I wanted to stay cool.

'No, it's not that, but, as you probably realize, I meet many people and can't remember them all. Was Susie a patient of mine?'

He laughed raucously and I took a step back from the alcoholic fumes. 'Well, you could shay that – 'cos you did order her to bed! Har har har!' I had to terminate this conversation quickly – it was going to ruin my whole evening. Who the hell was Susie anyway?

'Can I buy you a drink?' I asked him.

'Whishky,' he nodded.

'Chris, please give my friend here a whisky,' and I turned back to him. 'Thanks for the interesting conversation,' and I left him at the bar.

'He's drunk!' Karin laughed as I sat down.

'Yes – just ignore him or he'll never go away.'

'You were going to tell me something', she reminded me.

I took out a pen and a piece of paper and summoned up all the courage I could and wrote down a list as I spoke. 'Karin, in the next few months, I have to go down to my farm in Sedgefield, then to Johannesburg to judge the 'Miss South Africa' contest and then the Rattrays have asked me to Mala Mala to address a group of visitors they'll have staying there.'

She looked at me as if to say, What does all this have to do with me?

'I'd like you to come with me on these trips – it's awful to do them alone.' I answered her unspoken question.

I didn't know if I'd put it correctly. I hoped she didn't think I wanted her along just as a carnal companion. She was still so young and innocent, so I continued hurriedly, 'If, at any stage, you don't want to go any further with these engagements, then you'll have a return ticket and there'll be no fuss and bother – you can go back home whenever you like.'

She took a sip of the cappuccino before replying. 'I'll have to think about it.'

She went back home in her own car and I went back to 'Rockhaven' – Fritz and Maureen Brink's house in Bloubergstrand.

The next morning I went on one of my infrequent ward rounds at Groote Schuur and, later, another one at the Red Cross Hospital.

I didn't even know the patients' names any more and there wasn't a single one that I'd operated on.

How could I have turned my back on what had been such an integral part of my life for 25 years? A career that had given me so much joy and recognition. Was it because I no longer saw a challenge in heart surgery?

Routine surgery bored me – to do a by-pass or valve replacement day after day was like eating the same food meal after meal.

The economic deterioration caused by apartheid had put a brake on expansion and we now had to get permission before admitting foreign patients into our hospitals.

There was also a chronic shortage of nursing staff – especially intensive care nurses – which slowed down our routine work even further.

It's important to know when to quit. To be successful at your work, you must get up in the morning hungry for the day ahead and the tasks required of you. In my case, the hunger had gone – there was no thrill left.

The younger surgeons had to take over and, strangely enough, I wasn't jealous in the least. I was quite willing to bow out gracefully and without a single regret.

The pressures under which I'd worked since December 1967 and the arthritic flame, which at times had burned high, had taken their toll.

Only a winner is remembered – and one is remembered by the way one ends the last race. One is not remembered for what one did years ago – but for how one did things yesterday. My time to call it a day was very close.

The principal of the university and the dean of the faculty of medicine and some departmental heads were visiting various units at the medical school one afternoon, to find out what their needs were in terms of research money, equipment or staff.

They also visited my office and after some small talk, asked me what the department of cardiac surgery really needed.

'A new department head.' I replied without hesitation.

They were flabbergasted.

'He's joking – it's four years to go before his retirement,' one of them said.

But I think my expression convinced them I wasn't joking.

'Are you serious, Chris?' Professor Saunders asked after a minute of silence.

'Dead serious – I've had enough and I'm just not pulling my weight any more. It's time I handed over the reins to a younger, more energetic driver. In fact, I should have done so two years ago.'

When they were convinced I was serious, we talked about how I could retire earlier and still get my full pension. Eventually, it was decided I could do this on the basis of ill-health.

So the date was set. On 31 December 1983, I would leave my office at the medical school for the last time – an office where I'd spent so many years rejoicing in my successes and mourning my failures. I had only one request: no farewell parties where the guests would come for tea and sandwiches and listen to a few insincere speeches. I could do without all that shit.

When I went home that afternoon I felt relieved of an enormous load because now I could neglect my hospital work without my conscience worrying me.

I phoned Karin to ask if she'd thought about my offer and she said she'd decided to accept one invitation at a time and see how things developed from there.

'I'll fetch you at your house tomorrow morning and we'll drive to the farm.' It was over a weekend, so she didn't have to miss any classes at the technical college.

That evening I met Jacques le Roux and told him what good fortune his party had brought me as I was now dating Karin.

'You lucky bugger! There are so many young men after that girl and you get her!' We both laughed.

'Well, you know what they say: it's better to be an old man's darling than a young man's slave.'

'Behave yourself, Chris – she's still a virgin,' were his parting words.

I wonder how he knew?

I arrived at her home in Nederburg Avenue, Welgemoed, at 9 o'clock the next morning, driving a sports car which had been given to me by Datsun.

Karin and her mother came out of the front door and walked

down to the car as I stopped. Karin wore white stockings and flat shoes and her mother carried her small suitcase.

'Hello, Karin. Good morning, Mrs Setzkorn.' I greeted them as if this was no special event.

'Good morning, Chris,' they greeted me in unison. 'Look after her, Chris,' her mother added. 'She's my only daughter.' Then she produced a photograph of Karin, as a 6 year old, sitting on my lap – the one taken all those years ago in Buffelsbaai.

We were silent as we drove away.

Multimedia had joined up with a company called Goldcrest, to make a documentary on the normal functions of the various systems of the human body – the cardiovascular system, the gastrointestinal system, the central nervous system and so on.

They planned to use animation and the most modern audio-visual techniques to illustrate these programmes. The company invited me to do the narration.

I was under the impression that I could just study the programme, and do the narration off-the-cuff as a voice-over, but when I arrived they gave me a script written in a style completely foreign to me and alien to my own presentation technique, using words I'd never heard of before, let alone be able pronounce correctly.

An elocutionist came to my hotel to help me with the pronunciation. My Boere English wasn't acceptable for this sophisticated programme. I couldn't understand it – surely they must have heard me on TV programmes and were familiar with the standard of my English?

I had two days to memorize the script and spent hours in front of the mirror in the bathroom going over my lines.

The day for my acting début arrived. My first experience of being a movie star. There was someone to dress me, another to do my make-up and another one for my hair. There were cameramen, sound and lighting engineers, a director and someone to check my English – and my memory. Everything was ready. I had to appear through a door, walk seven paces into the garden, turn and look up into the camera and say three lines. Piece of cake.

'Quiet on set! Roll camera! And … action!'

Out I came, counted the seven paces, stopped and looked into the camera. The camera looked back at me. My mind was as blank as my expression.

I couldn't even remember the first word.

'Cut!' shouted the director and I had a sudden pain in my chest, which I'm sure was angina pectoris.

The director tried to calm me down. 'Don't worry, Prof, this happens to the most experienced actors – and it will happen again. Let's try again. Don't worry.'

It did happen – again and again and again.

I'm sure that the people watching me were saying, 'I'll never let that guy operate on me – he won't remember what to do next.'

After about the twentieth take, the director seemed to be happy with the garden scene.

Now the swimming pool. I had to swim the breadth of the pool underwater and surface to say, 'I've only been under the water for 10 seconds and I'm already out of breath. With training, there are people who can stay under water for several minutes.'

After fluffing these lines several times, I felt like staying under water permanently. But eventually, the very patient director was happy.

The cameraman gave a sigh of relief.

The next day was even worse. They had a beautiful female model lying on the couch and a special camera roaming over her nude body. I don't think I ever got those lines right.

That evening, my competence to do the narration was discussed by a few members of Goldcrest-Multimedia.

The following morning, they said they thought it would be much better if I would just introduce each programme with a few lines. It was their polite way of telling me I'd been written out of the script.

My acting career was short-lived.

Karin must have been satisfied with my behaviour on the trip to the farm, because she then joined me for the 'Miss South Africa' contest and also the trip to Mala Mala.

I was very taken with this young girl. Not only was she very, very pretty but she was always well groomed and at home in the company of people twice and even three times her age. She was wonderful company and we laughed a lot.

Fritz had miraculously recovered from multiple complications, after a motor car accident. We decided that he and his family should accompany me and my two children to Rhodos for a vacation. As Karin and I had a steady relationship by this time, I invited her as well; it would also be a good opportunity for her to get to know Frederick and Christiaan better.

Aris again reserved the Adam Suite for me at the Paradise Hotel. I'd now had the suite with three different women in three successive years.

As Fritz and his family wanted to see other parts of Europe, they left with Karin for a visit to London and Vienna, and I planned to catch up with them in Rome. Tony Ingala had invited me for a short cruise along the Yugoslavian coast.

I'd asked one of the girls from the Golden Door, who'd instructed aerobics on the *QE2*, to visit our development on Kos and advise us on the health centre. She arrived after the Brinks and Karin left and spent two days on Kos and Rhodos. But she didn't join me in the Adam Suite – although I was very tempted to ask.

After the short cruise with Tony and some friends and having judged a 'Miss Topless' competition in Yugoslavia, I met Karin in Rome and we stayed at the Hassler Hotel. Fritz and the family arrived the same evening and we had a great time in this wonderful city. Karin couldn't get enough of looking at the beautiful shops along the Via Condotti.

I now considered Karin to be my steady girlfriend and was very happy to have this extraordinary woman with me all the time – but she had to get back to Cape Town for a modelling contract she'd signed and I had to go to London for some more filming.

I just knew there was something wrong when I eventually arrived back in Cape Town and she wasn't at the airport to meet me. What could it be? We'd said goodbye to each other in Rome with great tenderness. Maybe she was waiting at Fritz and Maureen's house? Yes, that would be it – she'd gone there to put flowers in my room.

There were no flowers and no Karin.

I phoned her home and her mother answered. She said Karin was out and avoided my direct questions. She thought I should speak to her daughter myself.

After several attempts, I got hold of Karin on the phone. She told me that she was very busy with modelling engagements and couldn't see me for the next few days. But I insisted – and she eventually agreed to see me that evening.

It was one of the worst things that could have happened to me so soon after the divorce from Barbara. Karin said she'd thought about our relationship and decided that the age gap was just too big.

She said that it would never work out. When she was with me, she missed the company of her young friends and longed to do the things that she did before she met me.

I'd always feared old age. I knew that it would, sooner or later, come between me and my happiness – but I didn't think it would come that soon. There was so much I could give Karin that her young friends were unable to and, I thought, there were very few things, if any at all, that her young friends could give her that I couldn't.

After taking her home I went back to 'Rockhaven' a broken man. What could I do? Another battle to try and win her back? I couldn't go through all that scheming and heartache again.

The next morning, I phoned her mother who was also very upset. She said she thought Karin's friends had a big influence on her. They'd told her that she was making a terrible mistake, wasting her young life with an old man and that she'd regret it bitterly one day.

What could I say to that? Maybe they were right. I tried consoling myself that it wasn't possible to predict the future. Perhaps she'd change her mind and take a chance with me?

Karin had told her mother that she wanted to hear nothing more about Chris Barnard and if they kept on talking about me she was going to leave home.

So I started looking at my book with the old phone numbers and thought: 'I'll show that little bitch that there're many other young girls who would be over the moon to spend their young years with this old man.

I was particularly keen to see Sheila Etoe again – at least she was in her early thirties and the age gap wasn't so great. But Sheila had also learned a lesson. I'd dropped her before, when Karin became available, and she told me she had no intention of having a serious relationship with me because she didn't want to take the chance of being dumped again.

The time came to say goodbye to Groote Schuur. The superintendent insisted there be a small farewell party, which was held in the dining hall at the nurses' home. I remember thinking that the last time I'd been in that building was when I visited Louwtjie during our courting days. A lot had happened since then.

After tea and sandwiches and the obligatory speech by the superintendent I received my gift 'for 25 years of faithful service' which was wrapped in a long box. A Rolex watch, I thought as I impatiently ripped off the wrapping paper.

It was a hospital tie, the back label of which proclaimed it to be washable.

There was also a party at the Red Cross Hospital which André, who was now a paediatrician, also attended and I was very proud to have him standing next to me. I didn't receive any gift at all there – perhaps they'd decided that one tie between the two hospitals was enough.

My staff, with the financial assistance of Sandoz, a pharmaceutical firm, gave a party at La Vita. It was a really great evening – Karin came as my partner, which fuelled a few rumours too.

Their gift was far more appropriate – I was presented with a large box and when I opened it, a beautiful young girl jumped out. I thanked everyone very much and said I couldn't wait to get home and play with my new toy.

I received another invitation to be a guest lecturer on the *QE2*. This trip would be from Los Angeles to Singapore.

Karin still preferred the company of her young friends and I had just about given up hope of getting her back, but decided to give it one more try. I was about to leave for the Frankfurt Book Fair and then, via New York, to Los Angeles where I'd board the *QE2*.

I phoned Karin and said I'd like to see her and asked if she could meet me at Maureen's home. I told her about my travel plans and said that I would leave a first-class air ticket for her to New York. The booking had already been made and there would be a limousine to pick her up at Kennedy Airport – she'd be taken to the Carlyle Hotel, where I'd reserved a room for her. She didn't have to decide immediately.

If she did decide to come, I would meet her in New York and, from there, we could go to Los Angeles and join the *QE2* cruise.

I left for Frankfurt and all I achieved in Germany was to get a picture of myself with a nude girl published in one of the magazines. After all this time, I still hadn't learned that you can't trust journalists. Karin would probably see this picture in South Africa and I could say goodbye to any hope of her joining me – either then or at any time in the future.

As soon as the seat-belt sign went off, I reclined my seat, slipped the ear-phones on and selected the country-music channel. The lyrics always had a message and most of the time there was a lot of truth in what the music said. So I settled back comfortably and relaxed with a glass of champagne.

The first track was a song about a failed love-affair – I think it was called *Somebody done somebody wrong song*. The next was one that my father had liked very much, *Silver threads among the gold*. This was all very depressing and I thought about changing channels but decided to listen to one more. It was *Please daddy, don't walk so fast* – all about a father leaving his family and his son behind. This was too close to the truth for my liking. I left the earphones on (you don't get bothered by other passengers then) but turned the music off and closed my eyes. Was that what I'd done to my first son, André? Had I walked so fast that I'd left him behind?

I remembered the day I had a phone call from the professor of medical jurisprudence who asked me to see him in his office urgently. He told me that narcotic inspectors had reported to him that André frequently bought drugs like Wellconal and pethidine, which he'd prescribed himself, at various pharmacies.

Professor Smith said that because of our friendship he wouldn't take the matter further at that stage, but I had to promise him that I would speak to my son and persuade him to get treatment.

Actually, I'd noticed a few times, when he and his wife had dinner at my home, that he looked drowsy – and often drifted off to sleep during conversation. We all thought it was because he was on night duty or studying hard that made him so sleepy.

I didn't suspect anything at the time and have often since wondered, if it had been one of my patients, whether I would have dismissed it so easily – without further investigation.

Thinking back on his childhood now, as I was flying over the Atlantic Ocean, I was ashamed to realize that I remembered very little of where André had been on various important occasions. Where had my son been when I was given the 'Freedom of the City of Cape Town', where was he when Frederick and Christiaan were born? Where was he now, for that matter?

I remembered asking André to come and see me at the medical school.

'André, you have serious problems.'

He looked at me with his dark brown eyes – which were so much like his mother's.

'What do you mean, Dad?' But I could see that he knew I knew.

359

'This is what I mean.' And I read a list of pharmacies' names that had been given to me.

He slumped into a chair and said quietly, 'I'm so relieved that you know now, Dad. I've been trying so hard to scrape together the courage to come and speak to you. It started so innocently but now I can't control it. It was a stupid thing to do and I have to stop.'

He didn't try to find excuses for his addiction – although he'd been in a car accident and still had a lot of pain in his fractured leg. He could easily have said the drugs were for that. But he didn't – he understood that he was sick and needed treatment.

I phoned a psychologist and made an appointment for him, but I never bothered to check on his progress afterwards – my parental concern ended there.

Some months later, he was admitted to Groote Schuur Hospital, where I had to get special permission to visit him. It broke my heart to see my son in this neglected state – dressed in jeans, unshaven and with no pride.

After a few months the doctors were happy with his progress and he was discharged to face the harsh realities of life again.

The problem was that my poor son – probably because of lack of support from me – had grown up being unable to cope with the cruel world around him. So he'd chosen the easiest way.

Although he was married with two beautiful children, even that didn't mend the defects that had developed in his psyche during his childhood. He had to look at life through tinted glasses and got this tint by prescribing drugs for himself.

He was present in such a small part of my life. I *had* just walked too fast for him. I'd change all that and, sitting in the plane, I vowed that when I got back home to Cape Town after this trip, I would pay much more attention to my eldest son. We both had so much to share and so much to live for. It's never too late.

The air hostess came to ask me to put my seat upright as we were approaching Kennedy Airport. Quite contrary to the South African airports I was given VIP treatment on arrival and quickly dispensed with the formalities at immigration and customs.

A limousine driver met me and we took the now very familiar route to New York City and I booked into the Carlyle.

The assistant manager accompanied me to my room. He

unlocked the door and there was Karin waiting for me. I closed the door and walked to where she was lying on the bed.

'Make love to me, Chris,' she whispered.

Dr Nazih Zuhdi had also trained under Dr Lillehei in Minneapolis, although he'd started his programme at about the time I left. I'd read, with great interest, his work on what became known as haemodilution.

When the heart-lung machine was introduced in clinical surgery, all the surgeons took it for granted that it had to be primed with human blood compatible with that of the patient. It was therefore necessary to bleed four to six donors before surgery. This delayed emergency procedures and also put great strain on the blood bank, especially when surgical teams were performing ten to twelve operations a day.

Using such large amounts of human blood also increased the likelihood of complications which resulted from blood transfusions.

Dr Zuhdi, in his research, showed that heart-lung machines could be filled either with diluted donor blood, or just a bland physiological solution – such as Ringer's lactate. After by-pass, the blood in the heart-lung machine was slowly perfused back into the patient and his kidneys would get rid of the excessive amount of fluid in the body – especially with the help of diuretics.

Although haemoglobin dropped as a result of the dilution of blood volume, perfusion of the vital organs was much better. Open-heart procedures could now be performed using either no donor blood, or only a few hundred millilitres.

Since the publication of his studies, haemodilution has become widely used and is still preferred by surgeons all over the world.

When Nazih Zuhdi finished his training he settled in Oklahoma City, where he was one of the senior cardiac surgeons.

After I'd retired, he invited me to come to Oklahoma and assist him in starting a heart transplant programme.

Nazih and his wife, Annette, came to see us in New York. He explained that later that year, they were going to inaugurate the new Oklahoma Heart Centre at the Baptist Medical Centre, and invited Karin and me as their guests. This would also give us the opportunity to look around and see if we'd like to settle in Oklahoma, if only for a few years.

Karin and I discussed it and as she hadn't seen much of the United States, we thought this would give her the opportunity to do so.

The two of us left New York in great spirits. The old and the young had decided to give it a go.

Before boarding the *QE2* in Los Angeles, we paid a visit to Disneyland – the climax of Walt Disney's dream. We also saw the *Queen Mary* and the *Spruce Goose*. I'd always been a great admirer of Howard Hughes. In my mind he was a true genius, so I was very keen to see what everyone called his folly – the largest wooden aircraft ever built, with a 320 foot wingspan. It had been designed by Hughes himself in 1942 and had flown only once.

Our first stop on the cruise was Honolulu where we spent several hours at Pearl Harbor. It was eerie standing on the wreck of the *Arizona*, knowing that the remains of the sailors who perished with her were still floating around somewhere in her hull.

Karin wasn't a good sailor and was seasick at times. Fortunately the *QE2* called at several ports – Bali, Manila, Hong Kong and finally Singapore, where we were very sad to leave this wonderful old lady.

Karin was due to fly home the next day via Taipei, but I had to go on to London for some more work on the documentary, which they had now decided to call *The Living Body*.

The day in Singapore passed too quickly. We visited the world famous bird park and were both very impressed by the cleanliness of the city. It convinced me, again, what a difference discipline can make. There are so many cities in the world that could learn a lot from Singapore.

The following morning, I took Karin to the airport and, as my own flight was later in the day, I returned to the hotel. On the way back I reminisced fondly about the wonderful time we'd spent together. I had no cares in the world and it was good to be alive.

When I walked into my hotel room the phone was ringing.

There was a call from South Africa, the exchange operator told me, as she put the call through and I recognized the familiar voice.

'Chris? It's Fritz. I have very bad news for you,' and he paused. 'André committed suicide last night.'

I slumped into the chair next to the phone, shaking my head wildly as if I could make what I'd just heard go away.

'What happened, Fritz?'

'His wife found him sitting dead in the bath this morning when she came home from night duty. That's all I know, my friend.'

'Did he drown? Maybe it was an accident?'

'That's all I know, Chris. When can we expect you?'

'I'm not sure, Fritz – I'll let you know.'

'Sorry, Chris. We're all so deeply sorry – you know how much we loved André.'

'Thanks, Fritz.'

And I had recently thought it was 'never too late'. Well it was.

During the past three weeks, while I was wining and dining on a luxury cruise in a fantasy world, my poor son was struggling to get to grips with real life.

'I was going to show how much I loved him when I got back!' I sobbed into the empty room, 'and now it's too late.' My words sounded hollow and my hands began to shake uncontrollably.

If only I'd phoned him! Or at least sent him a card – it might never have happened. But it was too late now.

It was the second time I'd received bad news when I was in a strange country – without friends. The first time was when Noel Tunbridge phoned me about the divorce – and now this tragedy.

If I'd known an hour earlier, I could have left with Karin.

I willed myself into action and phoned Singapore Airlines. They told me that the quickest way to South Africa would be to fly to London that afternoon, where I would arrive the following morning, and then that evening, take the South African Airways flight to Johannesburg and a connection to Cape Town.

It was the saddest journey I've ever made. My thoughts kept wandering back to my son. How he'd played on the sidewalk in New York with a set of Cowboys and Indians I'd bought him. Based on the television programmes he'd seen in America, the Indians were always the 'baddies' and the Cowboys the 'good-guys'. I remembered how annoyed he was when I'd knocked down one of the Cowboys – pretending that he'd been shot by one of the Indians. In the psychology of this little boy the good always triumphed over the bad.

The 'good-guys' never lost – but last night one did. Alone in a bathroom.

As a proponent of euthanasia and suicide (which, in some cases, can be seen as 'active euthanasia'), I found great comfort in the thought that he'd gone to a far better place than that from which he'd come. The quality of his life had deteriorated to the extent where there was no joy in living. Nothing to celebrate.

Somehow I survived the long journey home. The press had already given much coverage to my sorrow and at Cape Town airport, there were hordes of photographers who'd come to see whether they could capture my grief on film.

Fritz came to fetch me and we drove straight to André's home – or what had been his home. His wife Gail, a woman with great courage, cried softly when I arrived. She couldn't understand why he'd gone to such an extreme. She was convinced that it was purely an accident.

She was a nurse and, to earn a little extra money, she did night duty three times a week at the Red Cross Hospital.

That evening had been her turn to work the night shift and she'd left André at home with the two children. He'd told Deirdre, when she phoned that evening, that he was writing an examination the next day and planned to have a bath and then go to bed early.

The next morning, when Gail came home, she found it strange that the two children were still asleep and the doors still locked. She'd walked around the ominously quiet house. She peered through the bathroom window and saw her husband lying dead in the bath. A syringe was lying on the floor.

Perhaps he couldn't face the realities of the examination the next day and had decided that death was the way to escape. Gail, on the other hand, thought he had just decided to relax and had used drugs to do so – that his death was an accident.

The cause of death was definitely by drowning, so either theory could have been correct. I didn't dwell on it too much. All I knew was that my son was dead.

But the question which has plagued me ever since is whether my son could have been cured by treatment. I doubt it very much. The opportunity for treatment had been lost. I should have given him the love and affection he needed when he was still a little boy. It was my fault.

The family sat in the front pew of the chapel next to the crematorium. Karin thought she would show her respect for André by not attending the service.

As soon as Barbara heard the news, she contacted Gail and offered her all the assistance she needed. She also came to the funeral.

I sat next to Deirdre and Louwtjie.

The coffin was carried in and set down at the front of the chapel. We sang *Nearer My God to Thee* and Deirdre's husband, Kobus, read Psalm 23. It was a simple service.

I stared at the coffin and could picture André lying there. He had finally escaped. As in the case of my father and mother, I didn't want to see him after his death. I remembered him as a proud young man at his father's farewell party and a hard-working student. I remembered the handsome charm of his warm smile.

The service ended and we left the chapel. I turned back and could see black smoke coming from the chimney of the crematorium. All that remained of my son was a handful of ashes.

9

George van Wyk, a farmer from the Loxton District, phoned me and said he planned to make a documentary on hunting and wanted to discuss the project with me. He and his beautiful wife, Sandra, came to see me at Bloubergstrand.

I told George that the killing of wild animals was a very touchy subject and we had to be careful about filming that kind of thing.

No. That wasn't the purpose of the film. What he wanted to portray was that hunters were great conservationists. I agreed with that because there were now not only more but also a greater variety of game in the Karoo than I remembered during my childhood.

This was because hunting safaris had become a lucrative business and farmers who'd never had animals on their farms before had introduced antelope such as springbok, blesbok, gemsbok and various other species.

George told me that he was going to capture a few hundred springbok and blesbok and put them up for sale. The filming would start at this event.

Karin and I visited George and Sandra at their beautiful farm called 'Kafferskraal' (the name will probably be changed in the new South Africa, being a derogatory Afrikaans word for 'Natives' Village').

This trip took me back to my roots as Beaufort West was only a hundred kilometres away. It rekindled the yearning in me to have a farm in the Karoo one day.

The dream did eventually materialize and I now have a farm of 13 000 hectares (132 square kilometres or 50 square miles) with 17 different species of game.

Next, George organized a safari to Botswana, where the hunting of bigger animals could be filmed.

Since the transplant, I'd had several invitations to shoot big game, such as elephant, lion and buffalo, but I'd never accepted. To boast that I'd shot an elephant, or to display the skin of a lion that I'd killed, held no attraction for me. From youth my father taught me only to shoot for the pot – animals such as rabbit, an occasional springbok, pheasant and partridge.

Unfortunately, our party in Botswana was joined by trophy hunters who were only out to kill for the fun of it. I was both fascinated and disgusted at how their characters changed when they found a herd of antelope to decimate.

One of our guides had spotted some lion spoor and that morning we set off to hunt them. The spoor led us to a gemsbok they'd killed the previous night. The half-eaten carcass had been left behind, probably because they'd heard or seen us, and run away.

We followed the tracks further and suddenly, the Bushmen trackers jumped onto the truck. There they were – two lionesses with three cubs.

The hunters said that the cubs were big enough to look after themselves, so the two lionesses could be shot.

These two animals reminded me of my visit to the bull-ring several years previously and I remembered how the last bull had fought. They had no fear – but no chance either.

Repeatedly, the lionesses charged at the trucks, despite the bullets tearing into them. Maybe they were trying to protect their young but one of them was fatally wounded – by six badly placed shots. And by accident, one truck ran over the other. Both were now wounded and obviously in great pain.

I was given the dubious 'honour' of delivering the *coup de grâce* and putting a merciful end to their agony. But I was scared stiff – even though they were dying – so I opened the window just enough to get the rifle barrel through and grimly finished them off.

I left the carnage with great respect for the animals and utter contempt for the 'hunters' who had cowered from the safety of their trucks, but who could now boast that they'd shot a lion.

George and his two brothers, who were also in the party, did not fire a single shot.

Although we had permits to shoot these two animals, I just felt there was something wrong with the way in which it was done. If the hunters had faced the animals on foot – and taken the risk of being killed themselves, then with a stretch of the imagination, one might possibly condone the hunt. But to shoot them in cold blood, when they had no chance to get at their killers, was disgusting.

I decided that this was the end of my big game hunting and the matter would have ended there. But Carol Hancock, a girlfriend of the cameraman, who had accepted and enjoyed the hospitality of my friends, saw that she could make money out of the death of these two lionesses – especially as Chris Barnard was also involved.

So, allowing greed to get the better of valour, she wrote a distorted and sensational article about the safari – illustrated with pictures she had been 'commissioned' to take for the promotion of the documentary.

The article was published. She was paid and disappeared from the scene. I think she left the country – but it took months for the dust to settle.

The unfortunate guides nearly ended up in jail and George, who hadn't fired one shot at the lions, received abusive phone calls and death threats.

It was the end of our documentary in support of hunting.

It left me philosophizing about which was worse – the despicable and bloodthirsty actions of the hunters who had no regard for the life of the animals, or the avarice of the girl who saw a way to make a quick buck without regard for the feelings of her friends. I decided that both were equally bad and God help the human race.

I accepted the position of scientist in residence at the Baptist Medical Centre. The salary I had been offered was so good that what I earned in a month would have taken me two *years* to have earned as a professor at the University of Cape Town.

Just before we left, I received a progress report from Schafer telling me that the experimental work had produced some exciting and encouraging results.

In one of the experiments, he'd taken some live cells and exposed them to a fixed dose of ultraviolet light irradiation, which would result in damage to the genetic material. These cells were then divided into two groups: The one that acted as a control he incubated further but added radioactive (labelled) amino acids – the building blocks of protein. The second group he incubated further with the radioactive amino acids, but he also added sphingolipids.

After a few days, he separated the cells from the culture medium and counted the radioactivity present in the cells. What he found was that the control group had very little radioactivity whereas the cells treated with glycosphingolipids (GSL) had significant activity present.

These results suggested that in both groups there was genetic damage caused by the ultraviolet light. In the controlled group little, or no, repair took place after the irradiation was stopped and the cells were unable to synthesize proteins, as shown by the absence of the radioactive building blocks.

However, in the second group, the addition of GSL must have stimulated repair and allowed protein synthesis to take place. This was indicated by the presence of a significant concentration of radioactive amino acids.

There was one aspect of the research that puzzled me though. The results of our experiments always seemed to turn out just as we wanted them to. As an old researcher, I knew that things never worked out as well as that – unless you were very lucky.

In Oklahoma we arrived to a large reception party, which included Nazih and Annette Zuhdi. We were taken to a beautiful suite at the Waterford Hotel, where we would stay until more permanent accommodation could be found.

In the meantime Nazih and his partners had started the transplant programme. He had big plans to accelerate the work when I arrived.

I was looking forward to the challenge but there was something worrying me. I'd suddenly developed symptoms of some obstruction in the large bowel. There was no pain – just noises of excessive bowel activity. Not only did these symptoms cause me sleepless nights, but they were also terribly embarrassing in company. As soon as the bubbling, gurgling noises started, everyone would stare at me.

A very dear friend of mine had just died of a carcinoma of the large bowel and I was sure I had the same thing. Night after night I lay awake planning my future, if this should be the diagnosis. In fact, I was afraid to consult a doctor in case he told me that I *was* suffering from this dreaded disease.

Eventually I did discuss it with Nazih, and he made an appointment for me to see the gastroenterologist at the Baptist Medical Centre.

Dr Richard Welch was one of those medical men who immediately imparted confidence to his patients. He was decisive and knew exactly how to handle the situation.

After giving me a thorough examination, he said that a very good sign was that there was no blood in my stool, but he thought we should make certain by doing a colonoscopy.

In the days when I was an intern, one could only examine a short segment of the large bowel as the scope used was a rigid metal tube, unable to traverse the twists and turns of the bowel when inserted through the anus.

But now, with fibre-optics, the scope was not only much thinner, but very flexible. So the whole of the large bowel and even a portion of the lower, small bowel could be inspected from the inside.

As the large bowel had to be completely empty, the preparation for such an examination was awful. It started with a big dose of senna and was followed by glasses and glasses of a purgative. I spent the whole night on the toilet until eventually only water was present in my bowel action.

The examination itself was done under sedation and wasn't much of an ordeal, except that the doctor couldn't advance the scope further than about 15 centimetres – even after he'd distended the bowel like a balloon by pumping air into it.

He told me there was a significant narrowing in the lower part of the large bowel, but he was sure it wasn't due to a tumour. As he couldn't see beyond this constriction, he suggested I should have a barium enema.

With my stomach tight and swollen like a drum, I set off for the radiology department – waddling like a fat duck.

The doctor who did the examination was different from Richard Welch. He didn't keep me informed on the progress of the examination – he just looked concerned and puzzled. When he examined the X-ray film, I heard him say, 'This guy's got big trouble.'

I nearly screamed, 'What *kind* of trouble, you asshole? Tell me!' But I kept quiet and waited patiently. Again I realized as a doctor, that you should never allow the patient to become enmeshed in a conspiracy of silence. The truth should never be veiled by medical jargon.

Finally he came back to me. Here it comes, I thought and prepared myself for the worst.

'Professor, you have a severe stricture in the large bowel – but I've studied it very carefully and it has no characteristics of a malignant lesion.

'There is severe diverticulitis and I presume that this narrowing is a result of the healing of these lesions – nothing to worry about.'

I could have kissed him! And for the first time in weeks, I slept through the entire night without mentally writing my will.

We quickly settled down to life in Oklahoma City and I spent a lot of time with Nazih Zuhdi. During the day we were at the hospital together and most evenings he took us out to one of the local restaurants.

The Zuhdis were Muslims and Nazih was a student of the Koran. Some Sunday evenings, he gave very interesting talks about this book.

The Koran, the sacred book of Islam, believed by Muslims to be the infallible word of God, dictated to Muhammad through the medium of the angel Gabriel, impressed me. It had an understanding of all religions that accepted God as the Supreme Power.

In the operating room, I soon recognized that Nazih was a superb surgeon. However, his management of patients in the ward was foreign to me. Vi, a trained nurse who worked full-time for him, did most of the work-up before surgery and was also responsible for most of the post-operative care. He was only called in for major complications. I never could get used to such extensive delegation.

They also made much more use of consultations and special investigations than I did. This approach was probably due to the constant fear of litigation – but it certainly escalated the cost of hospitalization as far as the patient was concerned.

I discussed my duties with Nazih and we agreed that I should act only in an advisory capacity, supervise the research programme and be a public relations officer for the transplant programme and the heart centre.

The team at the Baptist Medical Centre had, so far, performed three orthotopic transplants. Nazih discussed the advantages and disadvantages of the heterotopic operation and we decided that, in the next few cases, we would use this technique.

At Groote Schuur Hospital, after the death of Martin Franzot, we had routinely performed the piggy-back operation. But it was clear to me that, with the superior rejection control now possible with Cyclosporin and, especially having cut down very acute episodes of rejection, the need for this operation had been reduced – and it should no longer be done routinely.

It appeared that it should be mainly employed in cases where it had been determined that the donor heart, for some reason or another, was not capable of managing the circulation on its own after the operation.

As post-operative failure of the donor heart had become one of the major reasons for mortality in transplant programmes, the judicious use of the piggy-back operation could reduce this risk.

Dr Zuhdi used this technique for the next three patients, with one death (for reasons other than the transplant). But, just as I had experienced in Cape Town, the criticism and the pressure to stop the programme increased and we had no choice but to abandon cardiac transplantation – if only for a while.

Frederick and Christiaan came to visit us and to see something of the United States. After a two-week stay in Oklahoma City, Karin and I took them to see Disney World and Sea World in Florida. On our way back from Orlando we stopped for two days in Tampa to visit Dr Pupello, who was trying to get a heart transplant programme started there too.

From Tampa we had a connection in St Louis for Washington. I thought it was an excellent opportunity to show the children some of the wonderful museums in the capital of the United States. As we only had 15 minutes to change planes in St Louis, I asked one of the officials if our luggage would be transferred in time. He told me that if it didn't make that plane, it would 'probably' be on the next one. It was obvious that any inconvenience to us was of no concern to him.

We arrived in Washington and, as I expected, there was no sign of our luggage.

After filling in the necessary forms we took a taxi to the Washington Hilton – where the American Medical Association had generously made their suite available for me and my family.

The accommodation was wonderful – and made up for the disappointment of not having our luggage with us.

The following morning we woke up full of eager anticipation of spending an interesting and enjoyable day in the city.

Karin and the two boys were going downstairs and I said I'd meet them later in the foyer, after I'd made a few phone calls.

About 15 minutes later there was a knock on the door and a member of the hotel staff told me I had to vacate the room immediately as there was a fire in the hotel. He was very calm and reassured me that it would only be for a short time.

When I walked out of the hotel onto the street, a large crowd had gathered around the building and I couldn't find Karin or my sons. I was suddenly very worried – maybe they were still somewhere in the hotel, unaware of the fire? Maybe they were trapped in a lift or overcome by smoke?

I began searching frantically, calling out their names as I shoved through the morbidly fascinated mass of 'spectators' – many of whom were laughing and joking – as if it was a carnival. I grimly reflected that the human race hadn't changed very much since 19th century public hangings.

I couldn't find my family anywhere and finally elbowed my way through to a policeman who was standing in front of the building, casually drinking a Coke.

'Excuse me, officer – I'm looking for my wife and children – they might still be in the hotel. Could you please help me?' I tried to keep the cold fear from my voice.

He held up his hand, as if stopping the traffic and brought the can of Coke away from his mouth.

'Get back,' he said laconically. I'd obviously interrupted his powers of concentration as he seemed confused about which was more important – his Coca-Cola or me. The Coke won.

'But I'm worried about my family!'

'If you don't get back, buddy, I'll arrest you,' he grunted and, satisfied that he'd performed his official responsibilities over and above the normal call of duty, he concentrated on finishing the Coke.

I briefly remembered the British bobby who'd helped me when I'd lost my way in London once and couldn't help comparing the two. 'God help America,' I mumbled as I turned away from him, not knowing what on earth to do next.

At that very moment I saw Karin and the two boys running toward me.

They'd been equally worried, of course, as they thought I might still be on the phone in our room, and trapped inside the hotel. We hugged each other gratefully.

We stood around for several hours not knowing what was going on. In the meantime, the fire chief had made several announcements to the TV cameras. It occurred to me that, as the rest of America knew more about the situation than we did, we'd better find a television set somewhere.

We decided that it was pointless just standing around wasting our time, so we went to visit the Aerospace Museum and some of the monuments.

We returned to the hotel in the afternoon, but we still weren't allowed inside. Fortunately, they'd made alternative accommodation arrangements for us.

I phoned the airline to see if our luggage had arrived. It had, but as they'd tried to deliver it to the hotel and been unable to find me, it had been returned to the airport.

I asked them to please bring the luggage immediately – I'd wait for them. In the meantime, I sent Karin and the children to our new hotel.

After an hour, the airline van arrived again with the luggage. Explaining our predicament I asked the driver if he'd mind taking me and the luggage to our new hotel. No. He only had instructions to deliver our cases to the Hilton Hotel.

Rather than argue, I watched him unload the luggage onto the pavement and drive off. Luckily, I found a taxi almost immediately and joined my family.

But I was to have yet another enlightening experience with the Washington Police Department.

The next day we made an early start and visited the Arlington Cemetery, the graves of the two Kennedy brothers and the Ford Museum where Abraham Lincoln had been assassinated. Karin then took the boys back to the hotel and I went back to the Hilton to clear my safety deposit box. When I arrived another policeman stopped me from going inside.

I explained that my passport, air tickets and money were locked inside the hotel safe and that as I was leaving for an international flight the next day it was vital I be allowed to collect all my documents.

But American policemen are extremely resourceful. His wise counsel was that I should get a new passport, new air tickets and, presumably, some new money.

Desperately trying to control my temper, I said, 'Then perhaps you could help me, Officer – here's the key to my box – I give you my full permission to remove my things from the hotel safe.'

No. He wasn't allowed to do that. I noticed that there were numerous people going in and out of the hotel the entire time we talked. So I said to the officer that as I had the key but wasn't allowed to get to the box, and he could get to the box but wasn't allowed to take the key, could I ask someone else?

He thought for a few moments. 'Yeah' that would be okay, he guessed.

So I spoke to an assistant manager, who took me inside the building and allowed me to remove the contents of the safety deposit box.

The next day we couldn't get out of Washington quickly enough.

We stayed at the Pierre Hotel in New York for a few days. Karin and the kids enjoyed the city much more than Washington. Then we took the South African Airways flight back to Cape Town.

I decided to give Karin a wild 21st birthday party at La Vita and, as we did at Deirdre's wedding, we'd use the entire Dean Street Arcade.

When we discussed the programme for the evening, someone suggested that I should propose the toast on her birthday.

As I hadn't known Karin long enough to talk about the way she grew up and as these aspects of speeches are inevitably boring anyway, I had a novel idea.

Instead of a speech, I would collect slides illustrating the various stages of her life and when these were being shown I planned to play appropriate music.

Karin invited quite a few of her school friends and I invited some older guests.

Aldo and Gino arranged the tables in the arcade and, in the restaurant itself, they laid out the buffet. Hilton Ross and his band were there to provide live music.

When the time came for my speech, I walked up to the microphone and much to everyone's surprise, the lights went out and the first slide of Karin as a baby appeared on the screen. Louis Armstrong sang *Hello, Dolly*, which was Karin's father's favourite song.

Three slides later Karin appeared at the age of six, sitting on my lap (the photograph which had been taken by her mother at Buffelsbaai fifteen years previously). Maurice Chevalier sang *Thank Heaven for Little Girls*.

The last slide was of my girlfriend at the age of 21 again sitting on my lap. The Beatles sang: When I get older, losing my hair, many years from now – Will you still be sending me a Valentine, Birthday Greetings, Bottle of Wine ...Will you still need me, will you still feed me – when I'm 64?

Everyone roared with laughter and said it was one of my best speeches ever.

Then I announced that Karin would say a few words and as she stepped forward, the music started. When she reached the front she mimed to the words, 'Oh Doctor, I'm in trouble,' and I, in turn, mimed, 'Well, goodness gracious me.' We'd rehearsed this song by Sophia Loren and Peter Sellers for days; it was a perfect ending to the speech and the evening went on to be a huge success.

I'd rented a house in Buffelsbaai and we decided to spend two weeks of the Christmas holidays there with Frederick and Christiaan.

George van Wyk phoned me from Plettenberg Bay to say that his holiday home was going to be publicly auctioned. He asked me to go along to the auction and try to push up the bidding.

The auctioneer was aware of this, he said, and wouldn't accept any of my bids.

Karin and the boys joined me at the sale. The bidding started slowly and when it reached R230 000, I thought I should help my old friend a bit and said 'R235 000'.

There was silence.

'No further bids?' asked the auctioneer. 'Going once, twice,' and he banged his gavel on the desk and said, with a smile, 'sold to Professor Barnard!'

I didn't want a house in Plettenberg Bay!

When I spoke to George, he said he couldn't understand how it had happened, but if I wanted the house, I could have all the furniture and appliances as well. It turned out to be an excellent buy.

In the New Year, Karin and I returned to Oklahoma where I was going to continue my work as the scientist in residence.

Armin Mattli asked me to meet him in New York, as he had a proposition to put to me. We had become very close friends and he'd been very kind to me – especially with financial assistance.

I met him in New York and he told me he'd had great success with a cosmetic called La Prairie but that he'd sold it to another company some years previously. He'd now developed a new product which would contain glycosphingolipids – we had shown, in our experimental work, that ultraviolet light damage to cells would be repaired by GSL.

Also, as ultraviolet light damage to skin cells is one of the causes of ageing, this cosmetic could help a lot to delay, or even reverse, a part of the ageing process.

I pointed out to him that I didn't think one could conclude that because glycosphingolipids had worked in cultures, it would have the same effect on cells in the intact skin.

He told me that Dr Schafer had developed what he called a 'transdermal factor'. He had illustrated, in experimental work, by putting a label on the glycosphingolipids, that when this factor was present, a molecule penetrated the outer layer of the skin and its presence could be demonstrated as it became incorporated in the membranes of the skin cells deeper down.

They'd also done extensive clinical tests and the product was all they claimed it to be.

As I hadn't been involved in the production or the testing of the cosmetic, I refused to promote it.

Armin Mattli assured me that this wasn't what they wanted me to do. All they wanted from me was to talk about the experimental work I had been associated with at the Schafer laboratory.

I then made one of the greatest mistakes of my life – and I've regretted it a million times since. I said, 'Okay, I'll do it.'

The following morning we met Mr Alfin for breakfast. He was the managing director of a fragrance company and was interested in distributing this cosmetic world-wide. All I had to do was explain to him, in layman's terms, our research findings.

After our meeting, Mr Alfin appeared to be very excited about the cosmetic. Karin and I then left for Oklahoma City.

A few months later I received an agreement between Mr Alfin and the Christiaan Barnard Research Institute, in which it stated that my sole involvement with the cosmetic would be to talk about the research I had done with Dr Schafer – and that my name could only be used in its promotion after the text had been approved by the American Medical Association. For my services, the Christiaan Barnard Research Institute would receive $75 000.

When I read the agreement I felt uncomfortable, but thought all the loopholes had been closed and that my colleagues could not object if I only discussed research. But I was very much mistaken.

We arrived in Oklahoma and settled into a little guest house, generously offered to us by a cardiologist at the Baptist Medical Centre. He lived next door with his wife and four children. This was a much better arrangement than staying at the hotel, as Karin now had her own home to keep her busy during the day.

I travelled extensively, especially in the state of Oklahoma, to talk about the work being done at the hospital.

Unfortunately, the arthritis had flared up again and was so bad at times that Karin had to help me get dressed some mornings. Fortunately, I could still continue with my daily duties.

Mr Alfin phoned me and asked if I could come to New York for a few days for the launch of the product – which was going to be called 'Glycel'. They'd organized interviews with some of the top women's magazines.

With the permission of Nazih Zuhdi and the hospital, I was given the necessary leave.

When I arrived in New York I was met by Mr Alfin at the airport and was taken by limousine to the Pierre Hotel, where I was given a large suite. I was wined and dined like a king.

When the interviews started, I noticed that the reporters talked about Glycel as 'your cosmetic' and I went to great pains to explain, each and every time, that I hadn't developed the product, nor had I tested it and could therefore make no claims for it. I said that I was only qualified to talk about the research on glycosphingolipids.

But it was too good a story to drop, so Glycel became known as 'Barnard's cream'. My name also started appearing on the boxes and jars, but instead of putting my foot down there and then and telling both Alfin and Mattli that I was withdrawing from the contract because they hadn't kept to its conditions, I let it ride.

I realize now that I'd been seduced by the hotel suite, the French champagne and all the five-star wining and dining. I'd been a complete walk-over.

What Mr Alfin and his advisers hadn't counted on, however, was that they were making an enormous mistake giving my name such a high profile in their promotions. Claims such as 'anti-wrinkle', 'anti-ageing' and 'rejuvenation' were not considered to be cosmetic claims. The public and authorities regarded these claims as medical – as they were backed by a well-known doctor.

The initial sales were tremendous but they also attracted the big guns. The well-known major cosmetic houses angrily denounced the product.

All of a sudden, well-known dermatologists appeared on television programmes saying that *my* claims were false. They gave no scientific reason for saying so – they just said they weren't true. I was not invited to appear with them to defend myself or GSL – and, they cleverly did not tell their audiences that they were actually employed by competing cosmetic companies.

I'd heard rumours that Dr Bruno Reichart, who had been appointed head of the department of thoracic surgery when I left Cape Town, didn't get on well with some of the senior staff, so I wasn't really surprised when I heard from Dr Dimitri Novitzky and then Dr David Cooper. They wondered if I could find them positions in Oklahoma.

When I mentioned this to Nazih Zuhdi, and told them what highly qualified men these were, and how they would be a great asset to his team, he was sold on the idea. He had the uncanny ability to get what he wanted and within the next few years, both these surgeons had positions at the Baptist Medical Centre. It was probably one of the best teams in the world at that stage.

The clinical programme of the transplant unit now got into full swing and we were exploring facilities to continue some of the research projects that Dr Novitzky had been involved in when he left Cape Town.

I also contacted Professor Thomson of the department of zoology at the University of Oklahoma, to start some research on the glycosphingolipids.

He suggested that we should study the survival of single-cell organisms called Tetrahymena, after exposure to ultraviolet light – one group treated with GSL and the other to act as a control.

Karin had also been employed by Mr Alfin. She had to train the girls at the stores where Glycel was sold. She travelled more extensively at that time than I did and I really admired her – this girl, born and raised in a quiet suburb of Cape Town – for the way she coped in a strange country with all the high-powered hype of American marketing.

Mr Alfin was a kind man. His only mistake was to surround himself with poor advisers. Had Glycel been launched without the fanfare and had my name been used sparingly and professionally he would today be the owner of one of the most widely used cosmetics in the world, I'm sure. Glycel, at that stage, was one of the few products where at least some of the claims were based on published experimental findings.

What I found difficult to understand was that competitive products made more outrageous claims than Glycel had, but no one questioned their validity. With Glycel we had criticism from every quarter. Even the Federal Trade Commission started an investigation.

Both Dr Schafer and I gave evidence and, to my knowledge, they couldn't establish any irregularity. They did find fault with our experimental model, but our findings must have been correct, as Professor Thomson's research subsequently confirmed that glycosphingolipids provide protection from ultraviolet light injury in living cells.

But the witch hunt hadn't ended.

The Christiaan Barnard Research Institute was established by Mr Mattli. This was yet another mistake I made. I agreed that this foundation had the right to use my name in the sale and promotion of products, as long as it didn't interfere with my practice as a physician. For this I would receive 10 percent of the foundation's earnings.

Accusations had been made that my involvement in Glycel was only for money, which is, I suppose, what most of us work for. But those who thought I'd be a millionaire were very much mistaken. My total income from this foolish exercise was not more than $200 000. Armin Mattli was the one who received the millions. Not only did he sell the patent and the distribution rights to Mr Alfin but Alfin still had to buy the product and packaging materials from him. Mattli, being an astute businessman, also avoided all the subsequent mud slinging.

Now came the worst.

I received a letter from the American College of Surgeons informing me that, as a fellow, I had to appear before a disciplinary committee for 'unprofessional behaviour'. They based their claims not on scientific reports, but from stories in newspapers and lay magazines. I couldn't believe my eyes when I read this letter and phoned the college to find out what it was all about. A secretary answered my call and her advice to me was: 'Get a good lawyer'.

I told her I wasn't a criminal and that I couldn't afford a lawyer in the United States. I also told her that all the promotional material in which I had been involved had been passed by the American Medical Association (AMA). If I could provide proof of this, she said, it would be of great help.

I phoned Mr Alfin and reminded him that, according to the contract, they had to use material approved by the AMA and asked him if that had been done. He said he'd complied, as it was part of our agreement. So I asked him for proof and he told me that a doctor, belonging to the AMA, had passed the text.

I was stunned.

After giving the matter a lot of thought, I wrote a long letter to the college, telling them that I was surprised such a prestigious institution could charge a highly respected fellow with 'unprofessional behaviour' based solely on newspaper reports. I went on to substantiate the claims I had made with a full report of the research done at Basel, on which the claims were based. I ended the letter by saying I didn't have the time or the inclination to continue this ridiculous argument and that if they felt it should be dragged on they should accept my resignation.

I signed the letter and listed all my degrees, leaving out the letters FACS (Fellow of the American College of Surgeons). I suppose this was juvenile and asking for trouble – and I got it.

A few weeks later I received a very curt reply that they had accepted my resignation.

So I was no longer a Fellow of the American College of Surgeons and, strange as it may seem, I haven't missed it at all. It certainly didn't result in any personal disadvantage, but I suppose it taught me a lesson.

The American College of Cardiology had a more mature approach and I'm still a fellow of that college – an honour which I hold very dear.

Doctors Zuhdi and Novitzky had a turbulent coexistence. They were both very ambitious and Nazih had to keep a tight rein on Novitzky to prevent losing complete control of his department. Dr Cooper, a real English gentleman, acted as a calming influence.

But, despite these personality clashes, the heart transplant programme became one of the most successful in the United States.

They were also preparing to perform a heart-lung transplant. This operation was technically not difficult, but the problems in the joining of the windpipes and the diagnosis of the onset of rejection remained.

Fortunately, Dimitri Novitzky had had experience with this operation during the time he'd worked in Cape Town.

I discussed my future in Oklahoma and told Dr Zuhdi and the directors of the Baptist Medical Centre, that the heart transplant programme was now well established and that my presence was superfluous.

Nazih didn't want to see me go and I'd also grown very fond of Oklahoma City and its people. So we compromised – after a holiday I would come back for one more year and stay for the 20th anniversary of the heart transplant.

Karin and I came back to South Africa for a vacation – to get away from the Oklahoma winter and to see the children. She was also wondering what her future was with me, saying it was very unsettling to live between her parents' home and my one-roomed apartment at Bloubergstrand. This situation was exacerbated by the fact that we now had our own apartment in Oklahoma.

After the holiday in South Africa I went back to the United States. Mr Alfin wanted me to do some work for him; then I would return for my last term at the Baptist Medical Centre. Karin said she'd follow later.

When I met Mr Alfin in New York, I had a distinct feeling that he was having serious problems with Glycel. Sales had dropped significantly and there were rumours that the Food and Drug Administration (FDA) had started investigating the cosmetic.

When I arrived in Oklahoma, I found that my previous accommodation was not available, but the director of hospital services generously offered me rooms in a small hotel that the hospital managed for the relatives of patients.

This was very convenient, as I could then walk undercover from my room to my office.

I received a phone call from Karin in Cape Town to say that a townhouse near her parents' home and opposite a children's crèche (!) was for sale. She thought this would be an ideal place for us so I phoned Noel Tunbridge and asked him to make a ridiculously low offer. I think I was hoping the sale wouldn't go through.

He phoned me back a few days later to say my offer had been accepted. Now Karin had her own home.

I had always dismissed the topic of marriage and we hadn't discussed it until a few months previously, in Oklahoma, when Karin announced one evening that she had something she wanted to talk about. Close to tears, and with a trembling voice, she told me she wasn't prepared to go on living as we were. I couldn't have my cake and eat it too.

'I know how you feel,' she said, dabbing at her eyes, 'that you're worried about getting married for the third time. But you must see my point of view as well – I'm still very young and I just can't drift along without at least having some idea of where I'm going.'

'Of course I understand,' I said gently, 'just give me a while to sort myself out.'

This was a difficult situation. I was very much in love with this beautiful girl – who'd coped with my unsettled life and physical disabilities, without complaining once.

She'd help me put on my jacket, when the pain in my shoulder was so severe I couldn't lift my arms above my head. She did it in such a way that it appeared natural and required no special effort. I never had the feeling that she was actually *nursing* me.

It would be extremely difficult – if not unbearable – if she was no longer a part of my life.

When I arrived back in Oklahoma, I discussed my personal problems with Nazih Zuhdi and, being extremely fond of Karin, he had no hesitation in advising that we should get married.

'You should thank your lucky stars that a girl like Karin is prepared to marry an old fossil like you!' he laughed.

His first suggestion was that we should go out and look for an engagement ring. I had a little knowledge about diamonds and knew that, apart from size, colour and clarity were also important and that it was better to buy a stone which was certified.

Nazih was more inclined to go for the size. 'Shit, no one's going to see those flaws,' he said, as we looked at one particular stone – so I bought the 2,75 carat diamond and had it set as a solitaire.

Karin was on her way from Cape Town to join me in Oklahoma and I had a surprise for her – all wrapped up in a little velvet-lined box.

She phoned me from New York to say that one of her suitcases with all her best clothes was missing. But Swissair assured her that it would be on the next flight, which was due to arrive an hour later and that it would definitely be on the TWA flight she was taking to Oklahoma.

I met Karin at the airport and we waited and waited at the luggage carousel – but there was no suitcase.

She started to cry, so I gave her the box and she squealed with delight when she opened it. She flung her arms around my neck and we both laughed ecstatically. I slipped the ring onto her finger and we kissed. So we got engaged at Oklahoma airport.

The next day I was to discover the strange workings of the airlines. We knew that the suitcase had arrived in Zürich from South Africa as the girl in the first class lounge confirmed it. We also knew the suitcase hadn't arrived in New York because it wasn't there for her to clear customs.

Surely the loss should be the responsibility of Swissair? No – it was TWA's because they were the last carrier. It didn't seem to matter that TWA had never received the suitcase.

I'd never experienced such a 'couldn't-care-less' attitude.

Neither Swissair nor TWA offered to give Karin, who was now without luggage, as much as a toothbrush. It was as if they felt that once they had delivered her to her destination, that's where their responsibilities ended.

This ridiculous situation made one wonder what Karin would have done if no one had met her in Oklahoma. The airlines certainly weren't going to do anything – and she was a first-class passenger! I dread to think of what would have happened in economy-class.

The following evening, Karin was sitting in our lounge, looking at her engagement ring. I thought she was admiring the beautiful diamond under the light of a table lamp until she suddenly said, 'Chris, this stone is full of black specks!'

'Let me see!' I said, pretending to be surprised. There was no doubt. Even with my old eyes I could see the flaws. I knew she wouldn't be happy with the ring, so I went back to the shop where I'd bought it and they refunded my money.

A few weeks later we went to New York and this time I bought a smaller diamond – but the clarity and colour were certified.

We heard nothing further from the airlines. A week later, when I phoned, they said they thought the luggage must have been stolen. I spoke to a friend of mine and asked him how this could happen. He just laughed and said it wasn't unusual at all at Kennedy airport.

There was a still bigger shock waiting for us. The compensation that the airline was prepared to pay was according to weight – so it didn't matter if your case was full of rags or designer clothes, the amount was the same. The money Karin received wasn't even enough to replace the Gucci suitcase, which had been a present from Joska.

When I asked about this injustice, the girl told me that the conditions were all on the ticket – which was fine if you had a magnifying glass to read all the small print. When I did read the conditions I found that the scale of compensation was determined so long ago, that the amounts paid out were ridiculously low. No wonder nobody gave a damn – it was easier and cheaper to pay out this small amount than to take proper and effective security measures.

But I've learned a few lessons. It's better to fly with the oldest suitcase you have – so that the thieves at the airport think it belongs to a poor man and is not worth stealing. Also, take out additional insurance because if it's stolen or lost, at least that will pay for the loss. Whatever you do, don't rely on the airlines.

The arthritis had now virtually immobilized me so, on the advice of the rheumatologist at Oklahoma, I started taking gold tablets. As this medication could have toxic effects on both the kidneys and bone marrow, I had my blood and urine tested every month.

After a few months, I noticed that I was gradually becoming anaemic and it was the kind of anaemia that develops as a result of chronic blood loss. I immediately had my stool tested and there were traces of blood present. Now I was *positive* that I had cancer of the large bowel and again, I started mentally drafting my will every night.

Back I went to Dr Richard Welch, the gastroenterologist, who suggested that I have another colonoscopy and a gastroscopy – so the torture of the bowel preparation and the anxious waiting for the outcome began all over again.

On this occasion, the doctor first examined my stomach and then from the bottom he managed to get the scope past the stricture and was able to examine the whole of the large bowel.

They thought I was losing blood as a result of inflammation of my stomach lining – probably caused by all the anti-arthritic medication. There was no cancer. What a relief! I felt like someone who'd just had the death sentence commuted for the second time.

Our stay in Oklahoma was virtually at an end. One more major function: the 20th anniversary of the first heart transplant. Nazih Zuhdi and his colleagues didn't skimp on making this a very glamorous and memorable occasion.

They invited all the the members of the original surgical team that they could find, and also all the doctors who'd worked with me when I was training in Minneapolis.

There was some method in their apparent madness, because the event received wide media coverage. I was flown to New York to appear on the programme *Good Morning America*. I was also interviewed, via satellite, from South Africa – but Mariëtta Kruger wasn't really interested in the progress of transplantation – of much more importance, apparently, was my new, young girlfriend and also the rumour that I'd had a face-lift.

President Ronald Reagan sent me a beautiful letter of congratulations but there wasn't a whisper from the South African government.

On 4 December 1987, Karin and I left Oklahoma to get married in Cape Town. We first flew to Dallas, to catch a connection to Paris, where I had a television engagement. When we arrived in Dallas, a gentleman met us at the plane and said he had to stay with us until we boarded our flight to Paris. He even followed me to the toilet.

I never could find out exactly what this was all about, but I suspect it was due to a death-threat I'd received earlier, which the hospital had reported to the FBI.

We eventually arrived in Cape Town in the middle of our summer and, after a few days, left with Frederick and Christiaan for a holiday in my newly acquired house in Plettenberg Bay.

Karin was restless to get back to Cape Town though, as there was a lot of preparation to be done for the wedding. The two of us had already discussed some of the main aspects of this event. We'd decided to get married at La Vita and to ask our dear friend, Father Tom Nicholson – the same priest who'd christened Christiaan – to officiate at the ceremony.

Karin was determined that there was no other person to design her wedding dress than the brilliant Errol Arendz. Errol is the South African equivalent of Yves St Laurent – if not better. He'd actually used Barbara to model some of his earlier garments when he first started. I think she helped him considerably to become one of the most respected and sought-after couturiers in the country.

I decided that the media and others had made enough money out of the Barnards and it was now time for me to make some for myself. So I sold the exclusive rights of the wedding to *Rapport* and was pleasantly surprised at how much they were prepared to pay.

At the ceremony, we would have security guards to keep reporters and photographers out and only Roelof Vorster and Bernard Jordaan of *Rapport* would be allowed in.

Several friends from the United States and Europe were invited including Nazih and Annette Zuhdi, Armin Mattli, Aris Argyriou and Manny and Elizabeth Villafana. It wasn't possible to keep all these arrangements secret from the press and almost every day there was a new headline:

BARNARD BOMBSHELL! Chris, 72 (sic), to wed Karin, 22.

But I was in good company in that edition, as the other main story was about the 'Bizarre secrets of Charles and Diana's marriage'.

PROF IS NOT GOING TO GET MARRIED!

KARIN WANTS TO MARRY
Does Chris want to or not?

WEDDING BELLS FOR CHRIS AND KARIN? RUBBISH!

BARNARD TO WED – BUT WHEN?

CHRIS & KARIN TO MARRY IN JANUARY

NEW YEAR WEDDING FOR CHRIS AND KARIN

SECRET OF THE WEDDING DRESS

ERROL'S ALREADY FINISHED KARIN'S DRESS

THE GREAT EVENT!
Date: 23rd January
Time: 7 pm
Place: La Vita Restaurant
Occasion: Prof Chris and Karin's wedding

A few of the arrangements ruffled some feathers. First, Father Tom was contacted by the department of the interior and he was reminded that if we were married in the restaurant, it wouldn't be legal as a marriage service can only be performed in a church, or before a magistrate, or in a private home.

Father Tom also phoned the Bishop to confirm the legality of the marriage. He was very sympathetic, but pointed out that as I was divorced, the Catholic Church couldn't condone my marriage.

On Friday evening, the day before the ceremony at the restaurant, Karin and I, with Nazih and Annette as witnesses, went to Father Tom's apartment where the magistrate married us. We kept this very quiet as it could dull the romance of the following evening.

Karin insisted that I didn't spend the night before our 'real' marriage with her. So, after a party at Maureen's restaurant, I spent the first night of my honeymoon in the same room at the Brinks' hotel where I'd mourned the loss of Barbara, which seemed like centuries before. It's amazing how time heals such deep wounds.

The next afternoon, I went to Gloria Craig's flat in Sea Point where I got dressed and left for La Vita quite early to see that everything was ready for the big occasion.

Aldo, Gino and Rudi had spent the previous evening and the entire day preparing the arcade – as they'd done for Deirdre's wedding and Karin's 21st birthday party. In one corner, they had a bar fully stocked with every drink imaginable – even Moët et Chandon for the toast – my wedding present from Vito. In the restaurant proper, the buffet was laid out and included fresh oysters, lobsters and smoked salmon, in addition to a variety of hot dishes.

In the arcade all the tables and chairs had been set with white table cloths and white napkins – each table having a floral arrangement of lilies and pink and white roses.

As the time drew nearer, the crowd outside the restaurant swelled to several hundred and the guests started arriving – the men in black tie and the women in formal gowns.

I looked at my watch – it was already ten minutes past seven and there was still no sign of the bride. At seven-thirty there were cheers outside in the street. The band rushed to the door with their instruments and started playing the Wedding March. Father Tom and I took up positions at the front.

I watched the door but could only see the flashes of the cameras. Karin must have stopped to give the photographers a chance. Then all the guests stood and she appeared, like a beautiful apparition in a white gown on her father's arm. I realized, at that precise moment, that Nazih Zuhdi had been 100 percent right when he'd said I should consider myself lucky. He'd just underestimated exactly *how* lucky.

I thought that by this time I'd be quite a professional at getting married but when I saw Karin I was overwhelmed and my eyes burned with the tears I tried to hold back. I didn't even see her father put out his hand to wish me well as he handed her over to me.

During the ceremony, which was really only a blessing of the marriage already performed the previous evening, I choked up several times and also saw Karin wipe away a few tears.

We were finally pronounced husband and wife for the second time in 24 hours.

There was only one speech and that was mine – a very brief one. I wanted to get it over with as quickly as possible and enjoy the rest of the evening. I began by saying that this was my third, and last, marriage. I said that Karin was a very lucky girl because in one night, she'd become a wife, a mother and a grandmother – and I promised her parents that they, too, would soon become grandparents. There was surprised laughter from the guests – I think they thought Karin must already be pregnant.

The party then got into full swing and everybody joined in the festive spirit of the occasion. Even the waiters and the kitchen staff had a ball. I think that with the exception of my son, Christiaan, everyone stayed until the end. It was his first introduction to free-flowing booze and he passed out halfway through the evening!

The next morning, Sunday, the newspapers were delivered. *Rapport* called it 'the Wedding of the Year' with the headline:
THE MOST BEAUTIFUL, BEAUTIFUL BRIDE!

The *Sunday Times*, obviously eager to maintain their own, very distinct image, carried the headline:
BABY, LOOK AT YOU NOW!

This was accompanied by an almost full-page photograph of Karin, at the age of 6, sitting on my lap. They'd somehow acquired the picture and had no permission whatsoever to publish a personal photograph. They probably did it out of spite as their opposition, *Rapport,* had been given the exclusive rights.

With Noel Tunbridge's help, Karin's mother later received compensation for the illegal use of the picture and I just ignored the jibes in the *Sunday Times* story. It was one of their typically sensational reports and we used the paper to light the fire of our lunchtime barbeque.

On Monday morning, our guests from America and Europe accompanied Karin and me to Johannesburg on the Blue Train on the start of our honeymoon.

The Blue Train is one of the most luxurious trains in the world. Originally called the 'Zambezi Express' it linked Bulawayo and

Cape Town. At the beginning of the 20th century, this long journey was made comfortable by de luxe compartments, oak-panelled gaming rooms and a library of leather-bound books.

When the train glided into the station at Beaufort West that evening I was both amazed and delighted to see the platform packed with the local coloured people – who'd come to wish Karin and me happiness for the future.

Our stay at Mala Mala was a wedding gift from Norma and Mike Rattray. Armin Mattli had persistently asked us to find him a girlfriend for this trip. It's difficult enough to find company for anyone in those circumstances, but it was especially hard to find someone for a short 60 year old with a generous beer-belly. However, two of Karin's friends had agreed to come along.

Mala Mala has always been my favourite game park. It's exceptionally well managed by Norma and Mike, and a great variety of game can be seen there – and always the 'Big Five'.

It's the oldest and largest private game reserve in South Africa spanning 45 000 acres (18 000 hectares) and borders the famous Kruger National Park. It's regularly voted the 'top safari destination in the world' and is invariably included in the top ten resorts in the world. It's long been the destination of film stars and royalty.

It's literally a 5 star hotel in the African bush. I went there with Barbara before and after our divorce. I went there alone on my 60th birthday and also with Karin before, and after, our wedding.

For me there's no better place to 'find yourself' than at Mala Mala.

On the second day we came across a pair of lions mating. Our guide told us that lions mate for three days and couple approximately forty times in this period.

Our guests enjoyed the stay there – and we had a lot of fun with Aris who thought that every animal we saw was going to eat him.

Karin and I said farewell to our friends when we reached Johannesburg and returned to our townhouse in Welgemoed.

After about three months the press began speculating about when, or if, Karin would become pregnant. This started me worrying as well, especially as she'd stopped taking the Pill a month before our wedding. Again my dreaded enemy, old age, began stalking me. Maybe the passing of years had significantly reduced my sperm count? Or the mobility of the spermatozoa had become sluggish? But I was too proud to consult a urologist. I decided to study Karin's menstrual cycle to determine, more or less, the time she should be ovulating and to intensify our sexual activities during that period.

I left for my Karoo farm, 640 kilometres from Cape Town, because the farm workers couldn't get the electric game fence to work, which I'd had constructed at great expense.

As I had recently introduced some eland into my game stocks, it was vital to have a fence to restrict their wanderings; otherwise they'd soon be all over my neighbour's property.

Days passed quickly, as I tried to get the fence working properly. One day I was sitting in front of the metal box that housed the energizers for the fence, when suddenly I felt a sledgehammer blow to my head and I was hurled backwards into the dust, sprawled out in a barely conscious state.

After a few minutes, I recovered sufficiently to work out what had happened. I must have bent forward and as I did so, my forehead had touched the live metal box and 6 000 volts had gone through my brain for 30 milliseconds.

Maybe this jolted my memory, because I suddenly realized that this was 'D-day' – when I'd calculated that Karin would be in a state of ovulation. I raced back to Cape Town and arrived six and a half hours later, dashed up the stairs with Karin and pretended I was a male lion for two days.

But unlike the King of the Jungle, by the third day I was shagged out and had to rest.

Two weeks later, Karin and I left for Kos. It was time for her period and every time she went to the bathroom, I expected her to return with the bad news that it had arrived. But nothing happened.

From Kos we went to Wimbledon to watch the tennis and by then, some symptoms and signs of pregnancy had appeared. She complained of feeling bloated and said that her breasts were getting bigger.

I know that when women badly want a child they can develop 'phantom pregnancies'. All the signs of pregnancy occur, even the absence of menstruation – but without any conception having taken place.

Was this also the case with Karin?

We returned to Cape Town and she consulted a gynaecologist, Harry Mukheiber, a close friend of mine.

Frederick and Christiaan had come down from Johannesburg to visit us but I had to get back to the farm and see if the fence was working properly.

Karin phoned that evening and all she said was, 'It's positive.'

I could hear the two boys shouting and laughing in the background. Karin told me they were so delighted about the news that they were dancing around the room. This made me very happy, because there would be no sibling jealousy.

I walked out into the still evening air, and as I gazed up at the stars, I silently offered a prayer to God, thanking him for this little life which was now growing inside the woman I loved so much.

Karin had very few problems as her pregnancy progressed. Each new development caused great excitement: the first time we heard the baby's heart and when she could first feel movement.

I went with her for the ultrasound scan. I could make out the legs and arms and body as they were quite clear. The little thing was sucking its thumb already. Karin didn't want to know the sex of the baby, so I didn't tell her. But I developed a pathological fear that my child would be abnormal. The radiologist who did the scan assured me that as far as he could see, the baby was completely normal. But this examination couldn't detect Down's syndrome.

I phoned Professor Peter Beighton, the head of human genetics with whom André had worked for a year. We discussed the possibility of Karin having an amniocentesis to rule out mongolism, but he advised against this examination.

Peter told me that mongolism, as a result of an elderly father, was not really a problem and that the risk of abortion after an amniocentesis was far greater than the risk of the baby being congenitally abnormal. I was more at ease, but the nagging uncertainty remained.

Karin and I went to Plettenberg Bay with the children for Christmas and New Year. She still had two months to go.

One evening we were sitting in the lounge, when she said to me, 'Chris, I think I'm getting contractions!'

'Nonsense. It's just your imagination.' I tried to calm her, but ice-cold panic gripped my insides. We so badly wanted this baby and now, maybe, we were going to have to deal with a premature birth.

What were the chances of survival of a baby born eight weeks premature? I wracked my brains, trying to remember my paediatric lessons.

'Come and sit next to me and when you think you're having a contraction tell me, so that I can feel the uterus. I'd hardly spoken the words, when she sat down and said immediately, 'There it is!'

I placed my hand on her tummy. Oh my God, there was no doubt that she was having contractions! I could feel that the uterus was tense. She'd bumped the car in a parking lot outside the supermarket that morning and the shock had probably caused her to go into premature labour.

'I told you to take it easy!' I shouted – more from fright than anger, 'But no, you had to drive around! I don't even know a doctor in this bloody place – let alone a gynaecologist!'

'Phone Oom Gert – he lives here permanently – he'll know who to phone,' she said calmly. In fact I was amazed at how calm she was. ('Oom' is a polite Afrikaans word for 'uncle' and often used with respect for an older man.)

I ran upstairs to the phone and then the lights suddenly went out – one of the frequent power failures that happen in Plettenberg Bay. It was pitch dark and I couldn't find Oom Gert's phone number. Damn! Damn and bloody damn!

'Karin, you sit quietly – I'll run to his house quickly.' My heart was thumping wildly and I couldn't think straight. One would think that a doctor who'd dealt with so many life-threatening emergencies throughout his career would handle this one with ease. But it was different. It was my wife and the life of my unborn child.

I blundered through the bushes, cursing and swearing as I went and arrived at his front door. His lights were also out but I could hear him inside. I banged furiously on the door.

When he opened it he could obviously see I was in a state of shock, and covered with scratches from the bushes.

'What's the matter, Chris? Scared of the dark?'

'Don't joke, Gert – I've got big problems,' and I blurted out the story.

'But there's a gynaecologist from Johannesburg on holiday, staying right next door to you – why don't you get him?'

Jesus! I'd forgotten all about him – so I started running again.

'Wait!' Gert called after me, 'I'll get my torch and come with you.'

Fortunately, Dr André van der Walt was at home. He immediately came to my house and confirmed that Karin was having contractions. But he also suggested that he examine her internally, to see if the mouth of the womb was open.

As he had no equipment with him I raced to the pharmacy to get some gloves and some lubricant.

By the light of Gert's torch he examined Karin and gave us the good news that these were false contractions – because the uterus was closed and there was really nothing to worry about. In fact the contractions were even good for the baby.

Back I rushed to the pharmacy to get some Epradol tablets which André van der Walt had prescribed and which he said would stop the contractions.

By this time I was totally exhausted – both physically and mentally.

We had to get back home as quickly as possible.

Soon after we arrived back in Cape Town another catastrophe struck. Karin's brother phoned to say that he'd just driven past La Vita in Welgemoed and had seen smoke coming out of the restaurant.

I didn't think too much about it, as it wasn't uncommon for small fires to combust in the extractor fans as a result of accumulated fat deposits. These were easy to extinguish.

In any case, Chris Lesley would be there and would take care of the problem.

Five minutes later, I heard Karin shouting from the bedroom. I rushed up to find her staring through the window. The flames from the restaurant were leaping 30 feet into the air. There was no doubt that my restaurant really was on fire.

'Shouldn't you go there, Chris?' she asked urgently.

'To do what?' I said 'I can't put out the fire – and I can hear the fire brigade coming.'

The next morning I drove to the golf club. The restaurant with all its equipment was totally destroyed. I found Chris Lesley looking through the ruins.

'What happened, Chris?' I asked him.

'I don't know, Prof. My brother and I were sitting inside when the fire started. We tried to put it out with the extinguishers, but it spread so rapidly that there was just no chance.'

He looked exhausted – and there was nothing to be done now. 'Did you keep up the insurance?'

He stared back at me and said, 'Prof, you never had it insured – but don't worry because I took out some insurance myself.'

I thought that was very strange – I was positive I'd had it insured when he took over the management of the restaurant.

Karin and I drove to his house because Anne, his wife, was also expecting a baby and was extremely upset about the fire. 'Prof, it's all finished!' she wailed when she saw me. 'All gone and finished.'

'Never mind, Anne,' I put my arm gently around her shoulder, 'We'll build a new one – and a better one.' I was trying to calm her down, but she became worse.

'But everything we have – the house, the furniture, the two cars, the helicopter – it all came from La Vita and now it's finished.' She was sobbing almost uncontrollably by now.

I drove to the pharmacy to buy her some Valium and then back to her home to explain the dosage to her.

I was still bothered by what Chris had said about the insurance, so when I got home, I took out the contract that we'd had drawn up when he took over, and carefully studied the document.

Yes. I was right. It clearly said that he was responsible for continuing to pay the premiums of the *existing* insurance.

Later in the day I phoned him and explained the clause in the contract. He said he'd misunderstood me and that he *had* kept up the premiums – what he'd meant was that he'd increased the amount.

That put my mind at ease and I didn't worry about it again. As soon as the insurance company had paid out, I'd build another La Vita which Chris and Anne Lesley would manage for me again.

A week later, I heard that they were negotiating to buy a restaurant close by. When I asked Chris about it he said that he was looking into other properties, but that he'd never do anything without me.

Three weeks later I had a phone call from the president of the Welgemoed Golf Club, who asked whether I was aware that the insurance company had paid out – but that the cheque had gone to Chris Lesley.

What the hell's going on? I thought as I phoned the insurance broker. 'Yes, Professor,' he said 'the money was paid to Chris Lesley because the insurance was taken out in his name. In fact

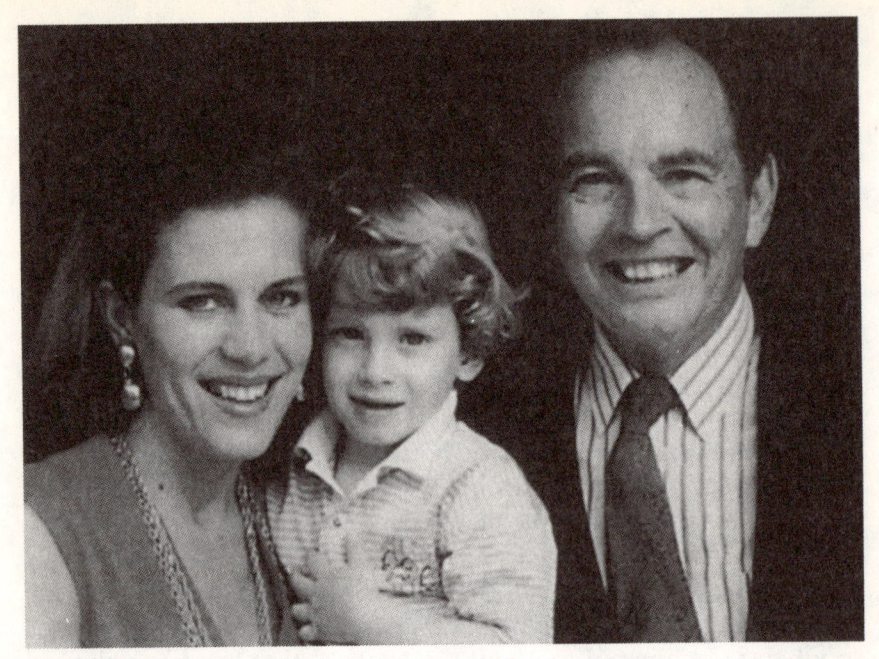

Together with Karin and Armin

about a year ago he cancelled the original policy and reinsured the restaurant in his own name.'

I quietly replaced the telephone and began putting all the pieces together in my mind.

Harry Mukheiber decided that our baby should be delivered by Caesarian section. Somehow the newspapers got hold of this and of course, it was followed by letters condemning me for 'not allowing' Karin to have a natural childbirth.

None of these people bothered to ask why the gynaecologist had decided to do the Caesarian section. Surely they must have realized there were medical reasons?

The date was set for the 25th February. I'd never attended the birth of any of my previous children. I never could see the purpose of the husband being at the side of his wife during the delivery. But Karin was insistent and wouldn't listen to my objections. I *had* to be there.

It was strange to change into a theatre gown again, after not wearing one for more than four years.

When I walked into the theatre, Karin was sitting up with her bare back facing me as Dr Prins, the anaesthetist, was putting the needle into her subdural space – she had decided to have an epidural Caesarian.

Once he found the space, he injected a local anaesthetic and then through the needle, threaded a thin tube which he left in place. This would serve for further injections to be given – either during the operation, or in the post-operative period to reduce the pain.

Karin lay back on the operating table and smiled at me. She was calm and almost serene. They covered her with several blankets, as she started to shiver when the anaesthetic took effect.

I hadn't heard Harry arrive, but he was now in the operating room – as jovial as always.

'Hello, Darling!' he greeted Karin, 'Would you like to see your little baby?'

'I can't wait,' Karin said with the broadest smile I've ever seen.

Only then did he notice me. 'Hi Chris! Have you come to check up on me?'

Harry gave the impression that we were about to start a Sunday School picnic. But I kept up my silent prayer – the same one I'd been repeating frequently ever since Karin told me the good news. Please God, let the child be normal.

Karin was draped and Harry made an incision just above the pubic hairline. 'When can we start, Dr Prins?' he called out, trying to deceive Karin into thinking that he hadn't yet begun.

'You've already made the cut,' Karin smiled. 'Don't try and bluff me.'

'Can you feel anything?' Dr Prins asked anxiously.

'No, I can't – but I can tell they're pushing on my stomach.'

Once through the skin, he separated the two stomach muscles vertically. I fumbled with a camera as I wanted to take a few pictures of the baby as it emerged.

Suddenly there was a gush of bloodstained fluid.

What the hell has he cut now! And then I realized he was already inside the uterus. Harry put his right hand inside, and then Dr Prins and the assistant surgeon pressed down on Karen's belly.

I stood there mesmerized. What were they doing? I hadn't seen a Caesarian section since my student days.

Black hair appeared in the uterus and Harry gently eased the head out. With both hands he took hold of the head and with slight traction, delivered first the right shoulder and then the left. The rest of the body slid out easily.

He held the baby upside down. Dr Vermeulen, a paediatrician, was waiting to examine the baby for any abnormalities – and he'd also continue the resuscitation.

'It's a boy.' Dr Prins said quietly to Karin and, as if he'd heard this, the baby started to cry to announce his arrival.

It was the most wonderful sound I've ever heard.

Both Karin and I wept tears of joy.

Armin was born.

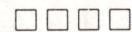

☐ ☐ ☐ ☐

Prof. Chris Barnard is now retired and lives in Cape Town with his wife, Karin, and son, Armin. He regularly gives talks and lectures round the world whilst pursuing his farming interests.

GLOSSERY OF MEDICAL TERMS

ACIDOTIC
An abnormal increase in the acidity of the blood and extracellular fluids.

AERUGINOSA
Producing gas. Bacteria that liberate free gaseous products.

ANASTOMOSE
To join two parts (blood vessels etc.) together.

ANAEMIA
Lack of blood.

ANENCEPHALIC
Congenital absence of the cranial vault, with cerebral hemispheres completely missing or reduced to small masses attached to the base of the skull.

ANEURYSM
A sac formed by abnormal dilation of the weakened wall of a blood vessel.

ANGINA PECTORIS
A sudden intense pain in the chest, often accompanied by feelings of suffocation, caused by momentary lack of adequate blood supply to the heart muscle.

ANGIOPLASTY
Removal of areas of narrowing in blood vessels.

ANOXIA
Lack or absence of oxygen. A deficiency of oxygen in tissues and organs.

AORTA
The main vessel in the arterial network, which conveys oxygen-rich blood from the heart to all parts of the body except the lungs.

ARRHYTHMIA
Any variation from the normal rhythm in the heartbeat.

ARTERIOSCLEROSIS
A pathological condition of the circulatory system characterized by thickening and loss of elasticity of the arterial walls. ('Hardening of the arteries'.)

ARTERIOLOSCLEROSIS
Thickening of the walls of the smaller arteries (arteroles)

ARTERITIS
Inflammation of an artery.

ARTERY
Tubular thick-walled muscular vessel that conveys oxygenated blood from the heart to various parts of the body. [q.v. Pulmonary artery.]

ATHEROMA
Fatty deposit on or within the inner lining of an artery.

ATHEROSCLEROSIS
Degenerative disease of the arteries characterized by patchy thickening of the inner lining of the arterial walls caused by fatty deposits.

ATRIUM
A cavity or chamber in the body. The upper chamber of each half of the heart.

AUTOLOGOUS
Relating to self; self-produced; originating within an organism itself.

BIOPSY
Examination, under a microscope, of tissue from a living body to determine the cause or extent of a disease.

CACHECTIC
A seriously and generally weakened condition of the body or mind resulting from any debilitating chronic disease.

CANNULA
A small tube for insertion into a body cavity for draining off fluid or introducing medication.

CEREBRAL EMBOLUS
An embolus (blood clot) transported to, and lodged within, the brain.

CORTEX
The outer layer of any organ.

CYANOSIS
To become blue. A bluish-purple discolouration of skin and mucous membranes usually resulting from a deficiency of oxygen in the blood.

DIATHERMIC (machine)
Local heating of the body tissues with an electric current.

DIASTOLE
The dilation of the chambers of the heart that follows each contraction, during which they refill with blood. [q.v. Systole.]

EMBOLUS
A blood clot or air bubble transported by the bloodstream until it becomes lodged within a small vessel and impedes circulation.

EMBOLISM
The occlusion of a blood vessel by an embolus.

ENDOCRINE GLAND
Any of the glands that secrete hormones directly into the bloodstream.

ENDOTHELIAL
A tissue consisting of a single layer of cells that lines the blood and lymph vessels, heart and some other cavities.

FEMORAL ARTERY
The artery in the thigh or femur.

FIBRILLATE
Irregular twitchings of the muscular wall of the heart, often interfering with the normal rhythmical contractions.

HAEMATOLOGY
The study of diseases of the blood and blood-forming tissues.

HAEMORRHAGE
Profuse bleeding from ruptured blood vessels.

HEPARIN
An anti-coagulant.

HETEROTOPIC
Abnormal displacement of a bodily organ or part.

ILIAC (artery)
The artery at the uppermost and widest section of the hip bone.

INFARCTION
The formation of dead tissues as a result of obstruction of the blood supply – especially an embolus.

INFUNDIBULA
Funnel-shaped stalk connecting the pituitary gland to the base of the spine.

INTRATRACHEAL
With, or through, the trachia; performed by passage through the lumen of the trachea.

ISCHAEMIA
Inadequate supply of blood to an organ or part, as from an obstructed blood flow.

KLEBSIELLA
A genus of bacteria not dependent on oxygen or air. Commonly

found in the intestinal tract. Frequently the cause of pulmonary infection.

LIPOPROTEINS
Fat or fatty proteins.

LOBECTOMY
Surgical removal of a lobe from any organ or gland in the body.

LUMEN
A passage, duct or cavity in a tubular organ.

MEDULLA
The innermost part of an organ or a structure. Short for *Medulla oblongata* – the lower stalk-like section of the brain, continuous with the spinal chord, containing control centres for the heart and lungs.

MORPHOLOGICAL
The form and structure of an organism.

MYOCARDITIS
Inflammation of the heart muscle.

MYOCARDIUM
The muscular tissue of the heart.

OEDEMA
An excessive accumulation of serous fluid.

OESOPHAGUS
The part of the alimentary canal between the pharynx and the stomach.

PATENT DUCTUS
An open and unobstructed passage.

PERCUTANEOUSLY
Introduced through the skin.

PERICARDIUM
The membranous sac enclosing the heart.

PNEUMONECTOMY
Surgical removal of a lung or part of a lung.

PSEUDOMONAS
A genus of gram-negative bacteria. *Pseudomonas aeruginosa* is a major agent of infection after hospital admission, causing severe/fatal infection.

PULMONARY
Relating to, or affecting, the lungs.

RINGER'S LACTATE
A solution containing the chlorides of sodium, potassium and calcium. Used to correct dehydration and, in physiological experiments, as a medium for *in vitro* preparations.

SAPHENOUS
Either of two large superficial veins of the legs.

SEPTUM
A dividing partition between two tissues or cavities.

STENOSIS
An abnormal narrowing of a bodily canal or passage.

SUBCLAVIAN
An artery or vein etc. below the clavicle (collarbone).

SUTURE
Catgut, silk thread or wire used to stitch two bodily surfaces together.

SYSTOLE
Contraction of the heart, during which blood is pumped into the aorta and the arteries that lead to the lungs. [q.v. Diastole.]

SEROUS FLUID
A thin watery fluid found in many body cavities, especially those lined with serous membrane.

TETRALOGY OF FALLOT
A combination of congenital cardiac defects (often/popularly: 'Hole in the heart') consisting of pulmonary stenosis and interventricular septal defect, where the aorta receives venous as well as arterial blood.

TRACHEA
The tube descending from the larynx and branching into the right and left main bronchi.

THROMBOEMBOLISM
The obstruction of a blood vessel by a thrombus that has become detached from its original site.

THROMBOSIS
The presence, or formation, of a thrombus – a clot of coagulated blood in the heart or blood vessel which remains at the same site and impedes the flow of blood. [q.v. Embolus.]

THROMBOPLASTIC
Causing or enhancing the formation of a blood clot.

TRICUSPID
Having three points, cusps or segments.

TRIGLYCERIDES
Any ester of glycerol and one or more carboxylic acids, in which each glycerol molecule has combined with three carboxylic acid molecules. Most natural fats and oils are triglycerides.

TROCAR
A surgical instrument for removing fluid from bodily cavities consisting of a puncturing device inside a tube.

UREA
A white water-soluble crystalline compound, often with an odour

of ammonia, produced by protein metabolism and excreted in urine.

URETERIC
Of, or relating to the urine.

VALVULITIS
Inflammation of a bodily valve, especially the heart valve.

VENA CAVA
Either one of the two large veins (superior or inferior) that convey oxygen-depleted blood to the heart.

VENESECTION
Surgical incision into a vein.

VEIN
Any of the tubular vessels that convey oxygen-depleted blood to the heart.

VENOUS
Of, or relating to the blood circulating in the veins.

VENTRICLE
A chamber of the heart, having thick muscular walls, that receives blood from the atrium and pumps it into the arteries.

(Based on definitions from *Dorland's Illustrated Medical Dictionary* – WB Saunders.)